The linear electric field effect in paramagnetic resonance

The linear electric field effect in paramagnetic resonance

W. B. MIMS

CLARENDON PRESS · OXFORD 1976

Oxford University Press, Ely House, London W.1

OXFORD LONDON GLASGOW NEW YORK
TORONTO MELBOURNE WELLINGTON CAPE TOWN
IBADAN NAIROBI DAR ES SALAAM LUSAKA ADDIS ABABA
KUALA LUMPUR SINGAPORE JAKARTA HONG KONG TOKYO
DELHI BOMBAY CALCUTTA MADRAS KARACHI

ISBN 0 19 851944 3

Printed in Great Britain
by J. W. Arrowsmith Ltd., Bristol

Preface

During the period of almost 30 years which has elapsed since its initial discovery electron paramagnetic resonance (EPR) has become a widely used experimental tool with applications in many areas of physics, chemistry, and biology. A number of related methods have also been developed, of which perhaps the best known is the electron nuclear double resonance (ENDOR) technique invented by Feher in 1956. More recently it has been shown that the resonance frequencies of many types of paramagnetic centre can be shifted by applying a d.c. electric field. These shifts result from the electrostatic polarization of the paramagnetic ion and its ligands and offer a new means for studying symmetry and bonding properties. Measurements of these shifts are indeed of unique value for the purpose of investigating non-centrosymmetric components of the ligand field since these components are not accessible to study by other EPR techniques.

In this book the experimental methods available for measuring electric field induced shifts in crystalline and non-crystalline materials are reviewed, and it is shown how the results can be stated in standard spin-Hamiltonian notation. Methods are outlined for analysing the internal electric fields generated when a voltage is applied across a sample and for rendering odd field effects amenable to treatment within the conceptual framework

PREFACE

which is commonly used in order to interpret other resonance observations. Several related matters are discussed, amongst them the nature of the electrostatic dipole moments associated with paramagnetic ions at non-centrosymmetric sites, the use of electric fields in conjunction with double-resonance ENDOR experiments, and the line-broadening effects which arise from internal electrostatic fields in solids. A mathematical appendix dealing with the effect of coordinate rotations on crystal field harmonics and on the terms in the spin Hamiltonian is also included. Mathematical complications of this kind can be avoided as long as one deals with model systems characterized by relatively high point symmetry but may have to be faced in applications of the technique, in particular those applications which lie in the realms of chemistry and biology.

W. B. M.

Bell Telephone Laboratories,
New Jersey
September 1975

Acknowledgements

It is a pleasure to acknowledge here my debt to Dr. A. Kiel who has helped to clarify my understanding of the linear electric field effect phenomenon during many years of fruitful collaboration and has also contributed directly to the material presented in this book. In addition to reading and commenting on various portions of the manuscript, Dr. Kiel has compiled Tables 5.8 and 5.9, where the multiplying factors required for the computation of the equivalent even field are given, and has derived the relevant equations. Many other portions of the manuscript have benefited from discussions with colleagues, in particular Drs R. J. Birgeneau, C. Herring, and L. R. Walker. In making the literature search I have been helped by Dr. A. R. Pierce of the Bell Telephone Laboratories library service, who compiled a bibliography of references to the linear electric field effect and to the magneto-electric effect. The review of linear electric field effect phenomena by A. B. Roitsin (1971) has also proved most useful. Table 10.8 is based on a table prepared by Dr. W. S. Moore of the University of Nottingham. The overall task of bringing the material together into a coherent form has been greatly facilitated by the excellent draft copies of the manuscript prepared by Mrs. S. Hughes and Mrs. J. M. Nichols.

For permission to use published diagrams either in their

original form or as a basis for textual figures I thank N. Bloembergen, W. E. Blumberg, S. Geschwind, G. W. Ludwig, J. Peisach, J. F. Reichert, J. P. Remeika, E. B. Royce, Z. Usmani, H. H. Woodbury, the American Institute of Physics, and the editors of *Biochemistry*.

Finally I should like to thank the management of Bell Telephone Laboratories for their support of this work and also the University of Konstanz and the Kultusministerium of Baden Wurttemberg for a visiting professorship during which part of the work was done.

Contents

CONTENTS

CONTENTS

1. Introduction

In 1961, approximately seventeen years after electron paramagnetic resonance was discovered by Zavoisky (1945), Ludwig and Woodbury published spectra showing the splitting of a resonance line in an applied electric field. At first it may seem surprising that such a long time should elapse before the observation of an effect resembling the well-known Stark effect in optics, the more so in view of the wide range of electron paramagnetic resonance (EPR) studies which were undertaken during this period. But the electric field induced shifts are quite small in most materials, and the application of sufficiently large electric fields to samples inside a microwave resonance cavity presents serious technical problems.

The essential reason why the shifts are small is that laboratory applied fields are generally several orders of magnitude smaller than the electrostatic fields (or equivalent ligand fields) generated by neighbouring ions in a crystal. It can, moreover, prove as difficult to make measurements on narrow resonance lines as on broad lines, since narrow lines tend to be associated with small shift parameters while lines with large shift parameters tend to be comparatively broad. Linewidth and sensitivity to applied fields are, in fact, often closely related properties (see Appendix B). The same practical problem is encountered in experiments aimed at measuring electric field induced shifts in the nuclear quadrupole resonance (NQR) frequencies and in the optical spectra of impurity ions in crystals. Electric effects of both these kinds were observed at about the same time as the electric effect in EPR, the quadrupole resonance shift by Armstrong, Bloembergen, and Gill (1961), and Kushida and Saiki (1961), and the optical shift by Kaiser, Sugano, and Wood (1961).

We shall be concerned here solely with electric field effects in paramagnetic resonance, although some of the discussion, for instance that which relates to the internal field in Chapter 4, may also be relevant to optical shifts and to NQR shifts (electric field effects in NQR have been reviewed by Lucken (1969)). We shall also be concerned almost exclusively with the 'linear electric field effect', i.e. shifts in the spin Hamiltonian parameters which are proportional to the applied field. Linear shifts can only be found for sites which lack inversion symmetry, i.e. 'non-centrosymmetric sites'.

Non-centrosymmetric sites occur in many of the materials commonly studied in paramagnetic resonance, including most of the hydrated crystals which served as host lattices in the earlier EPR experiments. Such sites often occur in pairs related by the inversion operation, i.e. 'inversion image pairs'. The two sites of the pair are indistinguishable in conventional EPR experiments but undergo equal and opposite shifts in an applied electric field resulting in an apparent splitting of the resonance line. Substitution generally occurs with equal probability at both types of site and both components of the split line are therefore of equal intensity.

The earliest electric field effect experiments were made with simple tetrahedral centres in silicon (Ludwig and Woodbury 1961), but for the most part the materials investigated in the first few years following the discovery of the effect contained sites of relatively low point symmetry. This was perhaps merely because samples consisting of paramagnetic ions in host lattices such as Al_2O_3 and $CaWO_4$ were readily available and gave shifts which were not unduly difficult to measure. But the results themselves were not easy to interpret in detail. Fortunately a number of more recent studies have involved sites of higher symmetry, such as the substitutional sites in zinc blende (T_d) and wurtzite (C_{3v}) and the charge-compensated tetragonal sites in halides and in the fluorite lattice (C_{4v}) (see §10.1 - §10.3). Several of these studies have also been accompanied by attempts to derive the shifts theoretically from first principles. Although such theoretical calculations do not always yield the experimental values, the agreement is not a great deal worse than it is when other parameters in the spin Hamiltonian are derived from first principles and is good enough to show that the basic features of the mechanism have all been recognized and taken into account.

Linear electric field induced shifts are calculated by applying perturbation theory within the same conceptual framework as that which is used to interpret EPR parameters such as the g-values and the crystal field splittings. The details vary a great deal according to nature of the ion concerned and it is difficult to proceed far without considering individual cases. There are, however, two problems of a general kind which arise and which must be dealt with before the methods of analysis described in standard EPR texts can be used. One concerns the nature of the internal electrostatic field seen by the paramagnetic ion when a voltage is applied across the sample; the other concerns the procedure to be adopted in treating the odd-parity portion of the crystal field.

The internal electric field problem has been extensively discussed in connection with the classical theory of dielectrics, but it requires some further refinement here in order to take account of the higher-order harmonics since these harmonics play a major part in determining the level splitting of paramagnetic ions in solids. The additional internal field components are estimated in Chapter 4 by making a point dipole analysis closely resembling the familiar point charge analysis of the crystal field. The resulting model of the internal field shares many of the defects of the point charge model and should not be relied on to give an exact description. But, in common with the point charge model, it has the cardinal virtue of providing a simple conceptual picture which can be modified later if necessary to bring it into closer agreement with the actual physical situation.

The odd-field problem falls properly within the domain of crystal field theory, but it is rarely dealt with in standard textbooks, where it is customary to parametrize the crystal field in terms of even harmonics only. This procedure is adequate from a qualitative standpoint since the phenomena observed in normal EPR studies are unchanged by a reversal of the probing fields. It can also be shown that in many instances the quantitative errors introduced by discarding the odd portion of the crystal field are relatively small. (§5.2). An applied electric field will however single out effects which depend on such deviations from inversion symmetry. According to the point charge model, in which the ligands generate an electrostatic field acting on the paramagnetic ion, the odd symmetry of the environment manifests itself in two ways. It makes possible the generation of new even harmonics when the lattice is polarized by the applied field, and it also gives rise to odd harmonics which, together with the applied field and the odd part of the induced crystal field enter into higher order perturbations which partially determine the values of the spin Hamiltonian parameters. In Chapter 5 it is shown how in some cases these higher-order perturbations can be simplified by contracting the two odd operators into an even operator which then effectively forms a part of the even field.

Aside from these two problems, the linear electric field effect can be dealt with by the same kinds of theoretical analysis as are used to interpret other phenomena observed in paramagnetic resonance experiments. Detailed discussion of the ways in which the Hamiltonian describing the interaction of an ion with its crystal field environment can be reduced to a spin Hamiltonian are given in a number of texts (see e.g. Griffith 1971; Abragam and Bleaney 1970) and are not reproduced here. To illustrate the use of the material in Chapters 4-5 and to demonstrate its connection with the material covered in standard texts we have, however, calculated one individual case in full. The case selected is that of the g-shifts for tetragonal Ce^{3+} centres in CaF_2. Although it is an unusually simple one from the computational point of view it conveniently serves to illustrate the general method and introduces a number of questions concerning interpretation and the validity of approximations which are encountered in dealing with more complex systems.

A review is given in Chapter 2 of the methods which have been used to measure linear electric field induced shifts. Most experiments have been performed by the straightforward method of comparing EPR spectra obtained with and without a d.c. applied electric field. In certain crystals at low temperatures, it has been found possible to generate fields of up to 10^6 V cm^{-1}, these fields usually being large enough to split the lines or to shift them by an amount which exceeds their width. This simple direct method has the merit of requiring few additions to an existing EPR spectrometer and may be the most suitable one in situations where an incidental measurement of the linear electric field effect is all that is needed (e.g. as a check on the point symmetry of a site). For more comprehensive studies it has a number of disadvantages, however. Not all samples will withstand large d.c. electric fields. Some undergo dielectric breakdown; some tend to discharge the applied field internally by means of leakage currents. Besides this, it is often necessary to make some of the measurements at field orientations where the shift is relatively small in order to complete the characterization of a site. Once the shifts are less than the linewidth the direct method becomes inaccurate and may be altogether impracticable. A modulation technique can be used to improve the signal-to-noise ratio in such marginal cases, but a better solution of the difficulty lies in the adoption of the electron spin echo method, which is limited by the width of individual spin packets rather than by the width of the overall line. The spin echo method is also well suited to study the linear electric field effect in powders and amorphous samples.

The extraction of a set of parameters describing the shifts is a more involved task than the determination of the g- or D- parameters and is not rendered any easier by the lack of a generally accepted notation. Special attention has, therefore, been devoted to questions of notation and data reduction which, although in themselves of little physical interest, are of essential importance if observations are to be presented in a convenient and useful form. Two systems of notation have been defined here, the one based on Cartesian spin operators and the other on normalized spherical spin operators. The Cartesian system is the one most commonly used and it has the merit of providing a formulation in terms of real coefficients and real spin operators, but it is not well suited to problems which require coordinate rotations, since the coefficients are third-rank tensor quantities which cannot be transformed by simple matrix methods. For this purpose, the spherical tensor system is preferable. The best course may therefore be to remain with the Cartesian system unless a rotation of coordinates is required and convert to spherical tensor form merely for this specific purpose, the necessary conversion being made by means of formulae and tables (§3.8; §§A.4.6-4.7). In the Cartesian system the shifts in the D-term have been rendered traceless by defining parameters R_{iD}, R_{iE}, which correspond to electric field induced shifts in the spin operators

$S_z^2 - \frac{1}{3}S(S+1)$ and $S_x^2 - S_y^2$.

One difficulty encountered in the description of linear electric field induced shifts concerns the symmetry of the g-matrix. It can easily be shown that the g-matrix g_{jk} used to describe EPR observations need not be symmetric in j,k. But the objection is academic in most EPR studies since the g-matrix can always be rendered symmetric by a suitable choice of spin matrices to represent the operators S_x, S_y, S_z, and its principal values can either be determined directly or found by diagonalizing the g^2-matrix. The linear electric field effect presents a new problem. If a spin operator representation is chosen so as to make the g-matrix symmetric in the absence of an electric field it will generally yield a matrix which has both symmetric and antisymmetric components in the presence of an applied electric field. These components can, in some cases, be measured separately by performing paraelectric resonance experiments (§7.2, §10.6). However, in the more common type of frequency-shift experiments they appear in combination with one another, the experimental data being effectively parametrized by a g^2-shift tensor which is always symmetric. (A set of 'equivalent symmetric' g-shift parameters can be derived from this g^2-shift tensor, if so desired, by solving the equations in Table 3.2.)

Chapter 10 consists of a summary of published data on the linear electric field effect. It will be apparent from the material assembled there that a great deal of ground remains to be covered before a truly comprehensive picture of the phenomenon can be drawn. Many ions, for instance the 4d group, have not been examined at all, and relatively little is known about the effect of different kinds of lattice environment on a given paramagnetic ion. It should not of course be assumed that a set of linear electric field effect parameters complementing the data already obtained by standard EPR methods would necessarily be very useful (although many of the systems concerned contain non-centrosymmetric sites and could probably be studied in this way). But some increase in the area surveyed would undoubtedly be helpful in providing a more solid foundation for the theory of the effect and would make it easier to use linear electric field effect measurements to solve problems arising elsewhere in physics, chemistry, and biology.

The likelihood that many readers will be interested primarily in applications of the effect has been borne in mind when planning the text and when assembling figures, tables, and mathematical expressions. Full attention has been given to low point symmetries and their properties. Cases of this kind tend to be avoided in basic physical investigations but are commonly encountered in other contexts. Much of the mathematical appendix, which includes notes on the principal axis transform and on other kinds of co-ordinate rotation, has also been prepared specifically to facilitate the handling of low-symmetry systems. For a comprehensive discussion of these topics a mathematical text should be consulted but it may nevertheless prove convenient to have a summary at hand which bears directly on problems arising in EPR and in the analysis of linear electric field effect results.

A brief review of possible applications is given in Chapter 9. The main purpose here is to indicate ways in which linear electric field effect measurements might be employed as a physical probe. Few experiments of this kind have been performed as yet, but more will undoubtedly be attempted as the effect becomes more widely known and better understood.

2. Experimental methods

2.1. ORDER OF MAGNITUDE OF ELECTRIC EFFECTS

The effect of laboratory electric fields on paramagnetic resonance transitions is usually quite small. This can be shown by making detailed calculations (see e.g. Chapter 6). Essentially, however, the reason is that the applied fields are much weaker than the electrostatic fields due to neighbouring ions in a crystal. The additional distortions of the electronic charge cloud, and alterations in the lattice spacing caused by the applied field, constitute a relatively small perturbation superimposed on the large crystal fields which are already present. A useful rough guess as to the order of magnitude can be made by dividing the applied field by 10^8 V cm^{-1} † and treating this parameter as the fractional change of the crystal field. An applied field of 10^5 V cm^{-1} can thus be estimated to produce linear electric shifts $\simeq 10^{-3}$ and quadratic electric shifts $\simeq 10^{-6}$. It is of course necessary when making such estimates to consider to what extent the resonance interval is affected by crystal fields at all. A free radical line will,

---

†The field due to a single electronic charge at 3 Å in vacuo is $1{\cdot}6 \times 10^8$ V cm^{-1}.

for example, show virtually no electric field induced shifts since its g-value is close to 2·0 for any crystal field environment. It is also essential that there should be a reasonably large departure from inversion symmetry in the vicinity of the paramagnetic centre if there is to be a linear shift of observable size.

2.2. LINEAR ELECTRIC EFFECTS: INVERSION IMAGE SITES

Many lattices which have overall inversion symmetry contain non-centrosymmetric sites. These sites normally occur in pairs, one member of the pair being related to the other by the inversion operation. Let us consider, for example, the arrangement of calcium and tungsten atoms in $CaWO_4$, as shown schematically in Fig. 2.1. Inversion of the calcium and tungsten coordinates with respect to site I yields an environment characteristic of site II (the same holds true for the coordinates of the oxygen atoms, which are not shown in the figure). An even simpler example is afforded by the tetragonal sites in CaF_2 (see Fig 6.2, p.172) for which the charge compensating F^- ion occurs with equal probability on either side of the trivalent substitutional ion. Sites a,d and sites b,c in Fig. 8.4 (p.225) are also related in this way. Sites of this kind can be termed 'inversion image sites'. In normal EPR experiments paramagnetic ions substituted at inversion image sites give rise to identical spectra and cannot be distinguished from one another. This follows from the fact that an interchange of the two sites is equivalent to reversal of the Zeeman field, an operation which has no effect on the resonance spectra. In an electric field effect experiment, however, interchange of the two sites is equivalent to a reversal of the applied electric field resulting in equal and opposite linear electric shifts for the two kinds of centre. Under most circumstances paramagnetic impurity ions substitute with equal probability at both types of site, and the effect of the electric

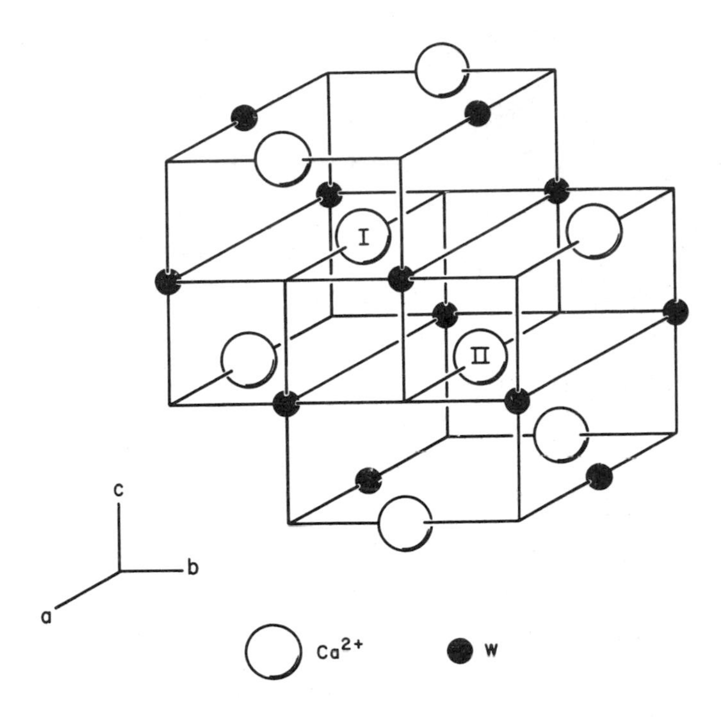

FIG. 2.1. Inversion image sites in the scheelite lattice $CaWO_4$. Paramagnetic ions commonly substitute at the Ca^{2+} site. For every W atom located at the position r with respect to an origin at site I there is an equivalent W atom located at -r with respect to an origin at site II. The same is true for the O atoms which are not shown in the diagram. The $CaWO_4$ lattice possesses overall inversion symmetry about a point midway between sites I and II. If it were possible to substitute a paramagnetic ion at this point it would not show any linear electric field effect.

field is to split the resonance line into a doublet whose components are of equal intensity.

Lattices containing inversion image sites have frequently been chosen as host lattices in EPR studies. The alums, the ethyl sulphates, and the double nitrates which figure prominently in the early EPR literature all contain substitutional sites distributed in this way. The same is true for many more recently studied materials such as the scheelites, the garnets, Al_2O_3, and $LaCl_3$. Some other lattices such as CaF_2, MgO, and the alkali halides which, in the pure state contain atoms at centrosymmetric sites only, can also yield pairs of inversion image sites for certain impurity ions as a result of charge compensating mechanisms. The property of containing pairs of centres which are indistinguishable in normal EPR experiments but which undergo equal and opposite linear electric shifts also extends to amorphous materials (see §3.7) consisting of randomly oriented crystallites, although some of these materials may not necessarily contain true inversion image sites.

Materials characterized by inversion image sites form convenient subjects for linear electric field effect studies since they are non-piezoelectric and not liable to undergo appreciable mechanical strains when a field is applied. Such strains would constitute an additional source of frequency shifts and would complicate the interpretation of results, although some studies for ions substituted in CdS and ZnS (Lambert, Marti, and Parrot 1970, Kiel and Mims 1972) suggest that piezoelectric effects may only be of secondary importance. Inversion image materials are also well suited to study by the electron spin echo method (§2.5). They may, on the other hand, be somewhat difficult to study by the direct method (§2.3) or the modulation method (§2.4) especially when the shifts are small.

2.3. LINEAR ELECTRIC SHIFT: DIRECT METHOD OF MEASUREMENT

The linear electric shift can be measured in a straightforward manner by applying a d.c. electric field to a sample and by finding either the shift of the resonance frequency or, in the case of an inversion image material, the splitting of the lines (Fig. 2.2). The shifts have been shown to be linear for fields

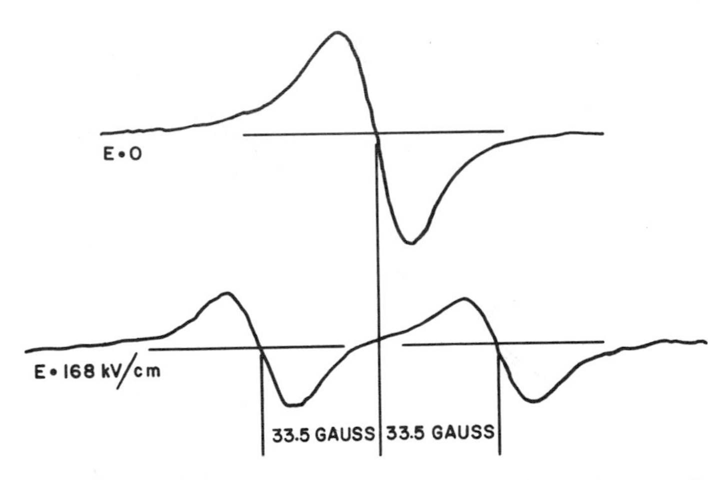

FIG. 2.2. Absorption derivative curves for the $M_S = +\frac{3}{2} \rightarrow +\frac{1}{2}$ transition of Cr^{3+} in ruby showing the splitting of the line due to inversion image sites in an applied electric field. $\underline{E}$ and $\underline{H}_0$ are both parallel to the crystal c-axis. (Royce and Bloembergen 1963.)

---

up to $\approx 10^5$ V cm^{-1} (Fig 2.3). Fairly high electric fields are usually needed, however, in order to cause an easily observed splitting (or a shift by an amount of the order of the linewidth), since lines which undergo large shifts are often broad initially and lines which are narrow tend to be shifted by only small amounts. One reason for this correlation of shift parameters and linewidth is that there are often large randomly oriented electric fields distributed throughout the interior volume of an ionic solid because of local fluctuations in the charge balance caused by point defects, vacancies, etc. (see Appendix B). These fields, which can reach values as high as 100 kV cm^{-1}, must be equalled by the applied field before a resonance line is shifted by an amount comparable with its inhomogeneous width. Such fields are likely to be especially large when the charge balance in the lattice has been disturbed by substituting ions of a different valency. Moreover, even in those cases where lattice strains

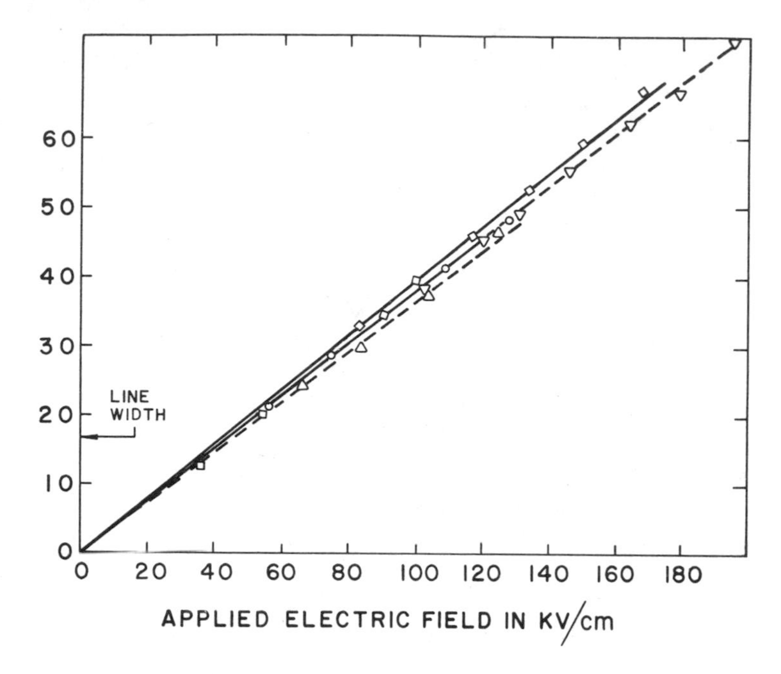

FIG. 2.3. Linear variation of the electric field induced line-splitting for the line shown in Fig. 2.2. Points were obtained using several different samples. (Royce and Bloembergen 1963.)

---

rather than random internal fields are the primary source of inhomogeneous line-broadening it still tends to be true that large shift parameters and wide lines are associated with one another. One might expect this to be so, since sensitivity to one kind of crystal field disturbance often implies sensitivity to others. Only occasionally, as, for example, in the case of the Fe^0 centre in silicon (Ludwig and Woodbury 1961) is this rule violated (see Fig. 2.4). Here the shift parameter is large but the line is narrow and is fully split in a field of only 10 kV cm^{-1}. The narrow line in these circumstances may result from the high degree of perfection of the silicon lattice and the ability of the material to screen out any large internal fields.

The 'direct method' can be used successfully to find the linear electric field shifts without necessarily applying a d.c.

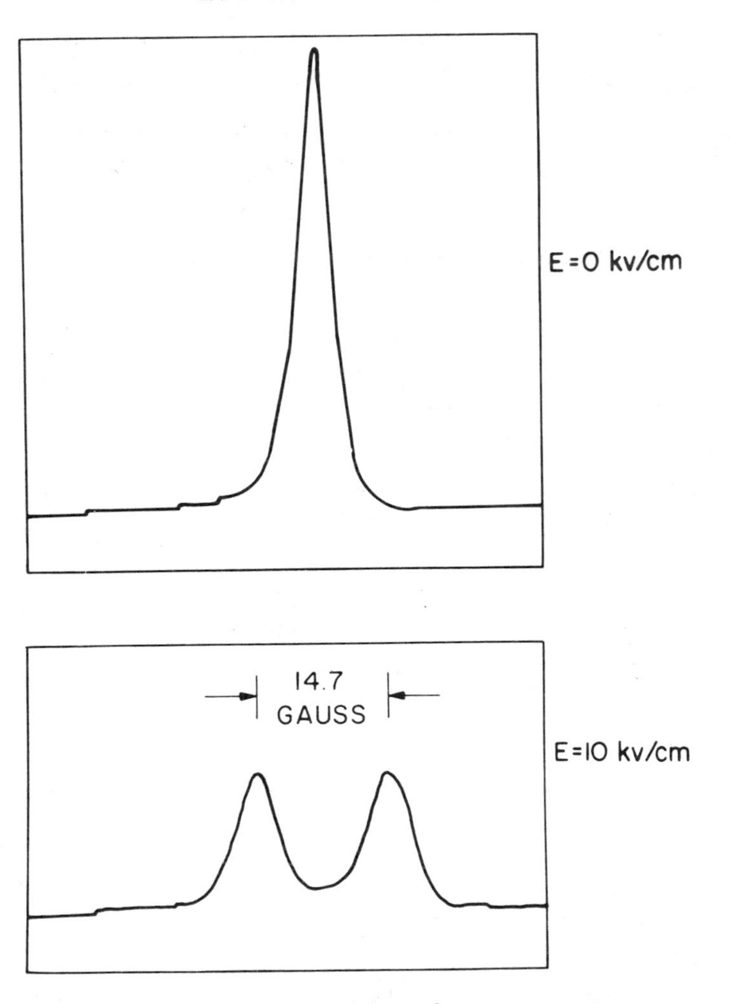

FIG. 2.4. Resolution of the line of Fe^0 in silicon into two lines associated with inversion image pairs of sites. $\underline{E}$ is along the [011] direction and $\underline{H}_0$ along the [110] direction. (Ludwig and Woodbury 1961.)

---

field large enough to shift the resonance line by a whole line-width, but the interpretation of the data then becomes a little less straightforward. The measurement is easiest to make when there is only one type of paramagnetic site. In this case the resonance line is moved to one side or the other by the applied electric field and the shift can be obtained either by measuring the displacement of its centre of gravity, or alternatively by recording the fractional change in the intensity $\delta I/I$ of the resonance signal at some suitable point on the side of the line. Thus if the function $f(\omega-\omega_0)$ representing the lineshape is displaced to $f(\omega-\omega_0-\Delta\omega)$ by an upward shift of $\Delta\omega$ in the centre frequency ω_0, then, to the first order in $\Delta\omega$,†

$$\begin{aligned}\frac{\delta I}{I} &= \{f(\omega-\omega_0-\Delta\omega) - f(\omega-\omega_0)\} \big/ f(\omega-\omega_0) \\ &\simeq -\Delta\omega\{\frac{\partial f(\omega-\omega_0)}{\partial\omega}\} \big/ f(\omega-\omega_0) \quad .\end{aligned} \tag{2.1}$$

For a Lorentz absorption line the lineshape function is

$$f(\omega-\omega_0) = (\frac{a}{\pi})/\{a^2+(\omega-\omega_0)^2\} \quad , \tag{2.2}$$

and the change observed at the half intensity points (i.e. where $\omega-\omega_0 = a$) is given by

$$\delta I/I = \Delta\omega/a \quad . \tag{2.3}$$

Since it is often easy to obtain large signal-to-noise ratios in paramagnetic resonance experiments this method can be used to measure shifts which are many times smaller than the linewidth.

---

† Throughout most of this chapter frequencies are expressed in radian units $\omega = 2\pi\nu$. The linewidth parameters a, ω, M_2, etc., must of course be expressed in these units wherever ω rather than ν appears in equations.

The situation is, unfortunately, much less favourable in the inversion image case. Since half of the ions undergo a shift $\Delta\omega$ and half a shift $-\Delta\omega$ there is no net movement in the centre of gravity of the line, and $\Delta\omega$ must be deduced from changes in the linewidth or in the lineshape. It has been shown that $\Delta\omega$ depends on the second moments $(M_2)_0$, $(M_2)_E$ before and after the application of the electric field $\underline{E}$ according to the relation

$$(\Delta\omega)^2 = (M_2)_E - (M_2)_0 \tag{2.4}$$

(Krebs 1964).† Thus in principle it is only necessary to plot M_2 as a function of E^2 to derive the shift parameter. In practice, however, it turns out to be quite difficult to measure the second moment accurately, since the result is strongly dependent on the intensity in the wings of the resonance line, a quantity which can only be determined if the baseline is accurately known.

An alternative method is to study the changes in signal intensity or in the width of the line at half height. These also turn out to be quadratic in $\Delta\omega$. The expression for the fractional change in signal intensity corresponding to eqn (2.1) is

$$\begin{aligned}\delta I/I &= \left[\tfrac{1}{2}\{f(\omega-\omega_0+\Delta\omega) + f(\omega-\omega_0-\Delta\omega)\} - f(\omega-\omega_0)\right]/f(\omega-\omega_0)\\ &= \{\tfrac{1}{2}(\Delta\omega)^2 \times \frac{\partial^2 f(\omega-\omega_0)}{\partial\omega^2}\}/f(\omega-\omega_0)\ .\end{aligned} \tag{2.5}$$

---

† This result is easily obtained by substituting $\tfrac{1}{2}\{f(\omega-\omega_0+\Delta\omega) + f(\omega-\omega_0-\Delta\omega)$ for $f(\omega-\omega_0)$ in the second-moment integral $\int \omega^2 f(\omega-\omega_0)d\omega$ and making suitable changes in the variable of integration .

For a Lorentz absorption line (eqn. (2.2)) observed at the half intensity point $\frac{\delta I}{I} = \frac{1}{2}(\Delta\omega)^2/a^2$. The change δW the full linewidth can be obtained by substituting $I = f(\omega-\omega_0)$ and $\frac{1}{2}\,\delta W = -\delta I/\{\delta f(\omega-\omega_0)/\delta\omega\}$ in (2.5), thus giving

$$\delta W = -\,(\Delta\omega)^2\,\frac{\{\partial^2 f(\omega-\omega_0)\}}{\partial\omega^2}\Big/\frac{\{\partial f(\omega-\omega_0)\}}{\partial\omega}\,, \qquad (2.6)$$

which reduces to $\delta W = (\Delta\omega)^2/a$ in the case of a Lorentz line observed at the half intensity point.[†] This simple formula is, of course, only valid if the line is Lorentzian, but an expression of the same form has been found adequate in a number of practical situations. For instance, it was found by Royce and Bloembergen (1963) that the empirical relationship $\delta W/W_0 = k(\Delta\omega/W_0)^2$, with $k = 0{\cdot}90 \pm 0{\cdot}05$, gave a good fit for the electric field induced broadening in ruby (Fig. 2.5). Approximate methods such as these may be needed in order to find some of the smaller shift parameters even when the shift is large enough to produce a clear splitting of the resonance line for the most favourable orientations of $\underline{E}$ and $\underline{H}_0$.

The instrumental problems of performing an experiment by the direct method can be considered under three headings: (1) the connection of a high-voltage supply to an electrode in the microwave cavity; (2) the generation of a large electric field in the sample without causing breakdown; and (3) the design of a cavity in which $\underline{E}$, $\underline{H}_0$, and $\underline{H}_1$ (the resonance field) can be appropriately oriented and in which the electrode does not unduly

---

[†] The result is perhaps easier to remember in the form $\delta W/W_0 = (\Delta\omega/W_0)^2$, where $W_0 = 2a$ is the width of the Lorentz line at half intensity in the absence of an applied field.)

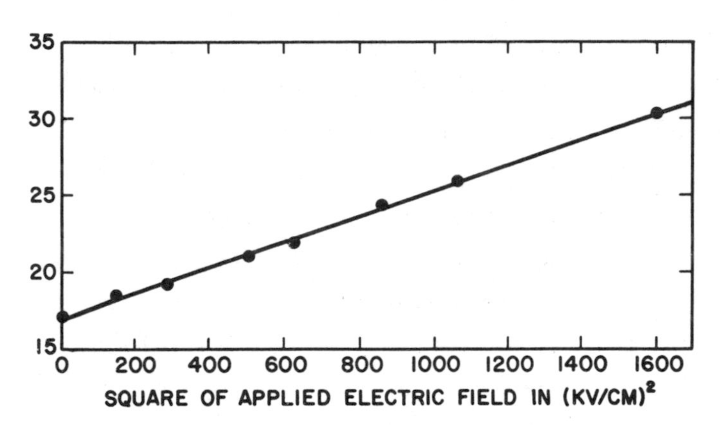

FIG. 2.5. Electric field induced broadening of the $M_S = -\frac{1}{2} \rightarrow M_S = -\frac{3}{2}$ resonance line in $Al_2O_3:Cr^{3+}$ (Royce and Bloembergen 1963) in the range where the electric field shift $\Delta\omega$ is less than the linewidth W_0. The results fit the semi-empirical relation $\delta W/W_0 = k(\Delta\omega/W_0)^2$, where δW is the increase in linewidth and where $k = 0{\cdot}90 \pm 0{\cdot}05$. The quadratic dependence of δW on the shift $\Delta\omega$ is a consequence of the fact that there are two kinds of site undergoing equal and opposite shifts.

disturb the microwave field. The first problem can be solved by connecting the power supply (typically a 20 kV supply) via a lead with a continuous Teflon insulating sheath to the cavity electrode. Breaks and solder connections should be avoided as far as possible, especially at points exposed to helium gas, which is a bad insulator. Where a connection has to be made it can be sealed with epoxy (Araldite), although this may not be necessary if the connection occurs beneath the surface of liquid helium.† Large fields are obtained by working with carefully

† Fields of the order of 10^6 V cm^{-1} can be attained in liquid helium with suitable electrode geometries (Goldschvartz, Ouwerkerk, and Blaisse 1970).

prepared thin samples sealed in epoxy to prevent surface breakdown. Remarkable field intensities can sometimes be reached without causing internal breakdown in the sample. Bugai and Roitsin (1967) describe an experiment in which fields of 10^6 V cm^{-1} were obtained by applying 20 kV across an Al_2O_3:Cr (ruby) sample 0·2 mm thick. It is also sometimes surprising to find how large a field can be sustained at liquid-helium temperatures by materials which are normally poor insulators. Peisach and Mims (1973) report the use of pulsed fields up to 70 kV cm^{-1} in frozen glasses consisting of proteins and water. The worst difficulties seem to occur in semiconductors and X-irradiated materials. Breakdown can sometimes be avoided in semiconductors by paying special attention to stoichiometry (Kiel and Mims 1972a). In X-irradiated materials, on the other hand, the only remedy may be to limit carefully the degree of irradiation (Usmani and Reichert 1969). In either case there is a risk that slow electrical leakage will result in a build-up of volume charges (Marti, Parrot, and Roger 1970) and make it difficult to perform measurements by the d.c. method.

There are two possible approaches to the problem of applying the potential to the sample in a microwave resonant cavity. One is to aim at a minimal disturbance of the microwave field by locating the sample, the electrodes, and the connecting leads well away from the region in the cavity occupied by the microwave electric field. In this case it may be helpful to use electrodes of less than a microwave skin depth formed by evaporating gold or silver directly onto the sample. An interesting technique of this kind is reported by Fedotov, Grachev, and Bagmut (1973), who use semiconducting films of SnO_2 deposited on thin glass plates as electrodes. The alternative approach is to design a cavity with the high-voltage electrode as part of the microwave resonant circuit. Reasonably thick electrodes can then be used and will indeed help to maintain the cavity Q. These two different approaches are illustrated by the cavities shown in Figs 2.6, 2.7, and 2.11. The electrode in the TE101 cavity in Fig. 2.6 is some distance from the microwave electric field maximum (which is located in the centre of the cavity at the lower end of the Teflon tuning plunger), and the connecting lead is taken out in a plane perpendicular to the microwave electric field. In the TE201 cavity in Fig. 2.7 the electrodes are placed close to the cavity walls and carry part of the microwave current. In the cavity shown in Fig. 2.11 the electrode itself constitutes the resonant element (see §2.6). In all cases the sample is located in a region of high microwave magnetic field, and in a region where this field is perpendicular to the Zeeman field. A further practical difficulty arises if it is necessary to rotate the sample so that the Zeeman field can be oriented arbitrarily with respect to the crystal axes. The arrangement shown in Fig. 2.6 is a convenient one from this point of view, but it does not lend itself to situations in which it is necessary to seal the connecting leads to prevent breakdown. The cavity has been used with pulsed potentials of 15 kV and with fields of 70 kV cm^{-1}, but its performance at higher fields is not known.

2.4. THE ELECTRIC FIELD MODULATION METHOD

Small shifts, which result in changes in intensity on the sides of the line, as indicated in eqn (2.5), can be measured by applying electric field modulation and using lock-in detection. The effects of apparatus drift and low-frequency noise can be largely eliminated in this way, thus making it possible to detect shifts which are considerably smaller than the linewidth. A field modulation experiment aimed at measuring the quadratic electric shifts for Co^{2+} in MgO has been described by Weger and Feher (1963). An EPR signal is traced out in the familiar manner, but with the sample subjected to an oscillating electric field instead of the customary magnetic field modulation. The frequency shifts are

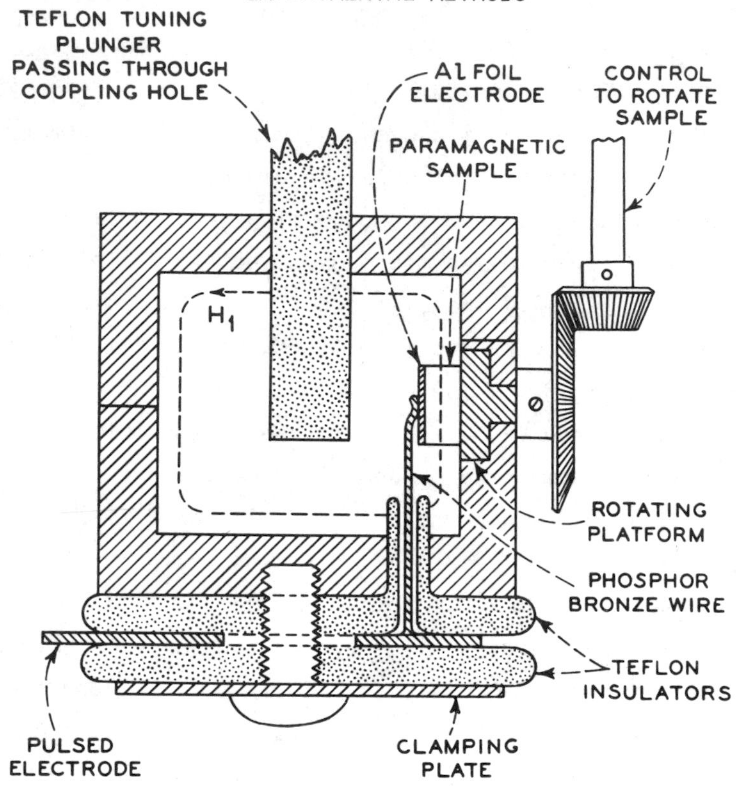

FIG. 2.6. Resonance cavity for the performance of linear electric field effect experiments. The electrode structure is designed to disturb the microwave field as little as possible. The connecting wire is perpendicular to the microwave electric field and the electrode is in a region where the microwave electric field is weak. The sample can be rotated about an axis perpendicular to the axis of rotation of the external magnetic field. (Mims 1964)

---

then inferred by comparing the effect of this electric modulation with the effect of a magnetic modulating field.

Modulation experiments are easiest to perform in the case of samples which possess only one type of site and which show a linear electric effect. Electric and magnetic modulating fields are then equivalent from an experimental point of view and the

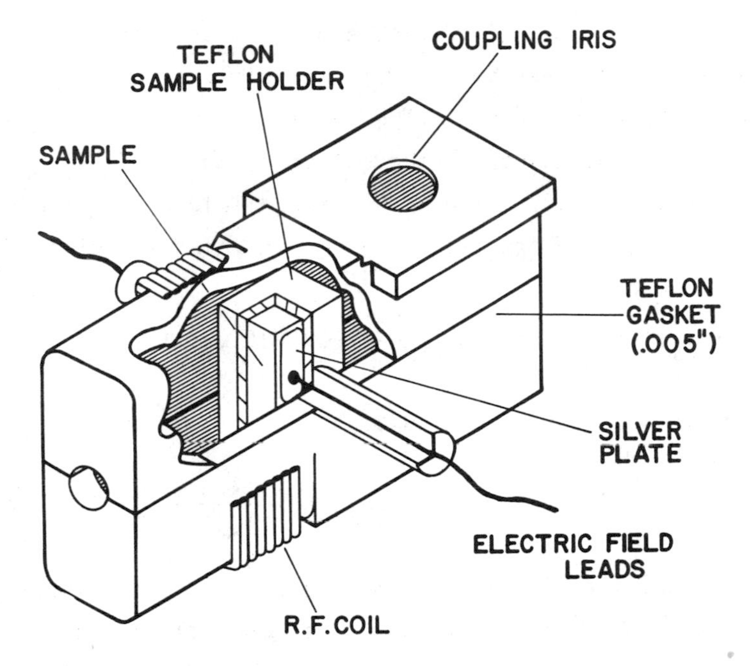

FIG. 2.7. Resonance cavity for the measurement of shifts in double resonance ENDOR transitions (Usmani and Reichert 1969; see also Chapter 8). The electrodes carry part of the microwave oscillating current which would otherwise travel along the inside wall of the cavity. For this reason they must be thick enough to ensure good high-frequency conduction. The Teflon gasket and the hole shown at the end minimize the extent to which the cavity screens out the field generated by the r.f. coil.

---

fractional change in intensity $\delta I(\Omega t)/I$ is given by the sinusoidal function

$$-(\Delta\omega_m \sin \Omega t)\left\{\frac{\partial f(\omega-\omega_0)}{\partial\omega}\right\} \Big/ f(\omega-\omega_0) \quad , \qquad (2.7)$$

where Ω is the modulation frequency and $\Delta\omega_m$ is the shift at the maximum value of the modulating field (this result follows at once from eqn (2.1). If, on the other hand, the sample contains inversion image sites the change in intensity is quadratic in the applied field (see eqn (2.5)), and the procedure will be essentially the same as the quadratic electric effect experiment described by Weger and Feher. The shifts can be examined in one of two ways: (1) by using the modulating field $E = E_0 \sin \Omega t$ and (2) by using a d.c. biased modulating field $E = E_0(1+\sin \Omega t)$. In the first case the fractional change in intensity will be

$$(\Delta\omega_m)^2\{\tfrac{1}{4} - \tfrac{1}{4}\cos 2\Omega t\}\{\frac{\partial^2 f(\omega-\omega_0)}{\partial\omega^2}\}/f(\omega-\omega_0)\ , \qquad (2.8)$$

and in the second case it will be

$$(\Delta\omega_m)^2\{\tfrac{3}{4}+\sin\Omega t - \tfrac{1}{4}\cos 2\Omega t\} \times \{\frac{\partial^2 f(\omega-\omega_0)}{\partial\omega^2}\}\ /f(\omega-\omega_0). \qquad (2.9)$$

The signals obtained in this way may be compared with the signal obtained by using magnetic field modulation. It should be noted however that in the inversion image case the ratio between the differential coefficients $\partial f(\omega-\omega_0)/\partial\omega$ and $\partial^2 f(\omega-\omega_0)/\partial\omega^2$ also enters into the comparison, and the measurement cannot be made by merely equalizing the two signals as it can in the simpler case where there is only one type of site. A careful measurement of the lineshape function is also needed.

The modulation method can be useful not only for the purpose of measuring shifts in broad lines but also when studying electric effects in materials with imperfect insulating properties, as mentioned at the end of the last section. Experiments performed by the direct method on such materials may show an initial splitting of the resonance line immediately on the application of the electric field followed by a relaxation as ions or electrons move and build up an opposing space charge. A 400 Hz modulating field was used by Marti, Parrot, Roger, and Herve (1968) and by Marti, Parrot, and Roger (1970) to overcome this difficulty in some semiconducting materials. The modulation method is also sometimes useful for discriminating between different kinds of paramagnetic centres present in a material (Parrot and Roger 1968).

2.5. THE SPIN ECHO METHOD

The experimental difficulties caused by inhomogeneous broadening of resonance lines can be overcome by using a method involving the generation of electron spin echoes. Inhomogeneous lines can be regarded as consisting of a continuous distribution of relatively narrow resonance lines, each interacting with the resonance spectrometer independently of the others. This structural property of the line is of no help when measurements are made by the d.c. method or the modulation method, since all observations concern the overall shape of the envelope, but it can be turned to advantage in a spin echo experiment where the echo phase memory time depends on the width of the individual component lines or 'spin packets'.

Electron spin echoes[†] can be generated by applying two microwave pulses in succession to a paramagnetic sample. If τ is the time between these pulses, then the sample emits a signal at a time τ after the second pulse. An echo decay function, or envelope of echoes, can be obtained by repeating the spin echo cycle of events for a number of different times τ and plotting the echo amplitude against τ (see Fig. 2.10(a)). This decay function can then be defined operationally as the Fourier transform of the lineshape associated with the spin packets. The resulting widths are often $\approx 10^3$ times narrower than the linewidths observed in c.w. resonance spectrometry. Thus an echo envelope decaying by e:1 in 5 μs corresponds to spin packets

---

[†] For a general discussion of the properties of electron spin echoes see Mims (1972).

≃30 kHz wide (≃10 mG at g = 2). Clearly it is much easier to measure shifts or line-splittings if observations can be made on the spin packets rather than on the overall inhomogeneous line. Some materials can then be examined with fields as small as 1 kV cm^{-1} and others, characterized by very broad lines or small shift parameters, are accessible to study without the risk of causing electrical breakdown.

To appreciate how this can be accomplished in practice it is necessary to consider in some detail the basic mechanism involved in the formation of spin echoes. This mechanism is illustrated in Fig. 2.8. The z-axis corresponds to the direction of the Zeeman field, and the coordinate system is assumed to be rotating about this axis at the microwave frequency $\omega_{r.f.}$. In the rotating coordinate system the microwave magnetic field vector $\underline{H}_1$ is stationary (along the x-axis in the figure) and the Zeeman field is eliminated save for a small residual component $(\omega-\omega_{r.f.})/\gamma$, corresponding to the amount by which the resonance frequency ω of an individual spin packet differs from the microwave frequency. To keep the explanation as simple as possible, we shall assume that these residual components of Zeeman field are negligible in relation to $\underline{H}_1$ and need only be taken into account during the intervals between microwave pulses (i.e. when $\underline{H}_1$ is absent). During the pulses themselves they will be ignored.

Fig. 2.8(a) denotes the initial state of the system with spins aligned along the Zeeman field giving a resultant d.c. magnetization $\underline{M}$. When pulse I is applied, the microwave field causes $\underline{M}$ to turn about the x-axis, the pulse being timed to last until $\underline{M}$ lies along the y-axis (90° nutation). This magnetization then begins to break up into a number of individual components during the interval τ between pulses I and II, since the different spin packets concerned see different residual Zeeman fields causing them to precess by different amounts, as shown in (c). (In practice the difference in precession angles may amount

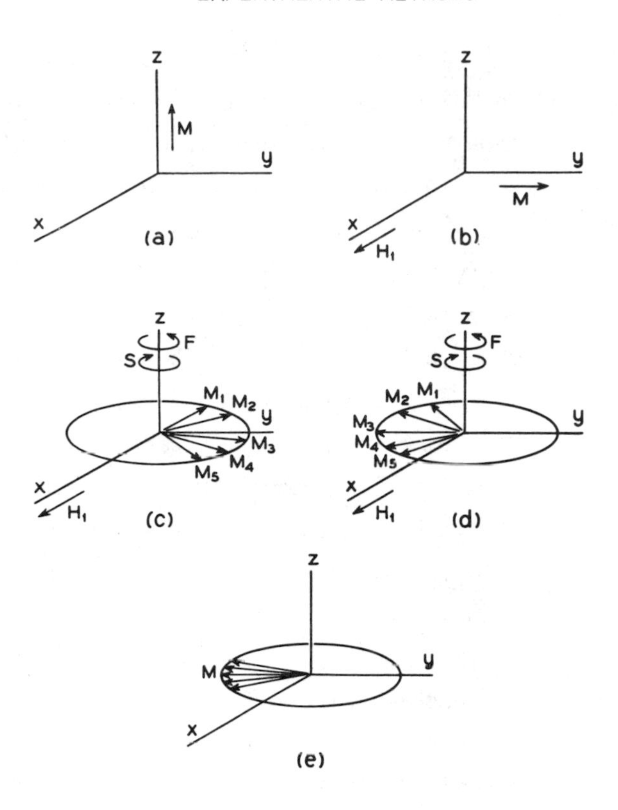

FIG. 2.8. Magnetization vectors associated with spin packets during the normal spin echo cycle of events shown in a rotating coordinate system. (a), (b) Before and after the 90° pulse. (c), (d) Before and after the 180° pulse. F denotes the direction of rotation of spin packets $\underline{M}_1$ and $\underline{M}_2$ which have free precession frequencies in excess of the microwave frequency. S denotes the direction of rotation of the slower spin packets $\underline{M}_4$ and $\underline{M}_5$. (e) Phase convergence of all spin packets at the time of the echo. Modification of this phase convergence by an applied electric field step is shown in Fig. 2.9(b),(c).

to many complete cycles, but it is shown as only $\simeq\frac{1}{4}$ cycle in the figure for simplicity.) The application of the second microwave pulse causes the spins to turn once more about the x-axis, the process being allowed to continue in this case until each magnetization component has turned by 180°, as shown in (d). The effect of this 180° nutation can be seen by comparing (c) and (d). The magnetization vectors corresponding to the spin packets are in the xy-plane in both cases, but the vectors which were leading in phase in (c) (e.g. $\underline{M}_1$) lag by an equivalent amount in (d), and those which were lagging in (c) (e.g. $\underline{M}_5$) lead in (d). During the remaining time between the second microwave pulse and the appearance of the echo, the spin packets precess once more in the residual Zeeman fields. Those which were retarded in phase by pulse II begin to catch up once again, and those which were advanced fall behind. After a further time interval τ all the spin packets are again in phase (along the -y-axis)(Fig. 2.8(e)), and the resultant magnetization $\underline{M}$, which in the laboratory co-ordinate system is rotating with angular velocity $\simeq \omega_0$, generates the spin echo signal.

The above represents a somewhat oversimplified version of the spin echo mechanism. Echoes can be obtained with nutation angles other than the 90° and 180° assumed here, and the restriction to residual Zeeman fields $|(\omega-\omega_{r.f.})/\gamma|$ which are less than H_1 is not essential. It should be noted, however, that the implicit assumption that each spin packet can be represented by a magnet-ization vector such as $\underline{M}_1$ with its own history of nutation about $\underline{H}_1$ and precession about the Zeeman fields is good only for a limited time, which we may call the 'phase memory time'. Random time-varying disturbances in the local magnetic fields eventually break up the magnetization vectors associated with the spin packets causing each vector in the diagram to spread out into a disc-like lobe which cannot be 'refocused' by pulse II. The echo signal will be attenuated accordingly. From this point of view each spin packet has a lifetime and an associated homogeneous width. Inverting our earlier definition we can say that the spin packet lineshape is the Fourier transform of the echo envelope decay function.

Let us next consider the effect of an electric field step as in Fig. 2.9(a) applied in synchronism with the second microwave pulse. The field modifies the spin echo sequence of events by

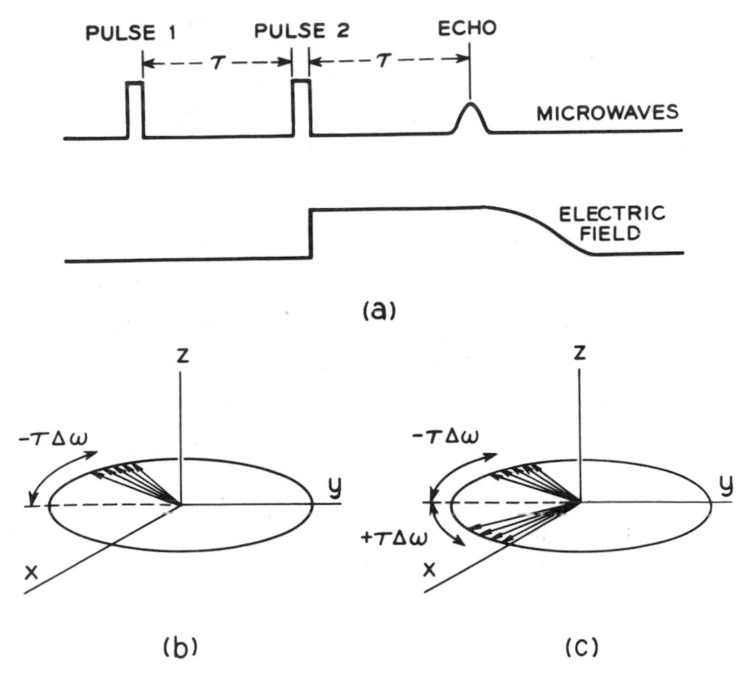

FIG. 2.9. (a) Timing of the electric field and the microwave pulses in an experiment to measure the linear electric field effect by the spin echo method. (b) Phase convergence of spin packets at the time of the echo when all frequencies are shifted monochromatically by $\Delta\omega$. (c) Phase convergence in an 'inversion image' material. The echo signal is eliminated entirely if $\tau\Delta\omega = \frac{1}{2}\pi, \frac{3}{2}\pi, \ldots$.

---

suddenly shifting the precession frequencies of all spin packets at a time half way through the cycle. Provided that the shifts are all the same this merely causes the resultant magnetization $\underline{M}$ in Fig. 2.8(e) to appear at a different orientation in the xy-plane as shown in Fig. 2.9(b). For instance, if there is a downward shift of $\Delta\omega$ $\underline{M}$ will be rotated away from the -y-axis by an angle of $-\tau\Delta\omega$, and the echo signal will be shifted in phase by this amount. The phase shift can be detected by using a phase-coherent pulsing and detection apparatus or by including a second sample which is not subjected to the applied field in the cavity to generate a comparison signal. For an inversion image sample, the problem of detection is even simpler. Two resultant vectors $\underline{M}$ are formed, one advanced by $\tau\Delta\omega$ and one retarded (Fig. 2.9(c)). If $\tau\Delta\omega = n\pi$, these two vectors will add coherently, but elsewhere there will be varying degrees of destructive interference. For $\tau\Delta\omega = \frac{1}{2}\pi, \frac{3}{2}\pi, \ldots$ the two magnetization vectors will cancel exactly and the effect of applying the electric field step will be to eliminate the spin echo signal entirely.

The argument is easily generalized to the case in which there is a continuous distribution of shifts $S(\Delta\omega)$. The ratio $R(E,\tau)$ between the echo decay envelopes $D_E(E,\tau)$ and $D(\tau)$ observed with and without the voltage step is then given by

$$R(E,\tau) = D_E(E,\tau)/D(\tau) = \int S(\Delta\omega)e^{i\Delta\omega\tau}d\tau \quad , \tag{2.10}$$

where $\int S(\Delta\omega)d(\Delta\omega) = 1$. The ratio can also be expressed so as to show the symmetrical roles of time τ and electric field E by substituting

$$\Delta\omega = \overline{\Delta\omega}\, E, \tag{2.11}$$

where $\overline{\Delta\omega}$ is the shift per unit field. Thus we have

$$R(E\tau) = \int S(\overline{\Delta\omega})e^{i\overline{\Delta\omega}E\tau}d(\overline{\Delta\omega}) \quad . \tag{2.12}$$

Measurements can be made by varying either E or τ, whichever is more convenient experimentally.

In the two simple cases illustrated in Fig. 2.9 $S(\overline{\Delta\omega})$ is represented by delta functions. Thus, when there is only one type of site and one monochromatic shift parameter we have

$$S(\overline{\Delta\omega}) = \delta(\overline{\Delta\omega} - \overline{\Delta\omega_0}) \tag{2.13}$$

and

$$R(E\tau) = e^{i\overline{\Delta\omega}E\tau} \quad . \tag{2.14}$$

The effect of the electric field is merely to shift the phase of the echo signal as shown in Fig. 2.9(b). In the inversion image case

$$S(\overline{\Delta\omega}) = \tfrac{1}{2}\{\delta(\overline{\Delta\omega} - \overline{\Delta\omega_0}) + \delta(\overline{\Delta\omega} + \overline{\Delta\omega_0})\} \tag{2.15}$$

and

$$R(E\tau) = \cos(\overline{\Delta\omega}E\tau) \quad . \tag{2.16}$$

The situation represented by Fig 2.9(c) and eqn. 2.16 is illustrated by the experimental echo envelopes in Fig. 2.10. This result was obtained with a superheterodyne detection apparatus sensitive to the absolute magnitude but not to the sign of the echo signal, hence the ratio of the two envelopes here yields the modulus $|R(E\tau)|$. There is, of course, no need to record the entire echo envelope in such a simple case but merely to find the product (or products) $(E\tau)_n$ which result in complete destruction of the echo signal. The shift can then be derived from the equation

$$\overline{\Delta\omega_0}/2\pi = \pm(2n-1)/\{4(E\tau)_n\} \quad , \tag{2.17}$$

where $(\Delta\omega_0/2\pi)$ is in hertz and n is the order of the null product of E and τ. Should it be impractical to determine the null product, it may instead be convenient to find the product $(E\tau)_{\frac{1}{2}}$

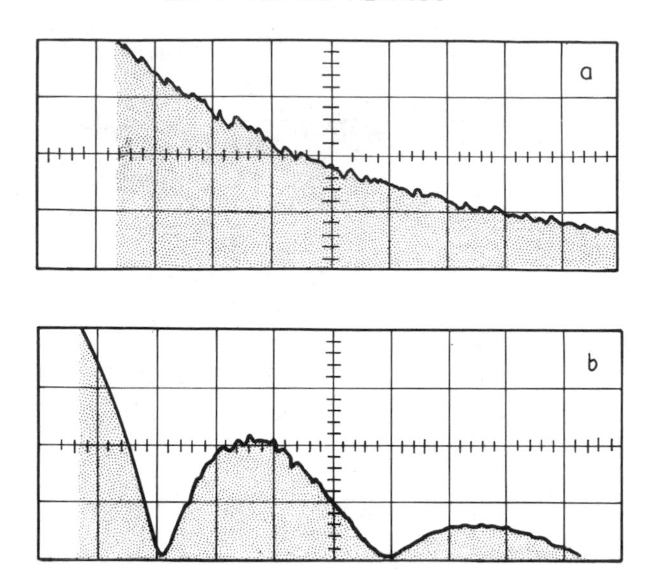

FIG. 2.10. Oscilloscope photograph showing the spin echo envelope for $CaWO_4:Ce^{3+}$: (a) without and (b) with the application of an electric field step as in Fig. 2.9. The field is 450 V cm^{-1} applied along the crystal c-axis. A phase shift of $\pm 90^{\circ}$ in the precessing magnetization vectors associated with the two inversion image sites occur at a time τ = 10 μs after the application of the electric field step and results in destructive interference of the echo signal. Destructive interference occurs again at τ = 30 μs, where the phase shift is $\pm 270^{\circ}$. The superheterodyne detector used in these measurements was insensitive to the sign of the echo signal. The figure therefore shows the absolute magnitude of the function $D_E(E,\tau)$. (Redrawn from Mims 1964).

which results in a 50 per cent reduction in the echo amplitude. In this case

$$\overline{\Delta\omega_0}/2\pi = 1/6(E\tau)_{\frac{1}{2}} \quad . \qquad (2.18)$$

It should of course be remembered that if the difficulty in finding a null point in the echo envelope is due to gross inhomogeneity of the shift a single measurement may not be adequate to describe the physical behaviour of the sample. A full determination of the function $S(\overline{\Delta\omega})$ obtained by measuring $R(E\tau)$ and taking its Fourier transform (the inverse of eqn (2.12)) may be required.

Practical problems may be encountered in devising an electrode geometry which will give a sufficiently homogeneous electric field, and in generating a clean step function which approximates to the ideal form assumed in the previous discussion. The performance of any given piece of equipment can be tested in these two respects and corrections can be determined by making spin echo measurements on suitable high-quality samples. An estimate can be made for the inhomogeneity introduced by the electrode structure by selecting an inversion image sample having a fairly large shift parameter and measuring $R(E\tau)$ through several null product points. A Fourier transform of $R(E\tau)$ will then give a distribution function $S(\overline{\Delta\omega})$ from which the homogeneity of the shift can be inferred. The observed inhomogeneity will be partly due to the electrode geometry and partly due to the intrinsic inhomogeneity of the sample and will therefore only give a limit for errors introduced by the former.

The timing of the voltage step can be adjusted by varying it so as to produce a maximum effect on the electron spin echo signal. A step which appears too late or too early will result in reduced effects. The finite transition time of the voltage step (and the finite duration of the second microwave pulse) can be allowed for by subtracting a correction time t_c from the observed value of τ. The simplest way to determine this time is again to select a good sample with reasonably homogeneous shift parameters $\pm\ \overline{\Delta\omega}_0$ and to locate the null products $(E\tau)_n$ by varying τ. The corrected values of τ should be in the ratio 1:3:5: - as indicated by eqn (2.17). An alternative method which does not depend on the quality of the sample or on the homogeneity of the electric field is described by Mims (1974). The correction time should be of the order of a quarter of the transition time of the step plus half the microwave pulse duration.

2.6. THE MEASUREMENT OF THE LINEAR ELECTRIC FIELD EFFECT IN AMORPHOUS SAMPLES

Paramagnetic centres in molecules of biological interest can often be studied only in amorphous samples or glasses containing a random distribution of orientations. Although the resonance lines are in such cases spread out over a wide range of magnetic fields (see e.g. Fig. 3.8, p.74) there need be no intrinsic difficulty in making linear electric field effect measurements if the spin echo method is used since the spin packets in an amorphous sample are no wider than they would be in a single crystal.

A number of additional practical problems arise in making experiments of this kind. Echo signals tend to be considerably weaker than they would be in a single crystal, and boxcar averaging or some equivalent data-collecting system may be required. It is also advantageous to increase the cavity filling factor over and above that which is obtained in conventional cavities such as the one shown in Fig. 2.6. The microwave magnetic field in the cavity in Fig. 2.11, which was designed for making measurements on frozen glasses, occupies a volume approximately ten times less than in the cavity shown in Fig. 2.6. The copper strip (≈ 1 cm long) in the centre of the resonator acts both as a $\frac{1}{2}\lambda$ dipole, coupled in the transmission mode to two tapered waveguide sections, and also as the high-voltage electrode. The microwave magnetic field is mostly confined to the region around the centre of the copper strip and interacts with the sample contained in two wells formed by cut-outs in the Teflon insulator.

By setting the Zeeman field at a given point in the EPR spectrum of the amorphous sample one makes a selection of paramagnetic centres oriented in certain ways. Since a range of

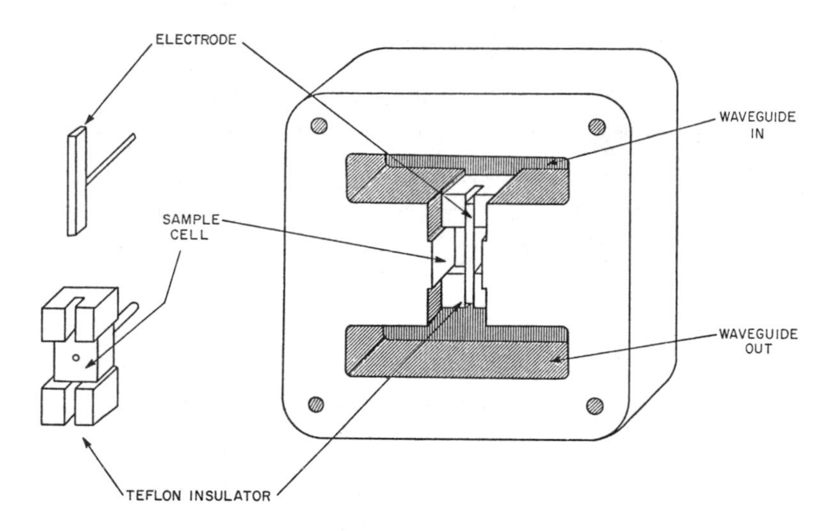

FIG. 2.11. Transmission cavity for studying electric field shifts in amorphous samples. The resonant element consists of a copper strip ≃ $\frac{1}{2}$ λ long which also serves as the high-voltage electrode. Microwave power is coupled in and out from tapered X-band waveguide sections. The sample lies adjacent to the centre of the copper strip, where the microwave magnetic field is maximum. It is contained in two wells formed by cut-outs in the Teflon insulator. (Mims 1974.)

different orientations are involved the shift is usually inhomogeneous. Whatever the range of shifts it can however be argued quite generally that the distribution $S(\overline{\Delta\omega})$ in a glass is an even function (§3.7). Hence $R(E\tau)$ (eqn (2.12)) is real, and the effect of the electric field is to change the amplitude but not the phase of the echo signal.

The behaviour of an amorphous sample can be characterized by making two sets of measurements, one with the electric field parallel to the Zeeman field and one with the electric field perpendicular to it. This can be accomplished by rotating the Zeeman field in a plane containing the applied electric field (e.g. in the plane of the figure of the resonator in Fig. 2.11).

The problem of extracting the g-shift or D-shift parameters in the spin Hamiltonian (eqn (3.2), p.39) from measurements made on an amorphous sample has not yet been fully explored. A brief discussion covering one or two relatively simple situations is however given in §3.7.

2.7. PARAELECTRIC RESONANCE

Transitions can be induced by a suitably polarized microwave electric field between the energy levels of a paramagnetic ion susceptible to the linear electric field effect. This possibility is implied by the form of the linear electric field effect spin Hamiltonian (egn (3.2)) and is explained by the interaction between the electric field and an electric transition moment associated with the ion and with its immediate environment. In an analogous manner the frequency shifts discussed in the previous section can be regarded as being due to the interaction of a d.c. electric field with a static dipole moment belonging to the paramagnetic centre.

The electric transition dipole moment can, when it is large enough, be measured by placing a sample in the microwave electric field in the resonant cavity instead of in the usual position in the microwave magnetic field. In principle this affords an alternative way of measuring the parameters in the linear electric field effect spin Hamiltonian and one which has the advantage that it can be used when the resonance lines are very wide. The breadth of the line is irrelevant here except in so far as it determines the signal intensity. There are, however, a number of practical difficulties (e.g. that of correcting for residual magnetic dipole interactions), and the method can only be applied in a very limited number of cases. A fuller discussion of paraelectric resonance phenomena in paramagnetic materials is given in Chapter 7.

3. Phenomenological description and reduction of data

3.1. THE LINEAR ELECTRIC FIELD EFFECT SPIN HAMILTONIAN

The interaction of the low-lying levels of a paramagnetic atom or ion with an applied electric field can be described by means of a spin Hamiltonian in much the same way as their interaction with applied magnetic fields. All that is required is the construction of terms having the appropriate symmetry. The resulting Hamiltonians are purely formal in the sense that they do not show the physical origin of the crystal field splittings, Zeeman splittings, electric shifts, etc., but they provide a useful and concise way of summarizing the results of microwave resonance experiments.

To begin with, let us consider the normal spin Hamiltonian†

---

† The terms 'normal spin resonance', 'normal spin Hamiltonian', etc. are used to indicate the absence of applied electric fields.

$$\mathcal{H} = \beta g_{jk}H_jS_k + D_{jk}S_jS_k + a_{jk\ell m}S_jS_kS_\ell S_m +$$

$$+ A_{jk}S_jI_k + \gamma_N \underline{H}\cdot\underline{I} + Q_{jk}I_jI_k \quad . \tag{3.1}$$

According to the 'dummy subscript convention' a summation is made over all repeated subscripts. In the present case this implies a summation in which j,k,ℓ,m successively take on the values 1,2,3 and where the subscripts 1,2,3 correspond to projections along the x-,y-,z-axes. For instance, $\beta g_{jk}H_jS_k$ expands to give terms $\beta(g_{11}H_1S_1+g_{12}H_1S_2+g_{13}H_1S_3\ldots)$ which might also be written in the forms $\beta(g_{11}H_xS_x+g_{12}H_xS_y+g_{13}H_xS_z\ldots)$ or $\beta(g_{xx}H_xS_x+g_{xy}H_xS_y+g_{xz}H_xS_z\ldots)$. $D_{jk}S_jS_k$, $A_{jk}S_jI_k$, and $Q_{jk}I_jI_k$ expand in a similar fashion. $\gamma_N\underline{H}\cdot\underline{I}$ contains only three terms, $\gamma_N(H_xI_x+H_yI_y+H_zI_z)$. The operator $a_{jk\ell m}S_jS_kS_\ell S_m$ would contain 81 terms if expanded in the Cartesian form indicated here, but the spherical tensor form is generally preferred as being more concise for all but the very highest point symmetries.

Under coordinate rotations the sets of coefficients g_{jk}, D_{jk}, A_{jk}, Q_{jk} transform contragrediently with the operators H_jS_k, S_jS_k, S_jI_k, I_jI_k as second-rank Cartesian tensors.† Coordinate rotations can be handled more easily however if these tensor quantities are written as 3×3 matrices (see §A.4). The matrices D_{jk}, Q_{jk} are always symmetrical in form, and the matrices

---

† Additional restrictions must be imposed to ensure that g_{jk} and A_{jk} transform as tensors if the S_j, I_j stand for the 'matrix representations' of the operators (see §3.4).

g_{jk}, A_{jk} can be made symmetrical by appropriate definitions (§3.4). Each term therefore contains a maximum of six parameters. A further reduction to five parameters can however be made in the case of D_{jk} and Q_{jk} by requiring that the trace expressions $D_{11} + D_{22} + D_{33}$ and $Q_{11} + Q_{22} + Q_{33}$, which have no effect on the level separations in EPR, should be set to zero (§3.3). The quartic spin operator term is described by a maximum of nine parameters in spherical tensor notation (§3.9).

An electric field applied to the paramagnetic sample may change any or all of the parameters in eqn (3.1). Restricting ourselves to changes which are linear in the applied fields E_i (and ignoring any shifts in γ_N)[†], we can thus write down the new spin Hamiltonian as $\mathcal{H} + \mathcal{H}_{elec}$, where

$$\mathcal{H}_{elec} = E_i(\beta T_{ijk}H_jS_k + R_{ijk}S_jS_k + F_{ijk}S_jI_k + q_{ijk}I_jI_k)$$

$$(i,j,k \text{ from } 1 \text{ to } 3) \qquad (3.2)$$

and where

$$T_{ijk} = \partial g_{jk}/\partial E_i, \quad R_{ijk} = \partial D_{jk}/\partial E_i, \quad F_{ijk} = \partial A_{jk}/\partial E_i, \quad q_{ijk} = \partial Q_{jk}/\partial E_i \;.$$

These coefficients represent the first term in the Taylor expansion of g_{jk}, D_{jk}, A_{jk}, Q_{jk} as a function of the applied electric field.

---

† The nucleus sees an effective field $H_{eff} = H_0(1+\sigma)$ rather than H_0 alone, σ being a paramagnetic shielding correction. Electric field induced shifts in γ_N could arise as a result of a shift in σ. Such shifts would be exceedingly small, however, and have not been observed.

The number of different coefficients can be inferred as follows, assuming for present purposes $T_{ijk} = T_{ikj}$ (see however §§3.4-3.5). Since there are six independent parameters in g_{jk}, A_{jk}, and five in D_{jk}, Q_{jk}, and since each of the three Cartesian components of the applied electric field can produce changes independently of the other components we have a maximum of eighteen parameters for the g-shift T_{ijk}, eighteen for F_{ijk}, fifteen for the D-shift R_{ijk}, and fifteen for q_{ijk}. Shifts in the quartic spin operator term $a_{jk\ell m}S_jS_kS_\ell S_m$ can be described by a maximum of twenty-seven independent parameters by rewriting the term in the spherical tensor form (see §3.9). The quantities T_{ijk}, R_{ijk}, F_{ijk}, q_{ijk} can be formally treated as third-rank Cartesian tensors transforming contragrediently with the operators which they qualify, but in practice it is usually easier to deal with the problem of coordinate rotations by converting at least partially into spherical tensor form as shown in §A.4. The transformation of the quartic spin parameters under coordinate rotation is discussed at the end of §A.4.4.

The phenomenology of the quadratic shifts can be treated in a similar fashion. There have, however, been comparatively few experiments involving quadratic electric shifts and we shall not therefore discuss the properties of the associate spin Hamiltonian in detail.† The quadratic electric g-shift term will suffice as an illustration. It can be written in the form

$$\beta T_{ijk\ell}E_iE_jH_kS_\ell \quad ,$$

where $T_{ijk\ell} = \partial^2 g_{k\ell}/\partial E_i \partial E_j$. Since terms in E_xE_y are indistinguish-

† The symmetry properties are essentially the same as for the piezoresistivity tensor (Smith 1958, p.237).

able from terms in E_yE_x there are six quadratic electric field modifications of the six g-components yielding a maximum of thirty-six independent parameters.

With such a wealth of independent parameters it might seem that the measurement and interpretation of the linear shifts would be an almost impossible task. Fortunately most experiments involve only one kind of shift and require the measurement of a relatively small number of coefficients. For example, if the linear electric effect is being measured for a Kramers ion such as Ce^{3+}, it is only necessary to consider the g-shift tensor T_{ijk} describing the behaviour of the lowest doublet. For an ion such as Cr^{3+}, on the other hand, the g-shift is negligibly small, and the observed shifts can be wholly attributed to R_{ijk}. Moreover, in any but the lowest symmetries, many of the coefficients vanish and relationships exist between others, thus reducing very considerably the number of independent parameters which have to be fitted to the observations.

3.2. THE g-SHIFT TERM

The properties of the third-rank tensors and the way in which the point symmetry of the paramagnetic site restricts the number of parameters can be illustrated by considering the term $E_iT_{ijk}H_jS_k$. This is in some ways not an ideal choice since g_{jk} is not necessarily symmetric in j,k, but we can for the moment assume that the T_{ijk} are a set of equivalent symmetric parameters for which $T_{ijk} = T_{ikj}$ (see §3.5). It is then possible to use the condensed notation introduced by Voigt in which the subscripts j,k are replaced by a single subscript j obtained by making the changes 11 → 1, 22 → 2, 33 → 3, 23 → 4, 13 → 5, 12 → 6. Thus $T_{111}E_1H_1S_1 = T_{111}E_xH_xS_x = T_{11}E_xH_xS_x$, $T_{112}E_1H_1S_2 = T_{112}E_xH_xS_y = T_{16}E_xH_xS_y$, $T_{113}E_1H_1S_3 = T_{113}E_xH_xS_z = T_{15}E_xH_xS_z$, etc. In this notation the g-shift term becomes

$$E_i T_{ijk} H_j S_k$$

$$= E_x\{T_{11}H_xS_x + T_{12}H_yS_y + T_{13}H_zS_z + T_{14}(H_yS_z+H_zS_y) +$$

$$+ T_{15}(H_xS_z+H_zS_x) + T_{16}(H_xS_y+H_yS_x)\} +$$

$$+ E_y\{T_{21}H_xS_x + T_{22}H_yS_y + T_{23}H_zS_z + T_{24}(H_yS_z+H_zS_y) +$$

$$+ T_{25}(H_xS_z+H_zS_x) + T_{26}(H_xS_y+H_yS_x)\} +$$

$$+ E_z\{T_{31}H_xS_x + T_{32}H_yS_y + T_{33}H_zS_z + T_{34}(H_yS_z+H_zS_y) +$$

$$+ T_{35}(H_xS_z+H_zS_x) + T_{36}(H_xS_y+H_yS_x)\} \quad . \qquad (3.3)$$

The first subscript of T refers to the electric field component and the second to the element of the g-tensor which is being modified. It should be noted that in (3.3) $T_{14}(H_yS_z+H_zS_y)$ replaces $T_{123}H_2S_3 + T_{132}H_3S_2$ according to the substitutions $T_{14} = T_{123} = T_{132}$, etc. This differs from the procedure which is commonly adopted in piezoelectricity where the third-rank tensors are constructed by setting $T_{14} = \frac{1}{2}T_{123}$, etc., but it is more convenient here in so far as it prevents the appearance of awkward factors of 2 and $\frac{1}{2}$ in subsequent formulae and tables. The Voigt coefficients can be assembled for inspection in a 3 × 6 matrix T_{ij} ($i = 1$ to 3, $j = 1$ to 6) as follows

$$
\begin{array}{c}
 \\ E_x \\ E_y \\ E_z
\end{array}
\begin{array}{cccc:ccc}
 & H_xS_x & H_yS_y & H_zS_z & \begin{matrix} H_yS_z+ \\ H_zS_y \end{matrix} & \begin{matrix} H_xS_z+ \\ H_zS_x \end{matrix} & \begin{matrix} H_xS_y+ \\ H_yS_x \end{matrix} \\
 & 11 & 12 & 13 & 14 & 15 & 16 \\
 & 21 & 22 & 23 & 24 & 25 & 26 \\
 & 31 & 32 & 33 & 34 & 35 & 36
\end{array} \qquad (3.4)
$$

Each Voigt coefficient is represented by its subscripts only. The portion to the left of the broken line refers to shifts in the diagonal elements of the original g-tensor. The portion to the right of the broken line, the shifts in the off-diagonal elements.

A complete array of six g-parameters occurs only in C_1 point symmetry. In other point symmetries the number of parameters is fewer (see Table 3.1). Likewise the complete array of eighteen g-shift parameters as in (3.4) is only found in C_1 point symmetry the number being greatly reduced in other cases. For higher symmetries it is sometimes easy to see which terms will vanish. For example, if there is a reflection plane containing the x-,y-axes (as for point groups C_{3h} and D_{3h}) then the electric effect will be invariant under a change of sign of the z-axis. Thus, $E_zT_{31}H_xS_x = (-E_z)T_{31}H_xS_x$, etc., and this term together with other terms containing a z-axis component E_z, H_z, or S_z an odd number of times must therefore vanish. The same type of argument can be used to show that in the case of a site possessing inversion symmetry all the coefficients vanish. For an ion at a centrosymmetric site, the shift $E_iT_{ijk}H_jS_k$ is the same as the

TABLE 3.1

The g and D parameters occurring for each of the 21 odd point groups. The format is similar to that used in eqns (3.4) and (3.10). Thus the row of numbers [1,2,3:4,5,6], for C_1 point symmetry, indicates that the parameters $g_1, g_2, g_3, g_4, g_5, g_6$ can all occur. The row [1,1,3:0,0,0] for D_2, etc. indicates that only the coefficients g_1, g_2, g_3 can occur and that $g_2 = g_1$. The first two D-parameters are the coefficients of $(S_x^2 - S_y^2)$, $\frac{1}{3}S(S+1)$; the remainder are the parameters D_4, D_5, D_6 as in eqn (3.5). The notation $C_2(z)$ signifies that the twofold axis is taken here to be the z-axis. (The corresponding table for the eleven even point groups can be derived by substituting even point groups which are related to the odd point groups listed below as in Table 5.1, p. 141).

Odd point groups	g-parameters	D-parameters
C_1	[1 2 3:4 5 6]	[E D:4 5 6]
$C_2(z), C_s$	[1 2 3:0 0 6]	[E D:0 0 6]
$C_2(y)$	[1 2 3:0 5 0]	[E D:0 5 0]
$D_2, C_{2v}, C_3, D_3, C_{3v}, C_4, D_4, C_{4v}, S_4, D_{2d}, C_6, D_6, C_{6v}, C_{3h}, D_{3h}$	[1 1 3:0 0 0]	[0 D:0 0 0]
T, T_d, O	[1 1 1:0 0 0]	[0 0:0 0 0]

shift $(-E_i)T_{ijk}(-H_j)(-S_k)$ which is obtained by reversing the x-,y-, and z-axes. Thus $T_{ijk} = -T_{ijk} = 0$.

For a residue of cases a cursory inspection is not enough and the symmetry transformations must be examined more carefully to find the relationships between the coefficients. Fortunately the analysis is the same as that which is required to determine the relationships between the coefficients used in piezoelectricity† and the results are already tabulated elsewhere (see e.g. Nye 1957; Smith 1958). Fig. 3.1 shows which terms are permitted for the twenty-one odd point groups. The general format is that used in eqn (3.4). A blank space indicates that the element is zero, a bar over a subscript indicates that a minus sign should be used, and duplication of a subscript denotes equality of two tensor elements. For example, the first two rows of the C_{3v} tensor in Fig. 3.1 denote the following relationships for the coefficients T_{ij}.

$$\{T_{11} = 0,\ T_{12} = 0,\ T_{13} = 0,\ T_{14} = 0,\ T_{15},\ T_{16} = -T_{22}\}$$
$$\{T_{21} = -T_{22},\ T_{22},\ T_{23} = 0,\ T_{24} = T_{15},\ T_{25} = 0,\ T_{26} = 0\}$$

The orientations of the Cartesian x-,y-,z-axes which are assumed in arriving at the third-rank tensors given in Fig. 3.1 are indicated in Fig. 3.2, together with a diagrammatic representation

---

† Piezoelectric strain is a quantity consisting of six components (three compression terms and three shear terms) for each of the electric field components E_x, E_y, E_z. The total number of parameters in the lowest symmetry case is thus 18 as for T_{ijk}.

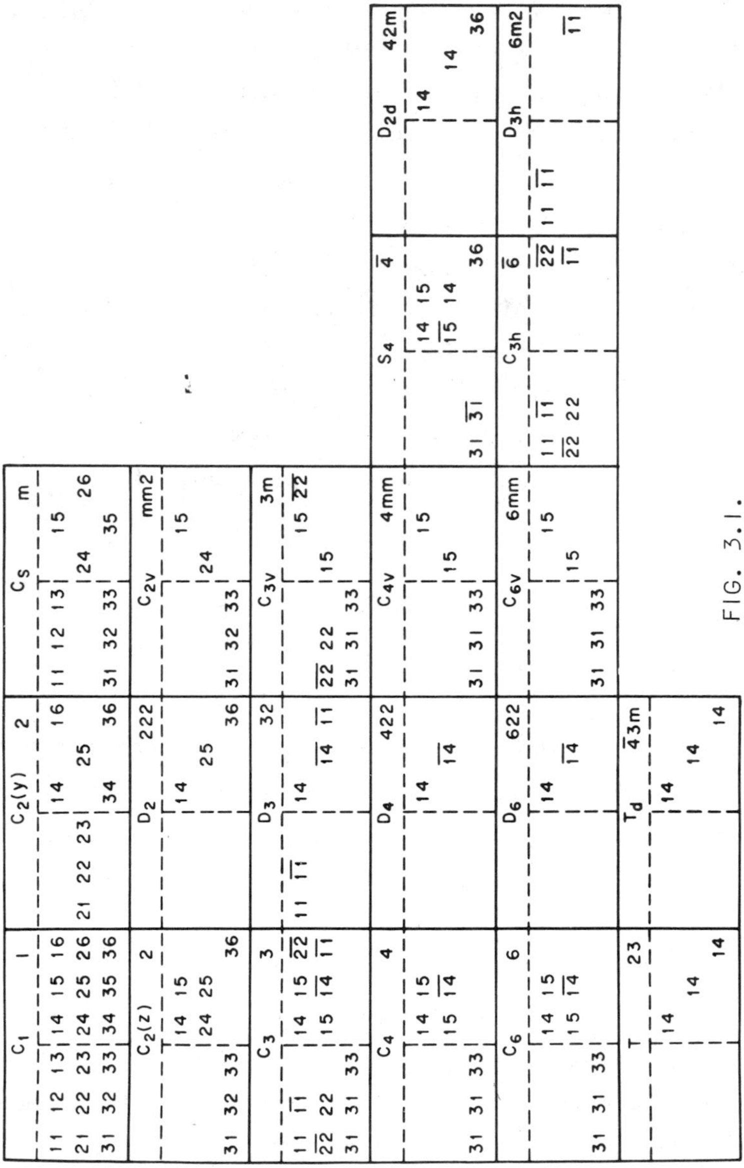

Class	Symbol	Row 1	Row 2	Row 3
C_1	1	11 12 13 14 15 16	21 22 23 24 25 26	31 32 33 34 35 36
$C_2(y)$	2	14 16	21 22 23 25	34 36
C_s	m	11 12 13 15	24 26	31 32 33 35
$C_2(z)$	2	14 15	24 25	31 32 33 36
D_2	222	14	25	36
C_{2v}	mm2	15	24	31 32 33
C_3	3	11 $\overline{11}$ 14 15 $\overline{22}$	$\overline{22}$ 22 15 $\overline{14}$ $\overline{11}$	31 31 33
D_3	32	11 $\overline{11}$ 14	$\overline{14}$ $\overline{11}$	
C_{3v}	3m	15 $\overline{22}$	$\overline{22}$ 22 15	31 31 33
C_4	4	14 15	15 $\overline{14}$	31 31 33
D_4	422	14	$\overline{14}$	
C_{4v}	4mm	15	15	31 31 33
S_4	$\bar{4}$	14 15	$\overline{15}$ 14	31 $\overline{31}$ 36
D_{2d}	$\bar{4}$2m	14	14	36
C_6	6	14 15	15 $\overline{14}$	31 31 33
D_6	622	14	$\overline{14}$	
C_{6v}	6mm	15	15	31 31 33
C_{3h}	$\bar{6}$	11 $\overline{11}$ $\overline{22}$	$\overline{22}$ 22 $\overline{11}$	
D_{3h}	$\bar{6}$m2	11 $\overline{11}$	$\overline{11}$	
T	23	14	14	14
T_d	$\bar{4}$3m	14	14	14

FIG. 3.1.

FIG. 3.1. Parameters appearing in the equivalent symmetric g-shift tensor T_{ij} for the twenty odd point groups (excluding O). The format is as shown in eqn (3.4). A blank indicates that the parameter is zero; the appearance of the same indices in two places indicates that the corresponding two parameters are equal; a bar indicates that the parameter is negative. The same sets of parameters occur for F_{ij} and for B_{ij} (see §3.5). For R_{ij} see Fig. 3.3.

of the symmetry operations belonging to each point group. It is important to know what axis system has been assumed in defining any given set of third-rank tensor coefficients as there is some variation in the conventions employed in published work (i.e. interchanges and rotations of axes). To help in eliminating one possible source of confusion we have here represented the point group C_2 twice: once $C_2(y)$ with the C_2-axis as the y-axis and again $C_2(z)$ with the C_2-axis as the z-axis.

The point group O has no third-rank tensor coefficients in spite of the fact that it is a non-centrosymmetric point group, and it is therefore omitted from the table. All third-rank tensors (including the piezoelectric tensor) associated with this point group have vanishing coefficients, the same being also true for the tensor used to describe shifts associated with the quartic spin operators. This property is related to the absence of lower-order spherical harmonics for the point group O (see Table 4.1, p.109).

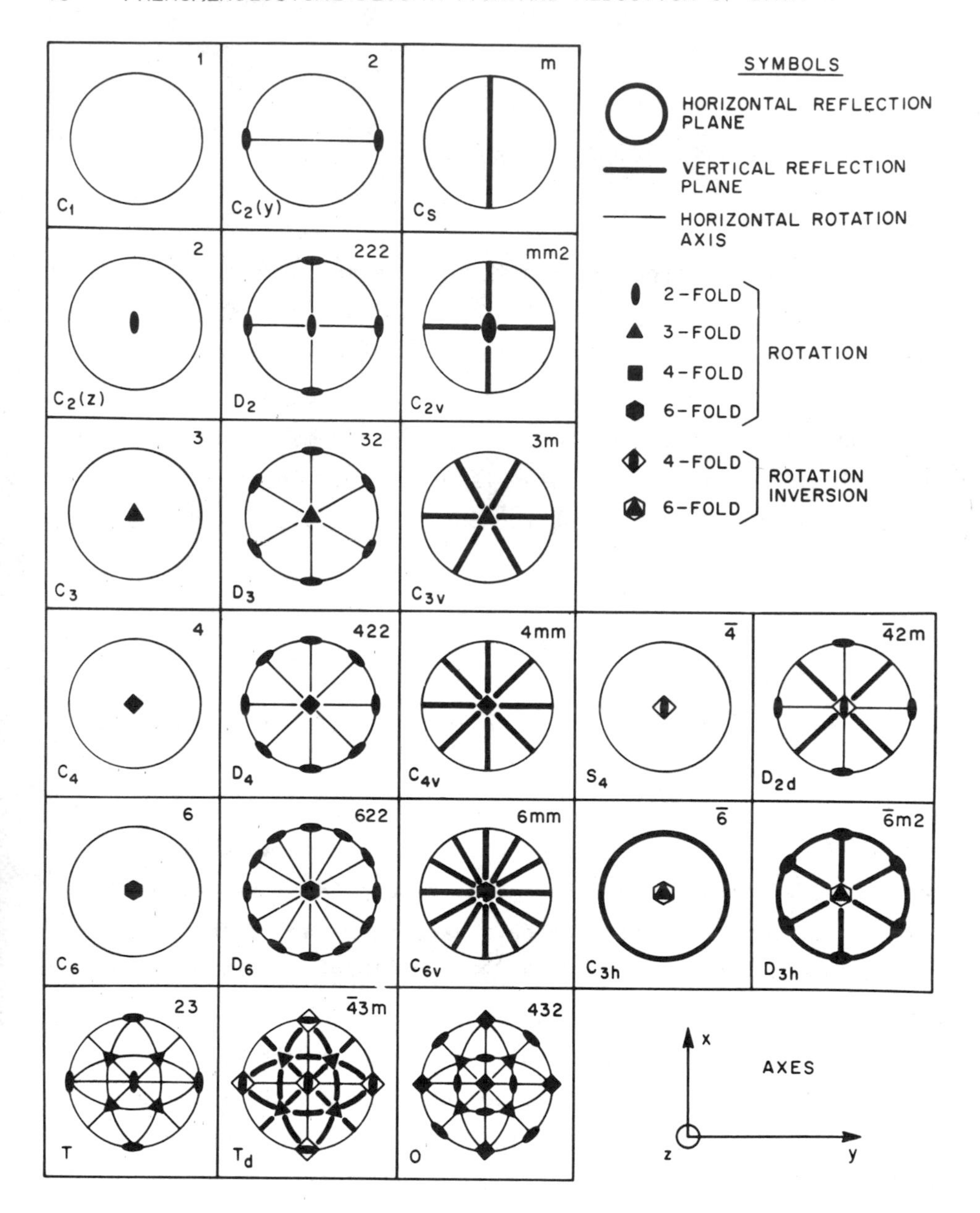

FIG. 3.2. Diagram showing the symmetry elements for the twenty-one odd point groups. (A similar diagram for the eleven even point groups is given in Fig. 5.2 (p.142).)

The conditions governing the parameters T_{ijk} are applicable to the parameters F_{ijk}. They are also applicable to R_{ijk} and to q_{ijk} although in these latter two cases the zero trace condition results in some further simplification. This matter is discussed next.

3.3. THE D-SHIFT TERM

The reasons for introducing the trace condition and the formal means used to incorporate it in the spin Hamiltonian can be understood by considering the D-term. Let us begin with the Cartesian expression

$$D_{jk}S_jS_k = D_1S_x^2 + D_2S_y^2 + D_3S_z^2 + D_4(S_yS_z+S_zS_y) + \\ + D_5(S_xS_z+S_zS_x) + D_6(S_xS_y+S_yS_z) \qquad (3.5)$$

in the Voigt notation. It can easily be verified that the addition of a constant parameter D_c to each of the diagonal terms in the matrix D_{jk} adds $D_c(S_x^2 + S_y^2 + S_z^2) = D_cS(S+1)$ to the Hamiltonian, and raises or lowers all the energy levels by the same amount making no difference to the resonance intervals observed in EPR. The parameters D_1, D_2, D_3 are thus unmeasurable to within an arbitrary constant. One way of removing this indeterminacy is to introduce the further condition $D_1 + D_2 + D_3 = 0$ in the definition (i.e. requiring that the trace of D_{ij} should vanish), as, for example, by subtracting

$$D_T = D_C = \frac{1}{3}(D_1+D_2+D_3) \qquad (3.6)$$

from each of the diagonal elements. This operation would lead to new coefficients

$$D_1' = \frac{1}{3}(2D_1 - D_2 - D_3) ,$$
$$D_2' = \frac{1}{3}(-D_1 + 2D_2 - D_3) , \qquad (3.7)$$
$$D_3' = \frac{1}{3}(-D_1 - D_2 + 2D_3) ,$$

which have the desired property. However, the D-term remains inconveniently clumsy unless we reformulate it to take advantage of the fact that there are only two independent quantities along the diagonal of D_{jk}. What is commonly done in EPR is to write the S_x^2, S_y^2, S_z^2 terms in the form

$$E\left(S_x^2 - S_y^2\right) + D\left\{S_z^2 - \frac{1}{3}S(S+1)\right\} . \qquad (3.8)$$

This corresponds to a Cartesian expression with zero trace as can be verified by making the substitution $S(S+1) = S_x^2 + S_y^2 + S_z^2$. A traceless expression for the overall D-term can be written down by replacing $D_1S_x^2 + D_2S_y^2 + D_3S_z^2$ in eqn (3.5) with (3.8). The traceless form is related to the Cartesian form by the equations

$$D_1 = E - \frac{1}{3}D,\ D_2 = -E - \frac{1}{3}D,\ D_3 = \frac{2}{3}D , \qquad (3.9a)$$

$$E = \frac{1}{2}(D_1 - D_2),\ D = \frac{1}{2}(2D_3 - D_1 - D_2) = \frac{3}{2}D_3 \ \text{(traceless set)}, \qquad (3.9b)$$

Eqn (3.9a) automatically yields a traceless set of coefficients. The first of the two expressions in (3.9b) must be used for D if the D_i are not traceless. The parameters permitted for each of the 21 non-centrosymmetric point groups in this notation are shown in Table 3.1.

The D-shift parameters R_{ij} should be reduced to traceless form for the same reason as the D-parameters. Since

$R_{c,i}(S_x^2+S_y^2+S_z^2)$ can be added to or subtracted from $\mathcal{H}_{elec}$ without introducing any changes in the linear electric shifts the quantities R_{ijk} in eqn (3.2) contain three experimentally indeterminate constants $R_{c,i}$. In the literature this indeterminancy has been eliminated in a variety of ways, perhaps the most elegant being via a redefinition of $R_{ijk}E_iS_jS_k$ in spherical tensor form. In order to keep the notation as close as possible to that used in normal spin resonance, we shall, however, adopt the convention of writing the term $R_{ijk}E_iS_jS_k$ in the form

$$E_i \times \left[R_{iE}\left(S_x^2 - S_y^2\right) + R_{iD}\left\{S_z^2 - \frac{1}{3}S(S+1)\right\} + R_{i4}(S_yS_z+S_zS_y) + \right.$$
$$\left. + R_{i5}(S_xS_z+S_zS_x) + R_{i6}(S_xS_y+S_yS_z)\right] , \tag{3.10}$$

where the parameters R_{iE}, R_{iD} denote shifts in the D- and E-terms induced by the electric field components E_i. There are obvious objections to this mixed notation which is neither Cartesian nor spherical but it has the advantage of being reasonably concise, especially in the case of the higher symmetry point groups, and it seems less likely than most to lead to confusion when employed alongside the standard notation (3.8) for the D-term. We refer to it here as the 'traceless practical notation'. The restrictions which apply to the coefficients in eqn (3.10) for the 20 non-centrosymmetric point groups (excluding O) are shown in Fig. 3.3 by the rows

$$(R_{iE},R_{iD}: R_{i4},R_{i5},R_{i6}) \ .$$

It is important to remember that the coefficients defined above do <u>not</u> transform as a third-rank Cartesian tensor and must be converted to Cartesian tensor form before any attempt is made to rotate axes. The conversion to Cartesian form is made by the equations

C_1 1	$C_2(y)$ 2	C_s m		
1E 1D	14 15 16 2E 2D	24 25 26 3E 3D	34 35 36		14 16 2E 2D	25 | 34 36	1E 1D	15 | 24 26 3E 3D	35		
$C_2(z)$ 2	D_2 222	C_{2v} mm2		
	14 15 	24 25 1E 1D	36		14 	25 	36		15 	24 3E 3D			
C_3 3	D_3 32	C_{3v} 3m		
1E	14 15 $\overline{2E}$ $\overline{2E}$	15 $\overline{14}$ $\overline{1E}$ 3D		1E	14 	$\overline{14}$ $\overline{1E}$		15 $\overline{2E}$ $\overline{2E}$	15 3D			
C_4 4	D_4 422	C_{4v}	S_4 $\overline{4}$	D_{2d} $\overline{4}$2m
	14 15 | 15 $\overline{14}$ 3D			14 | $\overline{14}$		15 | 15 3D			14 15 | $\overline{15}$ 14 3E	36		14 | 14 | 36
C_6 6	D_6 622	C_{6v} 6mm	C_{3h} $\overline{6}$	D_{3h} $\overline{6}$m2
	14 15 | 15 $\overline{14}$ 3D			14 | $\overline{14}$		15 | 15 3D		1E	$\overline{2E}$ $\overline{2E}$	$\overline{1E}$	1E
$\overline{1E}$
T 23	T_d $\overline{4}$3m			
	14 	14 	14		14 	14 	14			

FIG. 3.3

FIG 3.3. Parameters appearing in the D-shift tensor R_{ij} for the twenty odd point groups (excluding O). The five indices in each row correspond to the parameters $(R_{iE}R_{iD}:R_{i4}R_{i5}R_{i6})$ used in the traceless practical notation (eqn (3.10)). A blank indicates that the parameter is zero; the appearance of the same indices in two places indicates that the corresponding two parameters are equal; a bar indicates that the parameter is negative. The same sets of parameters occur for the nuclear quadrupole shifts q_{ij}.

$$R_{i1} = R_{iE} - \frac{1}{3} R_{iD} ,$$
$$R_{i2} = -R_{iE} - \frac{1}{3} R_{iD} , \qquad (3.11)$$
$$R_{i3} = \frac{2}{3} R_{iD} ,$$

and the contrary conversion to traceless practical notation by

$$R_{iE} = \frac{1}{2} (R_{i1}-R_{i2}) , \qquad (3.12)$$
$$R_{iD} = \frac{1}{2}\left(2R_{i3}-R_{i1}-R_{i2}\right) = \frac{3}{2} R_{i3} \quad \text{(traceless set)} ,$$

Eqn (3.11) automatically yields traceless sets of coefficients. The first of the two expressions must be used for R_{iD} in (3.12) if the R_{ij} are not traceless.

3.4. NOTE ON THE SYMMETRY OF g_{jk} AND T_{ijk}

It has been assumed so far that g_{jk} and T_{ijk} transform under axis rotations in the same way as Cartesian tensors and are symmetric in the subscripts j,k ($g_{12} = g_{21}$, etc). This assumption is often incorrect and can be a serious source of confusion in electric effect calculations. To see what is involved here let us first consider the transformation properties of the spin operators S_x, S_y, S_z and of the matrices by which they are represented in spin Hamiltonian calculations. A careful distinction must be made between the operators and the matrices. If the coordinate system is rotated, the operators themselves will always transform according to the equation

$$\underline{S}' = \underline{\underline{M}}\underline{S} , \tag{3.13}$$

where $\underline{M}$ is a real orthogonal 3 × 3 matrix (i.e. the matrix $\underline{M}$ in eqn (A.23)) and $\underline{S}$, $\underline{S}'$ are column vectors made up of the components S_x, S_y, S_z and S_x', S_y', S_z' in the two coordinate systems. When we turn to the representation by matrices, however, an element of arbitrariness enters into the problem. We can represent the spin operators by well-known standard matrices such as Pauli matrices

$$\underline{S}_x = \frac{1}{2}\begin{bmatrix} 0 & 1 \\ 1 & 0 \end{bmatrix} , \quad \underline{S}_y = \frac{1}{2}\begin{bmatrix} 0 & -i \\ i & 0 \end{bmatrix} , \quad \underline{S}_z = \frac{1}{2}\begin{bmatrix} 1 & 0 \\ 0 & -1 \end{bmatrix} . \tag{3.14}$$

Implicit in these matrices is a certain choice of basis functions ψ_+, ψ_- . But we could equally well take a different set obtained from ψ_+, ψ_- by means of the unitary transform

$$\begin{bmatrix} \psi'_+ \\ \\ \psi'_- \end{bmatrix} = [\underline{U}] \begin{bmatrix} \psi_+ \\ \\ \psi_- \end{bmatrix} ,$$

where $\underline{U}$ is a unitary matrix (§A.4.1). This new basis set will give new spin matrices

$$\underline{S}'_x = \underline{U}^\dagger \underline{S}_x \underline{U}, \quad \underline{S}'_y = \underline{U}^\dagger \underline{S}_y \underline{U}, \quad \underline{S}'_z = \underline{U}^\dagger \underline{S}_z \underline{U} \quad ,$$

which afford an equally valid representation, although one which is less simple in form. The new basis set may, if required, be considered to be a set of wavefunctions quantized with respect to a new set of axes x',y',z', instead of x,y,z. From this point of view the change of basis functions is equivalent to a rotation of the coordinate system used in defining the spin operators, even though no actual rotation of the coordinate system is involved.

Confusion can be avoided in situations where a coordinate rotation is in fact being made by insisting that the same basis set be retained throughout. The transformation of the spin matrices is then the same as the transformation of the spin operators, the overall transformation being performed as shown in §A.4.3. Thus the g-term in the spin Hamiltonian

$$\mathcal{H}g/\beta = g_{jk} H_j S_k$$

can be written in the form

$$\mathcal{H}g/\beta \quad \underline{\tilde{H}}\,\underline{g}\,\underline{S} \quad , \tag{3.15}$$

where $\underline{\tilde{H}} = \{H_x, H_y, H_z\}$ is a row vector, $\underline{S} = \{S_x, S_y, S_z\}$ is a column vector and $\underline{g}$ is a 3 × 3 matrix. Transforming to a new coordinate system we obtain new vectors $\underline{H}'$, $\underline{S}'$ and a new matrix $\underline{g}'$, where

$$\underline{H}' = \underline{\underline{M}}\underline{H},\ \underline{S}' = \underline{\underline{M}}\underline{S},\ \underline{g}' = \underline{\underline{M}}\underline{g}\tilde{\underline{M}} \ . \tag{3.16}$$

(The matrix $\underline{M}$ which defines the coordinate rotation is given in terms of Euler angles in eqn (A.23).) The requirement that the spin matrices should transform like the spin operators will of course change their apparent form. Thus the new operator $\underline{S}_x'$ is given in terms of the old by

$$\underline{S}_x' = M_{11}\underline{S}_x + M_{12}\underline{S}_y + M_{13}\underline{S}_z \ ,$$

and hence, if we use Pauli spin matrices for $\underline{S}_x, \underline{S}_y, \underline{S}_z$,

$$\underline{S}_x' = \frac{1}{2}\begin{bmatrix} M_{13} & M_{11}-iM_{12} \\ M_{11}+iM_{12} & -M_{13} \end{bmatrix}, \text{ etc.}$$

Under these conditions the commonly made assumption that description of the g-matrix transforms as a second-rank Cartesian tensor is correct, irrespective of whether $\underline{g}$ is symmetric or not.†

To see what happens when we do not impose these conditions let us consider the effect of changing the representation without rotating the coordinates. A requantization of the basis functions

---

† Strictly speaking it is still not correct to describe the quantities g,D,A etc. as tensors since they do not possess all the required properties. But they will transform as tensors under coordinate rotations.

with respect to new axes has, of course, no effect on the operator equations but when the components of the spin operator are written out in matrix form it becomes equivalent to a rotation of $\underline{S}$. There is no corresponding change in $\underline{H}$, and we therefore have the transforming relations

$$\underline{H}' = \underline{H},\ \underline{S}' = \underline{\underline{N}}\underline{S} \quad , \tag{3.17}$$

which result in the g-matrix transformation

$$\underline{g}' = \underline{g}\tilde{\underline{\underline{N}}} \quad , \tag{3.18}$$

Since orthogonal matrices are not generally symmetric it is easily seen that eqn (3.18) can turn an initially symmetric g-matrix into a non-symmetric one. It is also possible to convert a non-symmetric g-matrix $\underline{g}_N$ into a symmetric g-matrix $\underline{g}_S$ by the converse procedure. To demonstrate this let us tentatively suppose that $\underline{g}_N$ and $\underline{g}_S$ are related by the equations

$$\underline{g}_S^2 = \underline{g}_N\tilde{\underline{g}}_N,\ \underline{g}_S = \underline{g}_N\tilde{\underline{\underline{N}}} \quad . \tag{3.19}$$

It is then required to show that the transforming matrix N is orthogonal. Writing $\underline{N} = \underline{g}_S\underline{g}_N^{-1}$, $\tilde{\underline{N}} = \tilde{\underline{g}}_N^{-1}\underline{g}_S$ we have $\tilde{\underline{\underline{N}}}\underline{\underline{N}} = \underline{g}_N\underline{g}_S^2\underline{g}_N^{-1}$. Substituting (3.19) we obtain $\tilde{\underline{\underline{N}}}\underline{\underline{N}} = \underline{I}$, thus proving the result, provided that $\underline{g}_N$ is not singular.

We conclude therefore that a spin Hamiltonian with a symmetric g-matrix can always be used to describe EPR data provided that a suitable set of spin matrices is used to represent S_x, S_y, S_z. The g-matrix will then remain symmetrical under all coordinate transformations provided that the spin matrices are made to undergo the same set of transformations as the operators. This is equivalent to requiring that the axes of quantization should remain physically the same (relative to crystal axes, etc.) and that they should not undergo rotation along with the coordinate system. If, on the other hand, it is decided to use the Pauli spin matrix representation both before and after a coordinate rotation, (e.g. for computational convenience) then, by implication, the quantizing axes as well as the axes used to define the spin operators have been rotated. In this case, by (3.16) and (3.17),

$$\underline{S}' = \underline{N}\underline{M}\underline{S}, \quad \underline{g}' = \underline{M}\underline{g}\underline{M}\tilde{\underline{N}} \; . \tag{3.20}$$

Since $\underline{S}'$ is to have the same form as $\underline{S}$, $\underline{N}\underline{M} = \underline{I}$ and hence

$$\underline{g}' = \underline{M}\underline{g} \; . \tag{3.21}$$

The transformation in eqns (3.20) and (3.21) is not a similarity transform, and it will be incorrect to describe $\underline{g}$ as a second-rank Cartesian tensor if coordinate rotations are to be made in this manner.

The above argument has been illustrated with respect to a manifold consisting of two states only but the same considerations apply when this is no longer so, as, for instance, when the states belong to the lowest J manifold of a rare-earth ion. An unlimited number of representations in terms of magnetic eigenstates are possible, and calculations based on any arbitrarily chosen representation may be expected to yield an asymmetric g-matrix (see §6.1 and Table 6.2 for the case of half-integral J). A symmetric form of g-matrix can however be derived by quantizing along a new set of axes.[†]

[†] If the site under consideration has axial or simple octahedral symmetry then the first and most obvious choice of representation will often yield a symmetric g-matrix; see e.g. the treatment of Fe^{3+}, $S' = \frac{1}{2}$ in Griffith (1971)(p. 363) or in Abragam and Bleaney (1970)(p.481).

It is also possible to represent the term $A_{jk}S_jI_k$ in symmetric form by making a suitable choice of basis states. The basis states for S may have been determined in order to make g_{jk} symmetric, but the basis states for I can still be constructed in any way. Constraints begin to appear, however, when terms are added to describe the linear electric field effect, since it may not be possible to find a set of basis states which will make the g-matrix and the shifted g-matrix,

$$g_{jk}^{(E)} = g_{jk} + \sum_i E_i T_{ijk} , \qquad (3.22)$$

both simultaneously symmetric in j,k. Theoretical calculations of the g-shift parameters generally yield a non-symmetric set of T_{ijk} which can, if so desired, be resolved into a symmetric and an antisymmetric set. (see e.g. Ham 1963; also §6.2). In the usual kind of frequency-shift experiment the symmetric and antisymmetric portions of T_{ijk} combine to produce the observed effects and cannot be resolved. This is a consequence of the fact that frequency measurements yield parameters describing the g^2-tensor rather than the g-tensor, as shown in the following section. The parameters T_{ijk}, T_{ikj} can, however, be determined individually by means of paraelectric resonance experiments provided that such experiments are practical for the system concerned (see Chapter 7; also §10.6).

3.5. THE SHIFT IN g^2. EXTRACTION OF EQUIVALENT SYMMETRIC T_{ijk} PARAMETERS FROM EXPERIMENTAL DATA

In the following section we shall assume that the resonance transition takes place between the two levels of a Kramers doublet (for non-Kramers doublets see §3.10) and that the spin Hamiltonian, including the linear electric field effect term, is given by

$$\mathcal{H} = \beta(g_{jk}H_jS_k + T_{ijk}E_iH_jS_k) \quad .$$

The relationship between the parameters g_{jk}, T_{ijk} and the energy shifts can be demonstrated most easily by going back to first principles. Let us consider the term $\beta g_{jk}H_jS_k$. Diagonalizing the Hamiltonian matrix for this term in an $S = \frac{1}{2}$ manifold and equating the energies of the two eigenstates to $\pm\frac{1}{2}\, g\beta H_0$ we find that

$$g^2 = G_{11}\ell^2 + G_{22}m^2 + G_{33}n^2 + (G_{23}+G_{32})mn + \\ + (G_{13}+G_{31})\ell n + (G_{12}+G_{21})\ell m \,, \tag{3.23}$$

where ℓ,m,n are the direction cosines of $\underline{H}_0$ ($H_x = \ell H_0$, etc.), and

$$G_{jk} = g_{jq}g_{kq} \,. \tag{3.24}$$

In matrix notation (3.24) becomes

$$\underline{G} = \underline{g}\tilde{\underline{g}} \,. \tag{3.25}$$

Clearly it makes no difference whether $\underline{g}$ is symmetric or not. The matrix $\underline{G}$ will, in any event, be symmetric. Furthermore $\underline{G}$ will be unaffected by changes in the representation used for the spin operators and will transform as a second-rank Cartesian tensor. Using the Voigt notation we can rewrite (3.23) in the shortened form

$$g^2 = G_1\ell^2 + G_2m^2 + G_3n^2 + 2G_4mn + 2G_5\ell n + 2G_6\ell m \,. \tag{3.26}$$

In a resonance experiment at any given magnetic field setting the quantity measured is $|g|$ in the equation

$$\hbar\omega = |g|\beta H_0 \quad . \tag{3.27}$$

It will be noticed that the question of whether there may be an antisymmetric component of $\underline{g}$ does not arise in a typical measurement of the resonance interval and that a set of measurements of this kind will yield the g^2-tensor (3.24) rather than the g-tensor which appears in the spin Hamiltonian.

Eqn (3.26) is especially convenient for the purpose of plotting experimental values and fitting data. In terms of the polar and azimuthal angles θ,ϕ, which define the direction of the Zeeman field $\underline{H}_0$, $\ell = \sin\theta\cos\phi$, $m = \sin\theta\sin\phi$, $n = \cos\theta$ (Fig. 3.4.). Thus, if $\underline{H}_0$ is rotated in a selected plane and g^2

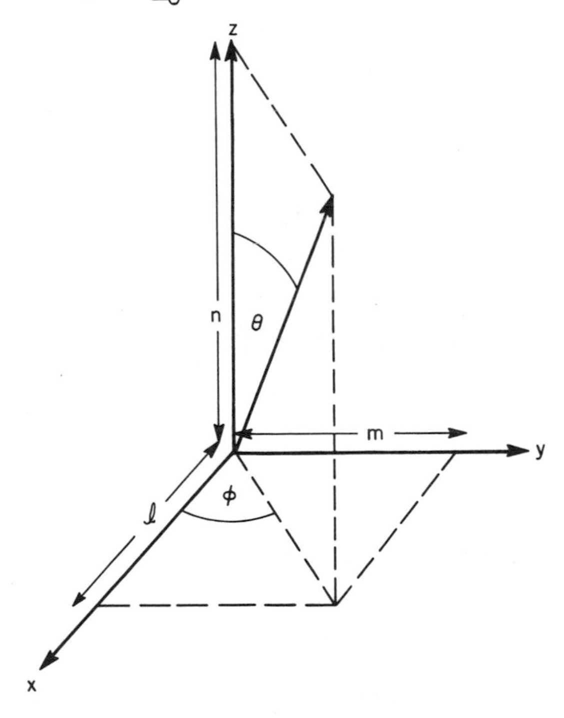

FIG. 3.4. Azimuthal and polar angles ϕ,θ and the corresponding direction cosines ℓ,m,n.

is plotted as a function of the angle of rotation, a simple sine-cosine function is obtained. For instance, if the Zeeman field is rotated in the xz-plane ($\ell=\sin\theta$, $m=0$, $n=\cos\theta$), then $g^2 = \frac{1}{2}(G_1+G_3) - \frac{1}{2}(G_1-G_3)\cos 2\theta + G_5\sin 2\theta$. Eqn (3.26) is related to a g-ellipsoid in the same way that the equation for the moment of inertia of a solid about a given axis can be related to an inertia ellipsoid (see e.g. Goldstein 1950). The g-factor assumes its three principal values when $\underline{H}_0$ is aligned along each of the principal axes of this ellipsoid. For some of the higher point symmetries these axes will coincide with the x-,y-,z-axes used in describing the symmetry operations of the point group (see Figs 3.2 and 5.2 (p.142)). In the general case, however, these orientations must be determined by making a principal axis transform of the matrix $\underline{G}$. Principal values of $\underline{g}$ can be derived by taking the square-roots of the principal values of the G-matrix (See §A.4.3).

Let us next consider the small changes in G_{jk} and g_{jk} which are induced by applying an electric field. Differentiating (3.26) with respect to the three components of electric field, we have the expression

$$\delta(g^2) =$$

$$E_x(B_{11}\ell^2 + B_{12}m^2 + B_{13}n^2 + 2B_{14}mn + 2B_{15}\ell n + 2B_{16}\ell m) +$$

$$+E_y(B_{21}\ell^2 + B_{22}m^2 + B_{23}n^2 + 2B_{24}mn + 2B_{25}\ell n + 2B_{26}\ell m) +$$

$$+E_z(B_{31}\ell^2 + B_{32}m^2 + B_{33}n^2 + 2B_{34}mn + 2B_{35}\ell n + 2B_{36}\ell m)\ , \qquad (3.28)$$

where

$$B_{11} = \frac{\partial G_1}{\partial E_x}\ ,\ B_{21} = \frac{\partial G_1}{\partial E_y}\ ,\ B_{31} = \frac{\partial G_1}{\partial E_z}\ ,\ \text{etc.}$$

The array of coefficients B_{ij} describe a physical property of the system as a function of its orientation and must therefore be invariant under the symmetry operations of the point group. In the present case this means that the relations between the B_{ij} are those indicated in Fig. 3.1, i.e. they are the same as the relations holding between the equivalent symmetric g-shift coefficients T_{ij} (§3.2). Eqn (3.28) is, like the g^2 equation (3.26), a convenient one to use when fitting data since it expresses the shifts $\delta(g^2)$ as simple sine-cosine functions of the polar and azimuthal angles of $\underline{H}_0$. The experimental frequency shifts $\Delta\nu$ can be readily converted into values of $\delta(g^2)$ by means of the relation

$$\delta(g^2) = 2g^2\Delta\nu/\nu \quad , \tag{3.29}$$

where ν is the microwave frequency, and where g^2 can either be calculated from eqn (3.26) or measured directly, as in eqn (3.27), during the experiment. A plot of $\delta(g^2)$ as a function of the polar or azimuthal angle can then be used to find the parameters B_{ij}.

Two examples of an experimental plot are shown in Figs (3.5) and (3.6). (Mims 1965). Fig. 3.5 shows the experimental values of $\delta(g^2)$ obtained for the Yb^{3+} Kramers doublet in $CaWO_4$ with the electric field applied along the z-axis and $\underline{H}_0$ rotated in the xy-plane. The point symmetry here is S_4 (see Figs 3.1 and 3.2), the x- and y-axes being identified with the crystalline a- and b-axes, and the material contains inversion image sites (§2.2). For this point symmetry and these field orientations eqn (3.28) reduces to

$$\begin{aligned}\delta(g^2) &= \pm E_z\{B_{31}(\ell^2-m^2) + 2B_{36}\ell m\} \\ &= \pm E_z(B_{31}\cos 2\phi + B_{36}\sin 2\phi) \quad ,\end{aligned} \tag{3.30}$$

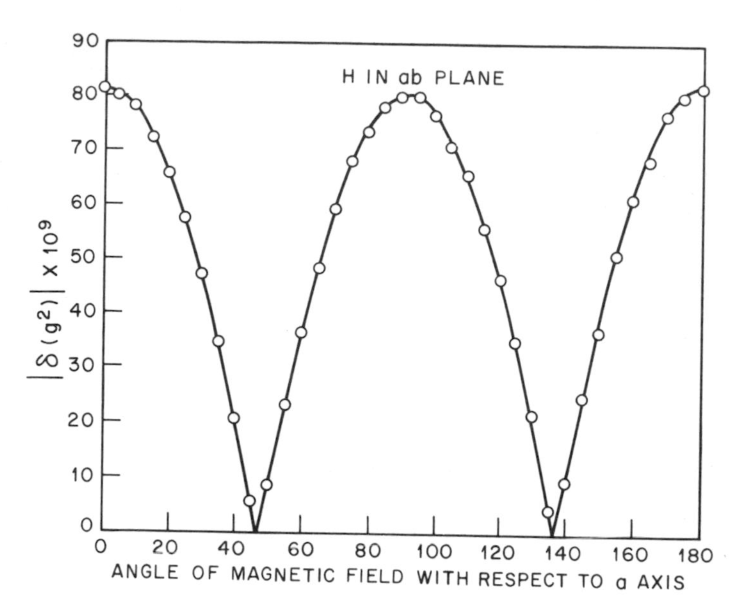

FIG. 3.5. $|\delta(g^2)| \times 10^9$ corresponding to an electric field of 1 V cm^{-1} applied along the c-axis in (Ca,Yb)WO_4. $\underline{H}_0$ is varied in the ab-plane. The curve can be fitted to the function given in eqn (3.30). The angle at which $\delta(g^2)$ is zero is given by $\phi_3 = \frac{1}{2}$ arc tan $(-B_{31}/B_{36})$. The maximum amplitude of the curve is $(B_{31}^2 + B_{36}^2)^{\frac{1}{2}}$. Equivalent symmetric g-shift parameters T_{ij} can be calculated from B_{ij} by using the results in Table 3.2.

the ± signs referring to the shifts undergone by the two kinds of site. The function has maximum and minimum values $\pm(B_{31}^2 + B_{36}^2)^{\frac{1}{2}}$, and crosses through zero at an angle ϕ_3 where $\tan 2\phi_3 = -B_{31}/B_{36}$. The angular dependence of $\delta(g^2)$ (represented by the absolute magnitude $|\delta(g^2)|$ in the figure) determines the relative signs of the coefficients, but the absolute signs cannot be found since there is no way of distinguishing between the inversion image sites.† Fig. 3.6 shows $\delta(g^2)$ for an electric

† The two inversion image sites have, however, been separately identified for Mn^{2+} centres in NaCl (see §10.4).

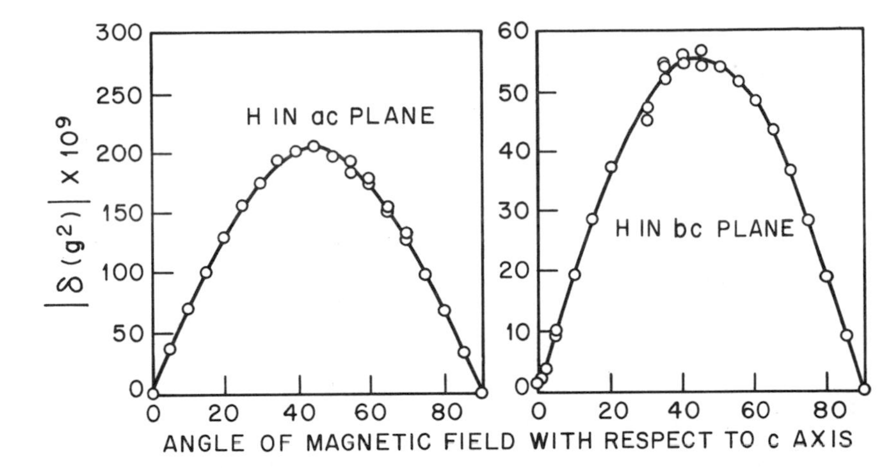

FIG. 3.6. $\delta(g^2) \times 10^9$ corresponding to an electric field of 1 V cm^{-1} applied along the a-axis in $(Ca,Yb)WO_4$. For $\underline{H}_0$ in the ac-plane the maximum amplitude of the curve gives B_{15}. For $\underline{H}_0$ in the bc-plane the maximum amplitude gives B_{14} (see eqn (3.31)). Equivalent symmetric g-shift parameters T_{ij} can be calculated from B_{ij} as shown in Table 3.2.

field along the x-axis and $\underline{H}_0$ in the xz- and yz-planes. Here the equations for $\delta(g^2)$ are

$$\begin{aligned} \delta(g^2) &= \pm 2E_x B_{15} \ell n = \pm E_x B_{15} \sin 2\theta \quad (\phi = 0^\circ), \\ \delta(g^2) &= \pm 2E_x B_{14} mn = \pm E_x B_{14} \sin 2\theta \quad (\phi = 90^\circ), \end{aligned} \tag{3.31}$$

and the parameters B_{15}, B_{14} can be obtained at once by measuring the peaks of the experimental sine curves.

The B_{ij} parameters are in themselves sufficient to describe the experimental data, and there is no need to re-express the results in terms of g-shift parameters T_{ijk}, thus raising the question of a possible asymmetry in T_{ijk} as discussed in the previous section. But it is sometimes necessary to be able to perform the converse operation of converting the T_{ijk} into B_{ijk}

coefficients in order to be able to compare theory and experiment. The general relationship can be found by differentiating eqn (3.24) and writing

$$T_{ijk} = \partial g_{jk}/\partial E_i \ .$$

We thus obtain the equations

$$B_{ijk} = \sum_q (g_{jq}T_{ikq}+g_{kq}T_{ijq}) \ , \qquad (3.32)$$

which can be used to derive the g^2-shift coefficients from theoretical g-shift coefficients. Since the theoretical values for the pairs of coefficients T_{ikq}, T_{iqk} may differ for the reasons indicated in the previous section, both coefficients will be required in order to calculate the B_{ijk}.

Eqn (3.32) can be used to derive a set of equivalent symmetric g-shift parameters from the experimental B_{ijk} by arbitrarily assuming that g_{jk} and T_{ijk} are both symmetric in j,k. These parameters will not generally correspond with the theoretical T_{ijk} parameters and merely have the property of leading to the correct frequency shifts. The conversion can be made by solving the equations from Table 3.2 after substituting the values g_j and T_{ij} appropriate to the point symmetry in question (see Table 3.1 and Fig. 3.1). As will be apparent from Table 3.2, this conversion is easiest to make if the coordinate system is chosen so that $\underline{g}$ is diagonal.

It is sometimes helpful to visualize the electric field induced changes E_iB_{ij} in the g^2-matrix G_j as geometrical modifications of the 'g-ellipsoid'. These modifications are most easily described in a coordinate system which gives $\underline{G}$ in principal-axis form. The terms E_iB_{i1}, E_iB_{i2}, E_iB_{i3} then represent changes in the principal values G_1, G_2, G_3, and the remaining terms

TABLE 3.2

Relationship between the g^2-shift parameters B_{ij} and the equivalent symmetric g-shift parameters T_{ij} (see §3.5). It is assumed here that the g-matrix has already been reduced to symmetric form and can therefore be expressed in Voigt notation. The true g-shift parameters as obtained in theoretical calculations or as measured in paraelectric resonance experiments are not as a general rule symmetric in j,k and cannot be expressed in Voigt notation. They are related to the B_{ij} as in eqn (3.32).

g^2-shift parameter	Function of g and equivalent symmetric g-shift parameters
B_{i1}	$2(g_1T_{i1}+g_6T_{i6}+g_5T_{i5})$
B_{i2}	$2(g_6T_{i6}+g_2T_{i2}+g_4T_{i4})$
B_{i3}	$2(g_5T_{i5}+g_4T_{i4}+g_3T_{i3})$
B_{i4}	$g_6T_{i5}+g_5T_{i6}+g_2T_{i4}+g_4T_{i2}+g_4T_{i3}+g_3T_{i4}$
B_{i5}	$g_1T_{i5}+g_5T_{i1}+g_6T_{i4}+g_4T_{i6}+g_5T_{i3}+g_3T_{i5}$
B_{i6}	$g_1T_{i6}+g_6T_{i1}+g_6T_{i2}+g_2T_{i6}+g_5T_{i4}+g_4T_{i5}$

E_iB_{i4}, E_iB_{i5}, E_iB_{i6} represent small tilts of the g-ellipsoid. In reference to a fixed axis system the g-ellipsoid is rotated by angles ψ_x, ψ_y, ψ_z about the x-, y-, and z-axes, where†

$$\begin{aligned} \psi_x &= E_iB_{i4}/(G_2-G_3) , \\ \psi_y &= E_iB_{i5}/(G_3-G_1) , \\ \psi_z &= E_iB_{i6}/(G_1-G_2) . \end{aligned} \tag{3.33}$$

It is of course assumed here that $G_1 \neq G_2 \neq G_3$ and that the angles ψ_x, ψ_y, ψ_z are small. This picture can not be used in the case of the true g-shift coefficients T_{ijk} since, even if $\underline{g}$ itself is symmetric, some of the terms are liable to contain an antisymmetric component and these terms cannot be generated by means of a rotation. The equivalent symmetric coefficients T_{ij} can, however, be regarded in this way. Substituting $B_{i4} = (g_2+g_3)T_{i4}$, $B_{i5} = (g_1+g_3)T_{i5}$, and $B_{i6} = (g_1+g_2)T_{i6}$ from Table 3.2 together with $G_1 = g_2^2$, $G_3 = g_3^2$ we have expressions

---

† The expressions for ψ_y and ψ_z can be obtained by setting $\alpha = 0$, $\beta = \psi_y$, $\gamma = 0$ or alternatively $\alpha = -\psi_z$, $\beta = 0$, $\gamma = 0$ in the matrix $\underline{M}$ in eqn (A.23) and equating the transformed matrix $\underline{G}' = \underline{M}\underline{G}\underline{\tilde{M}}$ (eqn (A.29)) to $G_j + E_iB_{ij}$. Negative values of ψ_y, ψ_z must be used since the transformations in §A.4 are defined for rotations of the axis system with respect to a fixed physical object. The result for ψ_x is not easy to derive in this way because of the convention used in specifying the Euler angles. It can be found by permuting axes, or by setting $\alpha = \pi/2$, $\beta = -\psi_x$, $\gamma = -\pi/2$ in $\underline{M}$ (see §A.4.2).

$$\psi_x = E_i T_{i4}/(g_2-g_3) ,$$

$$\psi_y = E_i T_{i5}/(g_3-g_1) , \qquad (3.34)$$

$$\psi_z = E_i T_{i6}/(g_1-g_2) ,$$

which are of the same form as eqns (3.33).

3.6. THE EXTRACTION OF OTHER LINEAR ELECTRIC FIELD EFFECT PARAMETERS FROM EXPERIMENTAL DATA: AN APPROXIMATE EXPRESSION FOR THE D-SHIFT

A straightforward, although often a rather tedious, method for fitting the parameters in $\underline{\mathcal{H}}_{elec}$ is to diagonalize the Hamiltonians $\underline{\mathcal{H}}$ and $\underline{\mathcal{H}} + \underline{\mathcal{H}}_{elec}$ numerically for the experimental Zeeman field settings and for suitable trial values of the parameters. In so far as the differences between the two sets of eigenvalues are linear in the electric fields E_i and in the shift parameters they can then be used to obtain a 'theoretical' curve which can be scaled to the experimental curve. When proceeding in this way, it is obviously necessary to choose trial values in $\mathcal{H}_{elec}$ which are large enough to avoid serious round-off errors in the computed differences, but care should also be taken to ensure that the trial values are not so large as to give frequency shifts with a quadratic dependence on E_i. (The range of safety can easily be found by making several computer runs.)

An alternative method, not requiring the calculation of small differences, is the following. The matrix $\underline{\mathcal{H}}$ is first diagonalized and its eigenvectors are assembled to form the unitary matrix $\underline{\mathfrak{M}}$. The required electric shifts are then found by making the diagonal elements of the transform $\underline{\mathfrak{M}}^{-1}\underline{\mathcal{H}}_{elec}\underline{\mathfrak{M}}$. To justify this procedure let us consider the transform

$\underline{\mathfrak{M}}^{-1}(\underline{\mathcal{H}}+\underline{\mathcal{H}}_{elec})\underline{\mathfrak{M}}$ of the full Hamiltonian. $\underline{\mathfrak{M}}^{-1}\underline{\mathcal{H}}\underline{\mathfrak{M}}$ is by definition diagonal and contains the eigenvalues of $\underline{\mathcal{H}}$. The remaining portion $\underline{\mathfrak{M}}^{-1}\underline{\mathcal{H}}_{elec}\underline{\mathfrak{M}}$ consists of both diagonal and non-diagonal terms. Of these the diagonal terms add to or subtract from the corresponding eigenvalues, and constitute the shifts, whilst the non-diagonal terms lead to small perturbations proportional to E^2, which can be ignored.

As we have seen in the previous section, numerical computations of this kind are not necessary for finding the g-shift parameters of a Kramers doublet ion since the experimental g^2-shift values can be fitted directly to a trigonometric expression. It is also sometimes possible to fit the frequency shifts associated with the parameters R_{ijk} to an analytic expression provided that the D term is small compared with the Zeeman term and g is nearly isotropic. This situation is relatively common at 35 GHz and can occur for some ions (e.g. Mn^{2+}) at X(≃ 10 GHz) Band. To derive the required expression, let us consider a rotation of the coordinate axes bringing the z-axis into alignment with the Zeeman field $\underline{H}_0$. Rotating the axes used to specify $\underline{S}$ and $\underline{H}$ (but not $\underline{E}$) in the spin Hamiltonian we have

$$\underline{\mathcal{H}}' + \underline{\mathcal{H}}'_{elec} = g\beta H'_z S'_z + D'_{jk} S'_j S'_k + E_i R'_{ijk} S'_j S'_k \,, \qquad (3.35)$$

where the terms $T_{ijk}E_iH_jS_k$, $A_{jk}S_jI_k$, etc. are ignored and where primes denote components in the new coordinate system. Since $D'_{jk}S'_jS'_k$ is assumed to be small compared with $g\beta H'_zS'_z$, the eigenstates of $\underline{\mathcal{H}}'$ can be taken as approximate eigenstates of $\underline{S}'_z$. Thus, in a matrix representation based on eigenstates of the rotated spin operator $\underline{S}'_z$, all the large terms in $\underline{\mathcal{H}}'$ appear along the diagonal together with the terms in S'^2_z from $\underline{\mathcal{H}}_{elec}$. The off-diagonal terms contribute perturbations ≃ $D'^2_{jk}/\hbar\omega$, $D_{jk}E_iR_{ijk}/\hbar\omega$, $(E_iR_{ijk})^2/\hbar\omega$, which we shall ignore in keeping with our assumption that the D-term is relatively small. The frequency shifts $\Delta\nu$ are derived from the diagonal matrix elements of linear electric field effect terms, i.e. from the matrix elements of the terms $E_i R'_{iD}\{S_z'^2 - 1/3\ S(S+1)\}$. For the $M_S \rightleftarrows M_S-1$ transition we thus have[†]

$$\Delta\nu = E_i R'_{iD}(2M_S-1) \quad . \tag{3.36}$$

The final step is to transform the R'_{iD} into a set of coefficients referred to the original coordinate system. This is the same as the operation of transforming the D-coefficient since only the spin operators were re-expressed in the primed system, the electric field components being left in the old system. Converting R'_{ID} to the Cartesian form R'_{i3} by eqn (3.12), then performing the orthogonal transformation (A.26) with Euler angles $\alpha = \phi$, $\beta = \theta$, $\gamma = 0$, (eqn (A.23)) we have

$$R'_{iD} = \frac{3}{2} R'_{i3}$$

$$= \frac{3}{2} (R_{i1}\ell^2 + R_{i2}m^2 + R_{i3}n^2 + 2R_{i4}mn + 2R_{i5}\ell n + 2R_{i6}\ell m) \ , \tag{3.37}$$

where ℓ, m, n are the direction cosines of $\underline{H}_0$. In the traceless practical notation eqn (3.37) becomes

---

† It is assumed here that the parameters R_{ij} are expressed in frequency units (e.g. Hz per V cm^{-1}). If the R_{ij} are expressed in energy units then $\Delta\nu$, or $\Delta\omega$ will replace $\Delta\nu$ on the left-hand side of this equation and on the left-hand side of eqns (3.37) and (3.38).

$$R'_{iD} = \frac{3}{2}\{(R_{iE} - \frac{1}{3}R_{iD})\ell^2 - (R_{iE} + \frac{1}{3}R_{iD})m^2 + \frac{2}{3}R_{iD}n^2 +$$

$$+ 2R_{i4}mn + 2R_{i5}\ell n + 2R_{i6}\ell m\} \quad . \tag{3.38}$$

The required approximate expression for the frequency shift is found by substituting (3.38) in (3.36) and by setting $i = 1,2,3$.

As an example, we can take the case of Mn^{2+} in $CaWO_4$ in magnetic fields ~3·5 kG (X-band resonance). Here $S = \frac{5}{2}$, the site has S_4 symmetry, the D-term and the term $A_{jk}S_jI_k$ have a relatively minor effect on the results, and the quartic spin operator terms are almost negligible. Selecting the appropriate R_{ij} coefficients from Fig. 3.3 and substituting in eqns (3.36) and (3.38), we have

$$\Delta\nu = \frac{3}{2}(2M_S-1)\{E_x(2R_{14}mn+2R_{15}\ell n) + E_y(-2R_{15}mn+2R_{14}\ell n) +$$

$$+ E_z(R_{3E}\ell^2-R_{3E}m^2+2R_{36}\ell m)\}$$

$$= \frac{3}{2}(2M_S-1)\{E_x\sin 2\theta(R_{14}\sin\phi+R_{15}\cos\phi) +$$

$$+ E_y\sin 2\theta(-R_{15}\sin\phi+R_{14}\cos\phi) +$$

$$+ E_z\sin^2\theta(R_{3E}\cos 2\phi+R_{36}\sin 2\phi)\}. \tag{3.39}$$

According to this approximate formula, the shifts for the $M_S = \pm\frac{5}{2} \rightleftarrows \pm\frac{3}{2}$ transitions will be twice the shifts for the $M_S = \pm\frac{3}{2} \rightleftarrows \pm\frac{1}{2}$ transitions, the shifts for the $M_S = +\frac{1}{2} \rightleftarrows -\frac{1}{2}$ transitions will be zero, and the shifts within each set of nuclear hyperfine lines will be the same. Fig. 3.7 shows the experimental electric field induced shifts for one of the $M_S = +\frac{5}{2} \rightleftarrows +\frac{3}{2}$ transitions (Kiel and Mims 1967). The electric field was applied along the crystalline a-axis, (i.e. the x-axis) here and $\underline{H}_0$ was rotated in the ac-plane. Under these conditions, the approximate

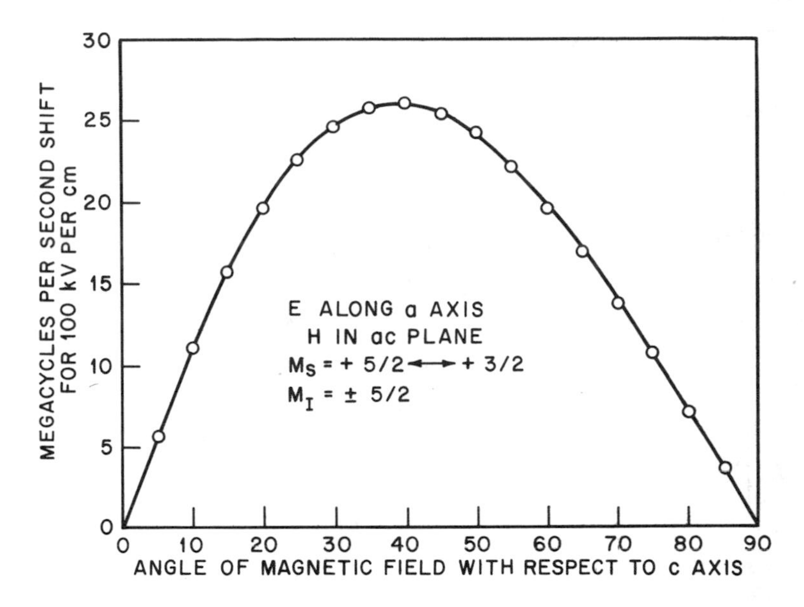

FIG. 3.7. Electric field induced shifts for the $M_S = +\frac{5}{2} \rightleftarrows +\frac{3}{2}$ transition of Mn^{2+} in $CaWO_4$. The electric field is applied along the a-axis, $\underline{H}_0$ is varied in the ac-plane. The curve can be roughly approximated by a sinusoidal function as in eqn (3.40), although it is not exactly sinusoidal as are the curves in Figs 3.5 and 3.6.

formula (3.37) reduces to

$$\Delta\nu = 6E_x R_{15} \sin 2\theta \tag{3.40}$$

It can be seen from Fig. 3.7 that the experimental curve closely resembles a sinusoidal function, although in this case the D-splitting corresponding to the $\frac{5}{2} \rightleftarrows \frac{3}{2}$ transition is by no means negligible ($4D \simeq 1{\cdot}65$ GHz). A sufficiently accurate value of R_{15} can nevertheless be obtained by measuring the height of the frequency-shift curve, thus avoiding the labour of diagonalizing the Hamiltonian for each setting of $\underline{H}_0$.

3.7. REDUCTION OF DATA FOR AMORPHOUS SAMPLES

Many materials which are of interest in chemistry and biology are not readily available in the form of single crystals and must be studied either as liquids or frozen glasses. We consider briefly here the problem of extracting g-shift parameters from measurements made on a frozen glass containing Kramers doublet ions.

A typical resonance absorption spectrum is shown in Fig. 3.8.

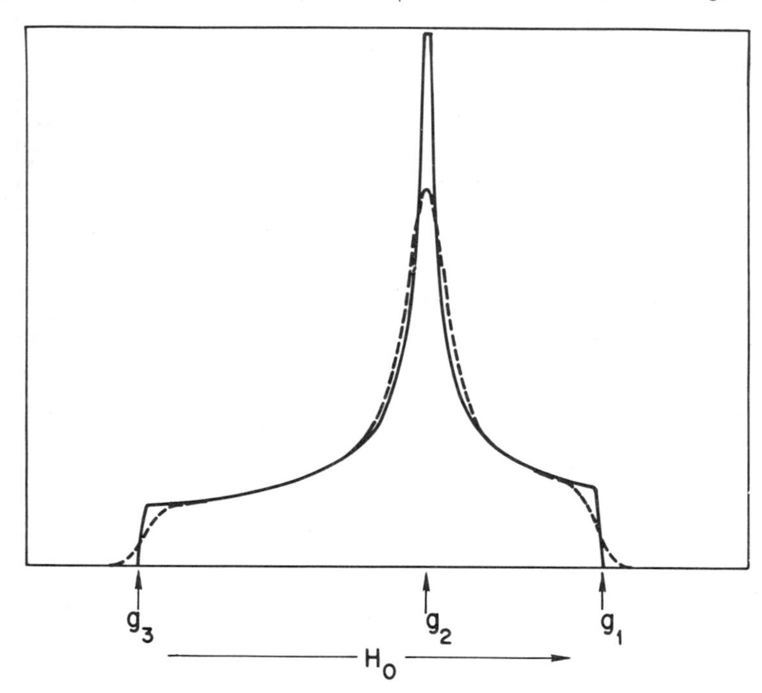

FIG. 3.8. Typical resonance spectrum for a glass-like sample or powder consisting of randomly oriented paramagnetic crystallites each characterized by three different principal g-values. The solid line shows the ideal spectrum which would be obtained if each orientation corresponded to an infinitely sharp resonance line. The broken line shows the spectrum which results after convolution with a line-broadening function. (Line-broadening may rise from strains, the proximity of nuclear magnetic moments, etc.)

At the bottom end of the spectrum the centres contributing to the resonance are those which are oriented in such a way that their g_{max} principal axes lie in the direction of the Zeeman field. At the top end of the spectrum the centres having their g_{min} principal axes along the Zeeman field are observed whilst in between these two limits each Zeeman field setting corresponds to a distribution of orientations. The peak in the middle of the spectrum corresponds to the intermediate principal g-value g_{mid}, and is partly due to centres for which the $g_{mi\bar{d}}$ axis lies along the Zeeman field, but centres with other orientations also contribute to the intensity here. The situation is discussed in more detail by Poole and Farach (1972), who gives some useful illustrations (see p. 95 and also Chapter 16.9 in this reference).

We shall be primarily concerned here with measurements made at the two ends of the spectrum where analytical expressions linking the frequency shifts with the B_{ij}-parameters can be derived. Let us consider the bottom end first and designate the Zeeman field orientation as the z-axis. The centres under observation are then characterized by the sets of axes shown in Fig. 3.9, the x- and y-axes being assumed for convenience to be the g_1 and g_2 principal axes. It should be noted that although all the centres have their $g_3 = g_{max}$ principal axis along the Zeeman field the g_1 ($= g_{min}$) and g_2 ($= g_{mid}$) axes are randomly distributed in a plane. If we now set the electric field parallel† to the magnetic field the field components are

---

† In practice $\underline{H}_0$ will probably be rotated into alignment with $\underline{E}_{app}$ rather than vice versa. Rotation of $\underline{H}_0$ makes no difference to the spectrum but merely changes the individual identity of the centres so that those with their g_{max} principal axes along $\underline{H}_0$ continue to be the ones which are observed.

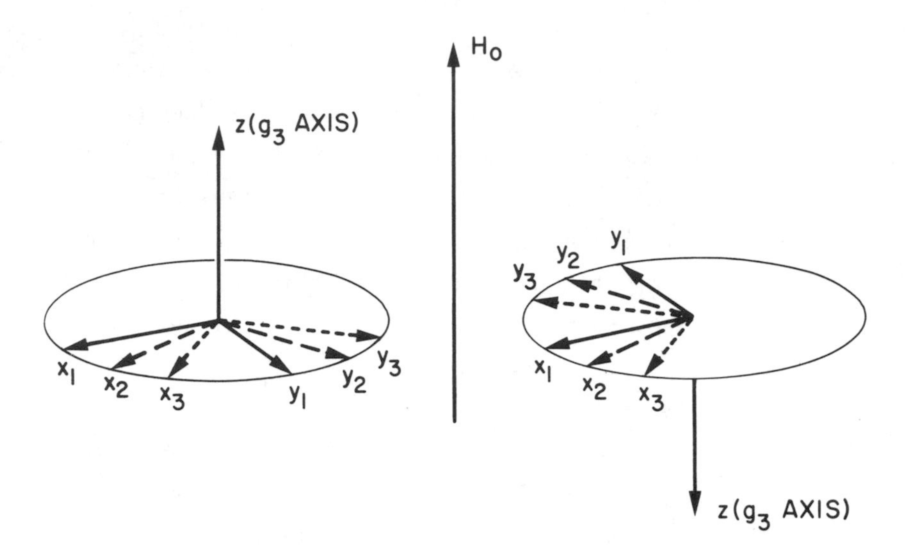

FIG. 3.9. The axes x, y, z etc. show the principal axes of the g-tensors for crystallites which contribute to the spectrum at the g_3 end (Fig. 3.8). Provided that the sites are non-centrosymmetric these crystallites can be divided into two groups with +z-axes parallel to and antiparallel to the direction of $\underline{H}_0$. These two groups undergo opposite linear electric shifts if $\underline{E}$ is parallel to $\underline{H}_0$. The x- and y-axes are randomly distributed in the plane perpendicular to $\underline{H}_0$. An electric field applied in this plane will give rise to a distribution of shifts (see eqns (3.48)-(3.49)).

$$H_x = H_y = 0,\ H_z = H_0\ ,$$
$$E_x = E_y = 0,\ E_z = E_{app}\ . \tag{3.41}$$

Thus by eqn (3.28)

$$\delta(g^2) = \pm\ E_{app}B_{33} \tag{3.42}$$

and

$$\Delta\nu = \pm\ E_{app}(\nu/2g^2{}_{max})B_{33}\ , \tag{3.43}$$

the frequency shift being determined as in eqn (3.29). Clearly the randomness of orientations in the xy-plane makes no difference in this experiment. If, on the other hand, we set the electric field perpendicular to the magnetic field, then

$$H_x = H_y = 0,\ H_z = 0\ ,$$
$$E_x = E_{app}\cos\phi_E,\ E_y = E_{app}\sin\phi_E,\ E_z = 0\ , \tag{3.44}$$

where ϕ_E is the angle between $\underline{E}_{app}$ and the g_1-axis for a particular centre. The experimental result will depend here on a distribution of frequency shifts determined by the distribution of angles ϕ_E. We can easily calculate this distribution by substituting (3.44) into eqn (3.28). Thus

$$\delta(g^2) = E_{app}(B_{13}\cos\phi_E + B_{23}\sin\phi_E) \tag{3.45}$$

or, alternatively,

$$\delta(g^2) = E_{app}(B_{13}^2 + B_{23}^2)^{\frac{1}{2}}\cos(\phi_E - \phi_0)\ , \tag{3.46}$$

where $\phi_0 = \arctan(B_{23}/B_{13})$. Applying eqn (3.29) to find the frequency shift we find that

$$\Delta\nu = E_{app}(\nu/2g^2{}_{max})(B_{13}^2 + B_{23}^2)^{\frac{1}{2}}\cos\psi\ , \tag{3.47}$$

where $\psi = \phi_E - \phi_0$. Since the angle ψ is, like ϕ_E, a random variable distributed uniformly over a range of 2π, we have the distribution (see e.g. Parzen 1960).

$$S(\Delta\nu) = (\Delta\nu_{max}^2 - \Delta\nu^2)^{-\frac{1}{2}}\ , \tag{3.48}$$

where $|\Delta\nu| \leq \Delta\nu_{max}$, and where

$$\Delta\nu_{max} = E_{app}(\nu/2g^2_{max})(B^2_{13}+B^2_{23})^{\frac{1}{2}} \qquad (3.49)$$

At intermediate values of the angle θ_{EH} between electric and magnetic fields the frequency-shift distribution will be given by a convolution of the results obtained from (3.42) and (3.46) with E_{app} replaced by $E_{app}\cos\theta_{EH}$ in the former and by $E_{app}\sin\theta_{EH}$ in the latter equations. There is, however, little reason for making measurements at these intermediate settings since the same data can be obtained more directly by setting $\underline{E}$ parallel to $\underline{H}_0$ and $\underline{E}$ perpendicular to $\underline{H}_0$.

The situation when the Zeeman field is set at the top end of the spectrum is essentially the same as that described above and the results can be derived from the results already given by interchanging the x- and z-axes (i.e. by changing g_{max} to g_{min} (=g_1) and interchanging subscripts 1 and 3). Thus for $\underline{E}$ parallel to $\underline{H}_0$ at g_{min}

$$\delta(g^2) = \pm E_{app}B_{11} \qquad (3.50)$$

and

$$\Delta\nu = \pm E_{app}(\nu/2g^2_{min})B_{11} \,. \qquad (3.51)$$

For $\underline{E}$ perpendicular to $\underline{H}_0$ the distribution of shifts is given by eqn (3.48) with

$$\Delta\nu_{max} = E_{app}(\nu/2g^2_{min})(B^2_{21}+B^2_{31})^{\frac{1}{2}} \qquad (3.52)$$

At intermediate Zeeman field settings numerical methods must be used to find the distribution of shifts. However, one useful general conclusion applicable at all field settings can be drawn regarding the distribution $S(\Delta\nu)$, namely, that the distribution of frequency shifts in an amorphous sample is always symmetric about zero, i.e. for each crystallite observed at a given value of H_0 and having a frequency shift $\Delta\nu$ there is another crystallite, observed at the same H_0, which has a shift $-\Delta\nu$. This can be shown as follows. Let us consider a particular crystallite oriented in a specific way with regard to $\underline{E}$ and $\underline{H}_0$. There is then another crystallite related to the first by a rotation of 180° about an axis perpendicular to $\underline{E}$ and to $\underline{H}_0$ which also contributes to the resonance absorption at the same point in the spectrum. This crystallite will have an equal and opposite frequency shift. The rotation is equivalent to a reversal of $\underline{H}_0$, which has no effect on the resonance, and also to a reversal of $\underline{E}$, which changes the sign of the shift. The two crystallites considered here are not inversion images. In the case of biological materials it may indeed be impossible to procure a sample containing true inversion image pairs, owing to the laevo-rotatory property of living matter.

If the electron spin echo method is used to make the measurements the distribution of shifts† $S(\Delta\omega)$ can be obtained by making a Fourier transform of the echo amplitude ratio function $R(E\tau)$ (see eqn (2.12)). This ratio function has a simple analytical form in the two cases considered above where the Zeeman field is set at either end of the spectrum. With $\underline{E}$ parallel to $\underline{H}_0$ at the bottom end of the spectrum $S(\Delta\omega)$ reduces to the sum of two delta functions, as in eqn (2.15), and $R(E\tau)$ is a cosine function, as in eqn (2.16). The parameter B_{33} is related to the half-full point $(E_{app}\tau)_{\frac{1}{2}}$ and the null points $(E_{app}\tau)_n$ of the function by

$$B_{33} = \pm\, g^2_{max}/\{3\nu(E_{app}\tau)_{\frac{1}{2}}\}$$
$$= \pm\, g^2_{max}(2n+1)/\{2\nu(E_{app}\tau)_n\} \quad , \qquad (3.53)$$

---

† Radian frequency units $\omega = 2\pi\nu$ are sometimes more convenient than hertz in discussions relating to the spin echo method.

where ν is the resonance frequency in hertz. With $\underline{E}$ perpendicular to $\underline{H}_0$ at the same setting $R(E\tau)$ is found by taking the Fourier transform of the function in eqn (3.48). We have

$$R(E\tau) = J_0(\Delta\omega_{max}\tau) \ , \tag{3.54}$$

where J_0 is the zero-order Bessel function and where $\Delta\omega_{max}$ depends on B_{13} and B_{23} as in (3.49). The half-fall point occurs when the argument of J_0 is 1·52, and the first and second nulls when the arguments are 2·41 and 5·52 respectively. The parameter $(B_{13}^2+B_{23}^2)^{\frac{1}{2}}$ is thus related to the observed half fall and the first two null points by the equations

$$\begin{aligned}(B_{13}^2+B_{23}^2)^{\frac{1}{2}} &= 0{\cdot}484\ g_{max}^2/\{\nu(E_{app}\tau)_{\frac{1}{2}}\} \\ &= 0{\cdot}767\ g_{max}^2/\{\nu(E_{app}\tau)_1\} \\ &= 1{\cdot}76\ \ g_{max}^2/\{\nu(E_{app}\tau)_2\} \ . \end{aligned} \tag{3.55}$$

The corresponding results at the high-field end of the spectrum can be obtained from (3.53) and (3.55) by changing g_{max} to g_{min} and interchanging the subscripts 1 and 3 in B_{ij} as indicated previously. It should be remembered that in practice $S(\Delta\omega)$ and $R(E\tau)$ will deviate from the ideal form owing to the fact that a finite portion of the spectrum is sampled in any measurement. There may also be some further broadening in the shift parameters due to strains, etc., rendering it difficult to determine the null points in (3.53), (3.55) accurately. In the case of non-crystalline samples it is therefore often more convenient to base the measurement on the half-fall product $(E\tau)_{\frac{1}{2}}$.

An example of the result obtained by making electron spin echo measurements on an amorphous sample is shown in Fig. 3.10. The quantity σ on the ordinate is $\{6\nu(E_{app}\tau)_{\frac{1}{2}}\}^{-1}$. At the low

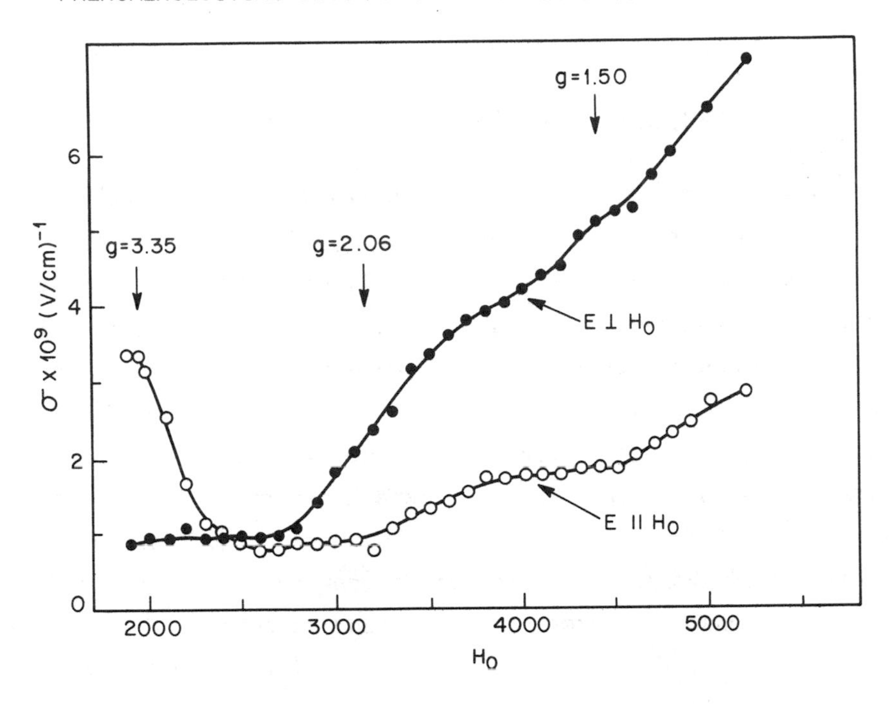

FIG 3.10 Electric field induced shifts for Fe^{3+} ($S = \frac{1}{2}$) centres in a sample of cytochrome c in the form of a frozen glass at pH 10. Measurements were made by the electron spin echo method. The parameter σ shown as the ordinate is equal to the quantity $\{6\nu(\tau E_{app})_{\frac{1}{2}}\}^{-1}$ (see eqns (3.53) and (3.55) et seq). For $\underline{E}$ parallel to $\underline{H}_0$ at the two ends of the spectrum $\sigma = (\delta g/g)/E_{app}$. (Mims and Peisach 1974.)

end of the spectrum with $\underline{E}$ parallel to $\underline{H}_0$ this corresponds to $B_{33}/2g^2_{max}$ (i.e. to $(\delta g/g_{max})/E_{app}$). At the high end with $\underline{E}$ parallel to $\underline{H}_0$ it corresponds to $B_{11}/2g^2_{min}$ (i.e. to $(\delta g/g_{min})/E_{app}$). At the low end with $\underline{E}$ perpendicular to $\underline{H}_0$ it corresponds to $(B^2_{13}+B^2_{23})^{\frac{1}{2}}/2{\cdot}90\ g^2_{max}$, and at the high end with $\underline{E}$ perpendicular to $\underline{H}_0$ to $(B^2_{21}+B^2_{31})^{\frac{1}{2}}/2{\cdot}90\ g^2_{min}$. Elsewhere, σ merely serves as a convenient experimental parameter. An elaborate curve-fitting procedure would be required in order to relate it more directly to the B_{ij} parameters of the system.

3.8. SPHERICAL TENSOR EQUIVALENTS FOR THE D_{jk} AND R_{ijk} TERMS

The Hamiltonians $\mathcal{H}$ and $\mathcal{H}_{elec}$ can be redefined by using spherical tensors in place of the Cartesian tensors g, D, etc. This form of spin Hamiltonian is not especially convenient for the purpose of describing experimental data. It has the merit of leading at once to traceless expressions for the D-term and the D-shift term, and it is considerably more economical for the purpose of describing the quartic spin operator terms (§3.9), but it involves a somewhat cumbersome resolution into isotropic and anisotropic components when it is applied to the Zeeman term or the electron nuclear coupling term. The reformulation of laboratory applied fields as spherical tensor operators may also tend to obscure the physical picture. The chief advantage of the spherical tensor notation is however that it is easier to handle in problems involving coordinate rotation (§A.4). It is therefore useful to be able to convert data in and out of this notation when required although the Cartesian notation may be preferable for the purpose of reporting measurements.

To begin with let us consider the electric field which has hitherto been treated as a Cartesian tensor of first rank, i.e. a vector. This can be re-expressed as a first-rank spherical tensor having the components

$$E_0^{(1)} = E_z, \ E_{\pm 1}^{(1)} = \mp \frac{1}{\sqrt{2}} (E_x \pm iE_y) \ , \tag{3.56}$$

The converse relation is

$$E_x = -\frac{1}{\sqrt{2}} (E_{+1}^{(1)} - E_{-1}^{(1)}), \ E_y = \frac{i}{\sqrt{2}} (E_{+1}^{(1)} + E_{-1}^{(1)}), \ E_z = E_0^{(1)}. \tag{3.57}$$

The Cartesian spin operators S_jS_k in the term $D_{jk}S_jS_k$ $(j,k = x,y,z)$ can be replaced by the spherical spin operators

$$S_0^{(2)} = \frac{1}{2}(2S_z^2 - S_x^2 - S_y^2) = \frac{1}{2}\{3S_z^2 - S(S+1)\} ,$$

$$S_{\pm 1}^{(2)} = \mp \frac{1}{2}\sqrt{\frac{3}{2}}\{S_z(S_x \pm iS_y) + (S_x \pm iS_y)S_z\} , \tag{3.58}$$

$$S_{\pm 2}^{(2)} = \frac{1}{2}\sqrt{\frac{3}{2}}(S_x \pm iS_y)^2 = \frac{1}{2}\sqrt{\frac{3}{2}}\{(S_x^2 - S_y^2) \pm i(S_xS_y + S_yS_x)\} ,$$

the converse relationships being

$$S_x^2 - S_y^2 = \sqrt{\frac{2}{3}}(S_{+2}^{(2)} + S_{-2}^{(2)}) ,$$

$$S_z^2 - \frac{1}{3}S(S+1) = \frac{2}{3}S_0^{(2)}$$

$$S_yS_z + S_zS_y = i\sqrt{\frac{2}{3}}(S_{+1}^{(2)} + S_{-1}^{(2)}) ,$$

$$S_xS_z + S_zS_x = -\sqrt{\frac{2}{3}}(S_{+1}^{(2)} - S_{-1}^{(2)}) ,$$

$$S_xS_y + S_yS_x = -i\sqrt{\frac{2}{3}}(S_{+2}^{(2)} - S_{-2}^{(2)}) . \tag{3.59}$$

The normalizing factors in eqns (3.56) and (3.58) are chosen so that the operators transform in the same way as the spherical harmonics $C_1^q(\theta,\phi)$, $C_2^q(\theta,\phi)$ (see §§ A.1–A.2.).

In spherical tensor notation the D-term becomes

$$D_j^{(2)}S_j^{(2)} \quad (j=0, \pm 1, \pm 2) . \tag{3.60}$$

The coefficients $D_j^{(2)}$ can be found in terms of the Cartesian coefficients by substituting eqn (3.59) into the identity

$$D_j^{(2)}S_j^{(2)} \equiv D_{jk}S_jS_k \tag{3.61}$$

and equating coefficients of $S_j^{(2)}$. The converse set of relations can be found in a similar way by substituting (3.58) into (3.61). We thus obtain the equations

$$D_0^{(2)} = \frac{1}{3}(2D_3 - D_1 - D_2) = D_3 \text{ (traceless set)},$$

$$D_{\pm 1}^{(2)} = \mp\sqrt{\frac{2}{3}}(D_5 \mp iD_4) \qquad (3.62)$$

$$D_{\pm 2}^{(2)} = \frac{1}{2}\sqrt{\frac{2}{3}}\{(D_1 - D_2) \mp 2iD_6\},$$

and

$$D_1 = -\frac{1}{2}D_0^{(2)} + \frac{1}{2}\sqrt{\frac{3}{2}}(D_2^{(2)} + D_{-2}^{(2)}),$$

$$D_2 = -\frac{1}{2}D_0^{(2)} - \frac{1}{2}\sqrt{\frac{3}{2}}(D_2^{(2)} + D_{-2}^{(2)}),$$

$$D_3 = D_0^{(2)}, \qquad (3.63)$$

$$D_4 = -\frac{i}{2}\sqrt{\frac{3}{2}}(D_1^{(1)} + D_{-1}^{(1)}),$$

$$D_5 = -\frac{1}{2}\sqrt{\frac{3}{2}}(D_1^{(1)} - D_{-1}^{(1)}),$$

$$D_6 = \frac{i}{2}\sqrt{\frac{3}{2}}(D_2^{(2)} - D_{-2}^{(2)}),$$

where the Cartesian coefficients are given in Voigt notation. It will be noted that in spherical tensor notation there are only five independent coefficients. Conversion from spherical tensor to Cartesian form will automatically ensure that $D_1 + D_2 + D_3 = 0$. If the Cartesian coefficients which are being converted in (3.62) are not traceless, however, the first expression on the right must be used for $D_0^{(2)}$. The D and E terms commonly used in the spin Hamiltonian $= D\{S_z^2 - \frac{1}{3}S(S+1)\} + E(S_x^2 - S_y^2)$ are related to the spherical tensor coefficients by

$$'D' = \frac{3}{2} D_0^{(2)} ,$$
$$'E' = \sqrt{\frac{3}{2}}\, \mathrm{Re}(D_2^{(2)}) = \frac{1}{2} \sqrt{\frac{3}{2}}\, (D_2^{(2)} + D_{-2}^{(2)}) . \tag{3.64}$$

Bearing in mind that the Hamiltonian is a scalar operator we see from the products in (3.61) that the operators $S_q^{(2)}$ and the coefficients $D_q^{(2)}$ transform contragrediently as first-rank tensors in five dimensions, whereas the corresponding Cartesian operators and coefficients transform as second-rank tensors in three dimensions. This matters little in the case of the D-term, where tensor methods need not be used for the purpose of rotating coordinate axes, other simpler methods being available (§ A.4.3). When it is required to rotate axes for the linear electric field effect terms the corresponding reduction in rank from third rank in the Cartesian form (3 × 3 × 3 dimensions) to second rank in the spherical tensor form (3 × 5 dimensions) does however result in an appreciable saving of effort (§ A.4.6).

The D-shift term $R_{ijk}E_iS_jS_k$ $(i,j,k = x,y,z)$ can be rewritten in spherical tensor notation in the form

$$R_{i,j}^{(2)}\, E_i^{(1)} S_j^{(2)} \quad (i = 0,\pm 1;\ j = 0,\pm 1,\pm 2) , \tag{3.65}$$

where the $E_i^{(1)}$ are the electric field spherical tensor components (3.56) and the $S_j^{(2)}$ are the spherical tensor spin operators (3.58). A mixed Cartesian-spherical notation is also sometimes convenient when rotating coordinates. In this mixed notation the D-shift term becomes

$$R_{i,j}^{(C,2)} E_i S_j^{(2)} \quad (i = x,y,z;\ j = 0,\ 1,\ 2) , \tag{3.66}$$

where the spin operator is in spherical form, but the field is given in Cartesian components. The equations converting the

Cartesian coefficients R_{ij} to the mixed form (3.66) can be written down at once since the $R^{(C,2)}_{i,j}$ are related to the R_{ij} in the sam way that the spherical coefficients $D^{(2)}_{j}$ are related to the Cartesian coefficients D_j. Thus by eqn (3.62) we have

$$R^{(C,2)}_{1,0} = \frac{1}{3}(2R_{13}-R_{11}-R_{12}) = R_{13} \text{ (traceless set)},$$

$$R^{(C,2)}_{1,\pm 1} = \mp\sqrt{\frac{2}{3}}(R_{16} \mp iR_{14}),$$

---------------------------- (3.67)

$$R^{(C,2)}_{2,0} = \frac{1}{3}(2R_{23}-R_{21}-R_{22}) = R_{23} \text{ (traceless set)},$$

$$R^{(C,2)}_{2,\pm 1} = \mp\sqrt{\frac{2}{3}}(R_{26} \mp iR_{24})$$

The coefficients $R^{(2)}_{i,j}$ can either be obtained from the mixed form by substituting eqns (3.57) and eqns (3.67) in the identity

$$R^{(C,2)}_{i,j} E_i S^{(2)}_j \equiv R^{(2)}_{i,j} E^{(1)}_i S^{(2)}_j \tag{3.68}$$

and equating coefficients of the operators $E^{(1)}_i S^{(2)}_j$, or more directly by expanding (3.65) in terms of the Cartesian operators and comparing the coefficients with those in eqn (3.10). Table 3.3 gives the coefficients $R^{(2)}_{i,j}$ in the traceless practical notation. The opposite conversion from spherical tensor coefficients $R^{(2)}_{i,j}$ to the traceless practical coefficients is shown in Table 3.4. It may be noted that the spherical tensor coefficients obey the relation

$$R^{(2)}_{-i,-j} = R^{(2)*}_{i,j}(-1)^{i+j}, \tag{3.69}$$

where $R^{(2)*}_{i,j}$ is the complex conjugate of $R^{(2)}_{i,j}$. This relation is

TABLE 3.3

Conversion from traceless practical coefficients R_{ij} (see eqns (3.10)-(3.12)) to spherical tensor coefficients (3.65)

Spherical tensor coefficients	Traceless practical coefficients
$R^{(2)}_{0,0}$	$\frac{2}{3} R_{3D}$
$R^{(2)}_{0,\pm1}$	$\sqrt{\frac{2}{3}}\ (\mp R_{35}+iR_{34})$
$R^{(2)}_{0,\pm2}$	$\sqrt{\frac{2}{3}}\ (R_{3E}\mp R_{36})$
$R^{(2)}_{1,0}$	$\frac{\sqrt{2}}{3}\ (-R_{1D}+iR_{2D})$
$R^{(2)}_{1,\pm1}$	$\frac{1}{\sqrt{3}}\{(\pm R_{15}-R_{24}) + i(-R_{14}\mp R_{25})\}$
$R^{(2)}_{1,\pm2}$	$\frac{1}{\sqrt{3}}\{(-R_{1E}\pm R_{26}) + i(R_{2E}\pm R_{16})\}$
$R^{(2)}_{-1,0}$	$\frac{\sqrt{2}}{3}\ (R_{1D}+iR_{2D})$
$R^{(2)}_{-1,\pm1}$	$\frac{1}{\sqrt{3}}\{(\mp R_{15}-R_{24}) + i(R_{14}\mp R_{25})\}$
$R^{(2)}_{-1,\pm2}$	$\frac{1}{\sqrt{3}}\{(R_{1E}\pm R_{26}) + i(R_{2E}\mp R_{16})\}$

TABLE 3.4

Conversion from spherical tensor coefficients $R_{ij}^{(2)}$ (eqn. 3.65) to traceless practical coefficients. (see eqns 3.10-12).

Traceless practical coefficients	Spherical tensor coefficients
R_{1E}	$\frac{\sqrt{3}}{4}\left(-R_{1,2}^{(2)} - R_{1,-2}^{(2)} + R_{-1,2}^{(2)} + R_{-1,-2}^{(2)}\right)$
R_{1D}	$\frac{3}{2\sqrt{2}}\left(-R_{1,0}^{(2)} + R_{-1,0}^{(2)}\right)$
R_{14}	$\frac{i\sqrt{3}}{4}\left(R_{1,1}^{(2)} + R_{1,-1}^{(2)} - R_{-1,1}^{(2)} - R_{-1,-1}^{(2)}\right)$
R_{15}	$\frac{\sqrt{3}}{4}\left(R_{1,1}^{(2)} - R_{1,-1}^{(2)} - R_{-1,1}^{(2)} + R_{-1,-1}^{(2)}\right)$
R_{16}	$\frac{i\sqrt{3}}{4}\left(-R_{1,2}^{(2)} + R_{1,-2}^{(2)} + R_{-1,2}^{(2)} - R_{-1,-2}^{(2)}\right)$
R_{2E}	$\frac{i\sqrt{3}}{4}\left(-R_{1,2}^{(2)} - R_{1,-2}^{(2)} - R_{-1,2}^{(2)} - R_{-1,-2}^{(2)}\right)$
R_{2D}	$\frac{i3}{2\sqrt{2}}\left((-R_{1,0}^{(2)} - R_{-1,0}^{(2)}\right)$
R_{24}	$-\frac{\sqrt{3}}{4}\left(R_{1,1}^{(2)} + R_{1,-1}^{(2)} + R_{-1,1}^{(2)} + R_{-1,-1}^{(2)}\right)$
R_{25}	$\frac{i\sqrt{3}}{4}\left(R_{1,1}^{(2)} - R_{1,-1}^{(2)} + R_{-1,1}^{(2)} - R_{-1,-1}^{(2)}\right)$
R_{26}	$\frac{\sqrt{3}}{4}\left(R_{1,2}^{(2)} - R_{1,-2}^{(2)} + R_{-1,2}^{(2)} - R_{-1,-2}^{(2)}\right)$
R_{3E}	$\sqrt{\frac{3}{8}}\left(R_{0,2}^{(2)} + R_{0,-2}^{(2)}\right)$
R_{3D}	$\frac{3}{2} R_{0,0}^{(2)}$
R_{34}	$i\sqrt{\frac{3}{8}}\left(-R_{0,1}^{(2)} - R_{0,-1}^{(2)}\right)$
R_{35}	$\sqrt{\frac{3}{8}}\left(-R_{0,1}^{(2)} + R_{0,-1}^{(2)}\right)$
R_{36}	$i\sqrt{\frac{3}{8}}\left(R_{0,2}^{(2)} - R_{0,-2}^{(2)}\right)$

sometimes useful for checking results.

The g-shift and g^2-shift parameters can also be re-expressed in spherical tensor form. This form is useful when making co-ordinate rotations, but it is never employed for the purpose of reporting measurements (see §A.4.5).

3.9. SPHERICAL TENSOR DESCRIPTION OF THE QUARTIC SPIN OPERATOR TERMS

The Cartesian expansion of the term $a_{jk\ell m}S_jS_kS_\ell S_m$ in eqn (3.1) contains eighty-one elements. It is easy to see, however, that this number is unnecessarily large and that there would be a great deal of indeterminacy in the coefficients $a_{jk\ell m}$. The quartic expression $C(S_x^2 + S_y^2 + S_z^2)^2 = CS^2(S+1)^2$, where C is any arbitrary constant could, for instance, be added to $a_{jk\ell m}S_jS_kS_\ell S_m$ without changing the <u>separations</u> between the energy levels derived from $\mathcal{H}$. Besides this, a large number of combinations of the type $C'(S_x^2 + S_y^2 + S_z^2)S_\ell S_m = C'S(S+1)S_\ell S_m$, $C''S_j(S_x^2 + S_y^2 + S_z^2)S_m = C''S(S+1)S_jS_m$, etc. are already represented in the second-degree spin operator term and should therefore be taken out of the quartic term. These problems can be avoided by using the nine spherical tensor spin operators related to the spherical harmonics $C_4^q(\theta,\phi)$ (see Table 3.5) to re-express the quartic term. These operators transform in the same way as the harmonics $C_4^q(\theta,\phi)$, and are consistent with the spin operators used in much recent work (see e.g. Smith and Thornley 1966), but it should not be taken for granted that they are the spin operators intended in any given reference, since notations may vary.

Linear electric shifts in the fourth-degree spin terms can be expressed either in the mixed Cartesian-spherical form (cf. eqn (3.63)),

$$R_{i,j}^{(C,4)}E_iS_j^{(4)} \qquad (i = x,y,z;\ j = 0,\pm1,\pm2,\pm3,\pm4)\ , \qquad (3.70)$$

TABLE 3.5

Fourth-degree spherical tensor spin operators $S_q^{(4)}$ in terms of the Cartesian spin operators S_x, S_y, S_z (Smith and Thornley 1966; see also §A.2).

Spherical tensor form	Cartesian operators
$S_{\pm 4}^{(4)}$	$\sqrt{\frac{35}{128}}\,(S_x \pm iS_y)^4$
$S_{\pm 3}^{(4)}$	$\mp\sqrt{\frac{35}{64}}\left\{S_z(S_x \pm iS_y)^3 + (S_x \pm iS_y)^3 S_z\right\}$
$S_{\pm 2}^{(4)}$	$\sqrt{\frac{5}{128}}\left[\{7S_z^2 - S(S+1) - 5\}(S_x \pm iS_y)^2 + (S_x \pm iS_y)^2\{7S_z^2 - S(S+1) - 5\}\right]$
$S_{\pm 1}^{(4)}$	$\mp\sqrt{\frac{5}{64}}\left[\{7S_z^2 - \{3S(S+1)+1\}S_z\}(S_x \pm iS_y) + (S_x \pm iS_y)\{7S_z^2 - \{3S(S+1)+1\}S_z\}\right]$
$S_0^{(4)}$	$\frac{1}{8}\left[35S_z^4 - \{30S(S+1) - 25\}S_z^2 + 3S^2(S+1)^2 - 6S(S+1)\right]$

or in the full spherical form

$$R_{i,j}^{(4)} E_i S_j^{(4)} \qquad (i = 0, \pm 1;\ j = 0, \pm 1, \pm 2, \pm 3)\ , \tag{3.71}$$

where the E_i are the spherical tensor field components defined in eqns (3.56) and (3.57). Eqn (3.69) with $R_{i,j}^{(4)}$ substituted for $R_{i,j}^{(2)}$ can be used to check for possible errors in the coefficients. In spite of the simplification introduced by the use of spherical tensor forms, the description of linear shifts in the fourth-degree spin terms is a complex matter, and it is fortunate that in practice this contribution to $\mathcal{H}_{elec}$ is usually small enough to be ignored (Kiel and Mims 1967; Sherstkov, Nepsha, Vagenin, Nikiforov and Krotkii 1968).

3.10. SPIN HAMILTONIANS FOR NON-KRAMERS DOUBLETS

Rare-earth ions with an even number of electrons are often impossible to study by means of microwave resonance because of the large zero field splitting of the levels. In axial fields, however, the degeneracy of the free ion states is not completely raised, and it may happen that the two lowest states form a time-reversed pair (Abragam and Bleaney 1970, p. 732). This pair may be termed a symmetry doublet, or a non-Kramers doublet. Its composition can be expressed in terms of the magnetic eigenstates $|J,M\rangle$ of the total angular momentum operator in the same way as a Kramers doublet, i.e. by the equations

$$|\psi^{+}\rangle = \sum_{J,M} \alpha_{J,M} |J,M\rangle \ ,$$
$$|\psi^{-}\rangle = \sum_{J,M} \alpha^{*}_{J,M} (-1)^{J-M} |J,-M\rangle \ , \qquad (3.72)$$

the axis of quantization being the C_n symmetry axis of the site (Abragam and Bleaney 1970, p. 650). Since M is integral there are in this case no matrix elements of the form $\langle\psi^{+}|S_{\pm}|\psi^{-}\rangle$ connecting the two states. A spin Hamiltonian for the doublet can in the ideal case therefore be written in the form

$$\mathcal{H} = \beta g_z H_z S_z + A I_z S_z \ . \qquad (3.73)$$

In practice there are small departures from axiality caused by crystal strains, the Jahn-Teller effect, etc., which lead to a small zero-field splitting. This splitting is often taken into account by including two additional terms in the spin Hamiltonian to give

$$\mathcal{H} = \beta g_z H_z S_z + AI_z S_z + \Delta_x S_x + \Delta_y S_y \,, \tag{3.74}$$

where the effective spin remains $\frac{1}{2}$ and where S_x, S_y are used algebraically to form matrix elements in the standard manner (although they are not time-reversing operators and do not have the usual transformation properties). Similar departures from axiality are caused by the application of an electric field perpendicular to the z-axis and can be represented in the spin Hamiltonian by adding the term

$$\mathcal{H}_{elec} = \delta_{xx}E_x S_x + \delta_{yy}E_y S_y + \delta_{xy}E_x S_y + \delta_{yx}E_y S_x + \delta_{zx}E_z S_x + \delta_{zy}E_z S_y \tag{3.75}$$

to $\mathcal{H}$. Electric field induced g-shifts and shifts in A can also occur, but they lead to much smaller effects and are for the present omitted.

The somewhat arbitrary rules used in setting up the Hamiltonians ((3.74)-(3.75)) can be rationalized by postulating a third state, well removed from the other two, and by considering an $S'=1$ manifold of states (Mueller 1968). The new Hamiltonian can then be written in a standard form as in eqns (3.1) and (3.2). Thus, taking only g- and D-terms in (3.1) and assuming provisionally that the symmetry is lower than axial, we have

$$\mathcal{H} = \beta g_{jk} H_j S_k + D_{jk} S_j S_k, \quad S' = 1 \quad , \tag{3.76}$$

The relationship between this Hamiltonian and the $S' = \frac{1}{2}$ Hamiltonian (3.74) can be seen by comparing the two matrices in Table 3.6. (In the matrix (b) the term $D_{jk}S_jS_k$ has been made traceless and rewritten with the diagonal terms in the form $D\{S_z^2 - \frac{1}{3}S(S+1)\} + E(S_x^2 - S_y^2)$. The quantities η_1, η_2 stand for the Zeeman terms

TABLE 3.6

Hamiltonian matrices for a non-Kramers doublet. (a) 2 × 2 matrix for the $S' = \frac{1}{2}$ Hamiltonian (3.74). (b) 3 × 3 matrix for the $S = 1$ Hamiltonian (3.76), where the states $|\pm 1\rangle$ refer to the doublet. When the axial splitting D exceeds the other terms by a sufficiently wide margin, the matrix (b) can be partitioned into a 2 × 2 matrix consisting of the rows and columns labelled $|\pm 1\rangle$ and a single diagonal element. The 2 × 2 matrix obtained by this partitioning is equivalent to the matrix (a).

(a)

	$\lvert +\frac{1}{2}\rangle$	$\lvert -\frac{1}{2}\rangle$
$\lvert +\frac{1}{2}\rangle$	$\frac{1}{2}\beta g_z H_z$	$\frac{1}{2}(\Delta_x + i\Delta_y)$
$\lvert -\frac{1}{2}\rangle$	$\frac{1}{2}(\Delta_x - i\Delta_y)$	$-\frac{1}{2}\beta g_z H_z$

(b)

	$\lvert +1\rangle$	$\lvert 0\rangle$	$\lvert -1\rangle$
$\lvert +1\rangle$	$\beta(g_3 H_z + \eta_1) + \frac{1}{3}D$	$\frac{1}{\sqrt{2}}(D_5 - iD_4 + \beta\eta_2)$	$E - iD_6$
$\lvert 0\rangle$	$\frac{1}{\sqrt{2}}(D_5 + iD_4 + \beta\eta_2^*)$	$-2/3\,D$	$\frac{1}{\sqrt{2}}(D_5 - iD_4 + \beta\eta_2)$
$\lvert -1\rangle$	$E + iD_6$	$\frac{1}{\sqrt{2}}(D_5 + iD_4 + \beta\eta_2^*)$	$-\beta(g_3 H_z + \eta_1 + \frac{1}{3}D$

$\eta_1 = g_5H_x + g_4H_y$, $\eta_2 = (g_1H_x+g_6H_y+g_5H_z) - i(g_6H_x+g_2H_y+g_5H_z)$.
Let us now suppose that D is much larger than all the other terms. The $|0\rangle$ state in (b) of Table 3.6 is then well separated from the $|\pm1\rangle$ states, and the relatively small perturbations connecting it with the $|\pm1\rangle$ states can be ignored. Rearranging the rows and columns, we can therefore partition the 3 × 3 matrix into a 2 × 2 submatrix (consisting of the rows and columns labelled $|\pm1\rangle$) and a single diagonal element $-\frac{2}{3}D$, which corresponds to the energy of the state $|0\rangle$. Introducing the further condition that $\eta_1 \ll g_3H_z$ (for almost axial symmetry) and subtracting the common diagonal term $\frac{1}{3}D$, we are left with a 2 × 2 submatrix which has the same form as the matrix in (a) of Table 3.6, the equivalent parameters being given by

$$\Delta_x = 2E,\ \Delta_y = -2D_6,\ g_z = 2g_3\ , \tag{3.77}$$

The effect of applying an electric field can also be understood in terms of the S' = 1 Hamiltonian (3.76). Let us suppose that the parameters D_j in (b) of Table 3.6 are replaced by $D_j+E_iR_{ij}$, where the R_{ij} are the Voigt coefficients appropriate to the axial point symmetry concerned (see Fig. 3.3). (The ideal point symmetry may be assumed when selecting the coefficients R_{ij}. Small deviations from axial symmetry such as those considered in connection with the parameters Δ_x,Δ_y correspond to shift terms which are smaller by several additional orders of magnitude and can be ignored here.) Inspection of (b) of Table 3.6 will show that the D-shifts E_iR_{iD} have no effect on the separation of the $|1\rangle;|-1\rangle$ states, the shifts E_iR_{i5} and E_iR_{i4} have an effect which can be neglected if the energy denominator D is large enough, and only the shifts E_iR_{iE} and E_iR_{i6} actually couple the $|1\rangle$, $|-1\rangle$ states. In the 2 × 2 matrix partitioned from (b) of Table 3.6, which represents these states, the off-diagonal terms $E \pm iD_6$ are increased by an amount

$$(E_xR_{1E}+E_yR_{2E}+E_zR_{3E}) \mp i(E_xR_{16}+E_yR_{26}+E_zR_{36}). \tag{3.78}$$

This corresponds to the term

$$\frac{1}{2}(E_x\delta_{xx}+E_y\delta_{yx}+E_z\delta_{zx}) \pm \frac{i}{2}(E_x\delta_{xy}+E_y\delta_{yy}+E_z\delta_{zy}) \tag{3.79}$$

in the $S' = \frac{1}{2}$, 2×2 matrix description.

Both these expressions can be further simplified by considering the point group of the site. From Fig. 3.3 we see that for the axial point groups C_4, C_{4v}, C_6, C_{6v}, the coefficients R_{ij} which appear in (3.78) are all zero. There is therefore no linear shift in the interval separating the $|1\rangle$ and $|-1\rangle$ states, and all the coefficients vanish in (3.75). For the axial groups C_{3v}, D_{3h} (3.78) reduces to $R_{1E}(E_x \pm iE_y)$, and hence in (3.79) $\delta_{xx} = \delta_{yy} = 2R_{1E}$, $\delta_{zx} = \delta_{xz} = \delta_{xy} = \delta_{yx} = 0$. In this case the Hamiltonian (3.75) can be rewritten in the form

$$\mathcal{H}_{elec} = \delta(E_xS_x+E_yS_y) , \tag{3.80}$$

where $\delta = 2R_{1E}$. For the axial groups C_3, C_{3h} (3.78) becomes $(E_xR_{1E}-E_yR_{2E}) \pm i(E_xR_{2E}+E_yR_{1E})$, hence $\delta_{xx} = \delta_{yy} = 2R_{1E}$, $\delta_{xy} = -\delta_{yx} = 2R_{2E}$, $\delta_{zx} = \delta_{zy} = 0$, and

$$\mathcal{H}_{elec} = \delta_1(E_xS_x+E_yS_y) + \delta_2(E_xS_y-E_yS_x) , \tag{3.81}$$

where $\delta_1 = 2R_{1E}$ and $\delta_2 = 2R_{2E}$. For the remaining axial groups S_4 and D_{2d} (3.78) reduces to $E_zR_{3E} \mp iE_zR_{36}$ and to $\mp iE_zR_{36}$. Hence for S_4, $\delta_{zx} = 2R_{3E}$, $\delta_{zy} = -2R_{36}$, and for D_{2d}, $\delta_{zy} = -2R_{36}$, all the remaining δ parameters being zero. The Hamiltonian (3.75) for S_4 becomes

$$\mathcal{H}_{elec} = E_z(\delta_1S_x+\delta_2S_y) , \tag{3.82}$$

where $\delta_1 = 2R_{3E}$, $\delta_2 = -2R_{36}$ and the Hamiltonian for D_{2d} is obtained by setting $\delta_1 = 0$.

The addition of electric field effect terms $E_i(\delta_{ix} + i\delta_{iy})$ to the parameters $\Delta_x + i\Delta_y$ in the matrix shown in (a) of Table 3.6 results in an off-diagonal perturbation

$$\tfrac{1}{4}\{|(\Delta_x + i\Delta_y) + \sum_i E_i(\delta_{ix} + i\delta_{iy})|\}^2/\beta g_z H_z \ .$$

The electric field effect term will therefore only result in a linear frequency shift if there is already some departure from axial symmetry. In the absence of such distortions $\Delta_x = \Delta_y = 0$ and the electric field induced shift is proportional to E^2_{app}. If distortions are present the shift in the resonance interval is

$$h\Delta\nu = \tfrac{1}{2}\{\sum_i E_i(\Delta_x \delta_{iy} + \Delta_y \delta_{ix})\}/\beta g_z H_z \qquad (3.83)$$

(where Δ and δ are expressed in energy units). Electric shifts arising in this way will obviously be very inhomogeneous on account of the randomness of the strain parameters Δ even if the shift parameters δ are themselves well defined. The shift parameters can, however, be studied directly independently of Δ in para-electric resonance experiments (see Chapter 7).

4. The internal electric field

The electrostatic field seen by the paramagnetic ions when a voltage V_{app} is applied across a sample of thickness d differs in several respects from the macroscopic field V_{app}/d. It is generally larger and it also contains higher-order harmonics. The lowest-order odd harmonics in this field can be calculated as described under the heading of the 'internal electric field' in texts dealing with the theory of dielectrics (e.g. Böttcher 1952 (p. 177); Kittel 1971 (p. 454)). But the harmonics of next higher order, which may be of comparable importance in determining the energy-level spacings of paramagnetic ions require a now approach. Here we shall review the classical theory of the Lorentz internal field and show how it may be extended to include the electrostatic field terms which are needed in order to calculate the linear electric field effects. The discussion will be based for the most part on a simple 'point dipole' model (Kiel and Mims 1972a) in which it is assumed that the effect of the applied electric field is to generate an array of new dipole moments at the lattice points in the crystal. These induced dipoles then give rise to an electrostatic potential in the same manner as the array of point charges considered in the familiar 'point charge' model for the crystal field.

To save excessive repetition, we shall refer to the local electrostatic potential, or 'crystal field', seen in the absence of a laboratory applied field as the <u>normal</u> field and denote it by V. (The same terminology was used in Chapter 3 where the Hamiltonian $\mathcal{H}$ which describes the behaviour of the paramagnetic ion in the usual type of EPR experiment without applied electric fields is referred to as the <u>normal</u> spin Hamiltonian.) The changes in the local electrostatic potential which occur as a result of applying the laboratory field will be termed the <u>induced</u> field and denoted by δV. Both normal and induced fields can be described in two ways. We can write down harmonic series for the normal crystal field potential,

$$V = \sum_{K,Q} A_K^Q r^K C_K^Q(\theta,\phi) \ , \qquad (4.1)$$

and for the induced crystal field potential,

$$\delta V = \sum_{k,q} a_k^q r^k C_k^q(\theta,\phi) \ , \qquad (4.2)$$

by expanding the electrostatic field about the centre of the paramagnetic ion as origin.† In spectroscopic calculations, however, it is often more convenient to express the amplitudes of the harmonics in the crystal field as parameters with the dimensions of energy. To see how these parameters are related to the A_K^Q, a_k^q in eqns (4.1)-(4.2) let us consider the formation of matrix elements $e\langle\psi_1|V|\psi_2\rangle$, $e\langle\psi_1|\delta V|\psi_2\rangle$ from the potentials V, δV. Factoring the wavefunctions ψ_1, ψ_2 into radial portions $\mathcal{R}_1$, $\mathcal{R}_2$, and angular-

---

† The $C_K^Q(\theta,\phi)$ are the spherical harmonics defined in §A.1. Since the potentials V, δV are real it follows from eqn (A.2) that $A_K^{-Q} = (-1)^Q(A_K^Q)^*$ and $a_k^{-q} = (-1)^q(a_k^q)^*$.

dependent portions $\psi_1^{\theta,\phi}$, $\psi_2^{\theta,\phi}$, we obtain the result

$$e\langle\psi_1|V|\psi_2\rangle = \sum_{K,Q} eA_K^Q\langle r^K\rangle\langle\psi_1^{\theta,\phi}|C_K^Q(\theta,\phi)|\psi_2^{\theta,\phi}\rangle ,$$

where $\langle r^K\rangle$ stands for the radial integrals $\int \mathcal{R}_1\mathcal{R}_2 r^{K+2}dr$ and $\langle\psi_1^{\theta,\phi}|C_K^Q(\theta,\phi)|\psi_2^{\theta,\phi}\rangle = \int (\psi_1^{\theta,\phi})^*\psi_2^{\theta,\phi}C_K^Q(\theta,\phi)d(\cos\theta)d\phi$ are matrix elements involving angular-dependent functions only. Similar expressions can be written down for $e\langle\psi_1|\delta V|\psi_2\rangle$. The electronic charge, the radial integral, and the potential amplitudes A_K^Q, a_k^q, can then be combined to yield the spectroscopic crystal field parameters

$$A_K^Q(s) = eA_K^Q\langle r^K\rangle \qquad a_k^q(s) = ea_k^q\langle r^k\rangle , \tag{4.3}$$

in terms of which eqns (4.1) and (4.2) become†

$$V = \sum_{K,Q} A_K^Q(s)C_K^Q(\theta,\phi) ,$$

$$\delta V = \sum_{k,q} a_k^q(s)C_k^q(\theta,\phi) . \tag{4.4}$$

Further calculations need only involve matrix elements of the spherical harmonics C_K^Q which are given in tables (see references

---

† The notation $A_K^Q(s)$, $a_k^q(s)$ (and later in Chapter 5, $a_k^q(E,s)$) is used in order to indicate unambiguously wherever the electrostatic potential amplitudes have been replaced by the corresponding spectroscopic parameters. The superscripts θ,ϕ, in $\psi^{\theta,\phi}$ can be dropped when writing down maxtrix elements of $C_K^Q(\theta,\phi)$ since it is clear that only the angular dependent portion of the wavefunction is involved.

in §A.2). The parameters $A_K^Q(s)$, $a_k^q(s)$ are generally expressed in cm^{-1}, spectroscopic energy units ($1\ J = 5{\cdot}034 \times 10^{22}\ cm^{-1}$).

4.1. THE LORENTZ FIELD

We begin the analysis of the induced potential by making an estimate for the first-degree potentials $a_1^q r C_1^q(\theta,\phi)$ according to the classical internal field theory of Lorentz. The field E_{int} at a point inside a parallel-sided dielectric sample is due to the field $E_{app} = V_{app}/d$ applied across the sample and also to the fields generated by dipoles induced in the sample. It can be expressed as the sum

$$E_{int} = E_{surf} + E_R + E_{<R} \quad , \tag{4.5}$$

where E_{surf} is the net field due to charges on the electrodes and on the outer surface of the dielectric, E_R is due to the charge on the inside of the imaginary sphere surrounding the impurity ion, and $E_{<R}$ is due to the configuration of dipoles inside the sphere (see Fig. 4.1). E_{int} is then estimated by treating the dipoles outside the spherical surface as a uniformly polarized medium with polarization P and considering the contribution due to dipoles inside R separately. The quantities E_{surf}, P, and E_R can be obtained from elementary electrostatics. Thus, $E_{surf} = E_{app} = V_{app}/d$. The polarization P is derived from the expression $\varepsilon_r E_{app} = E_{app} + 4\pi P$. where ε_r is the relative permittivity (assumed to be isotropic), and the field component $E_R = \frac{4}{3}P$ is found by integrating the components due to charges $\delta q = 2\pi PR^2 \sin\theta\cos\theta\, d\theta$ on the ring-shaped elements indicated in Fig. 4.1. Thus

$$E_{int} - E_{<R} = E_{app} \times \tfrac{1}{3}(\varepsilon_r + 2) \tag{4.6}$$

The quantity $E_{app} \times \frac{1}{3}(\varepsilon_r+2)$ is termed the Lorentz field. Under

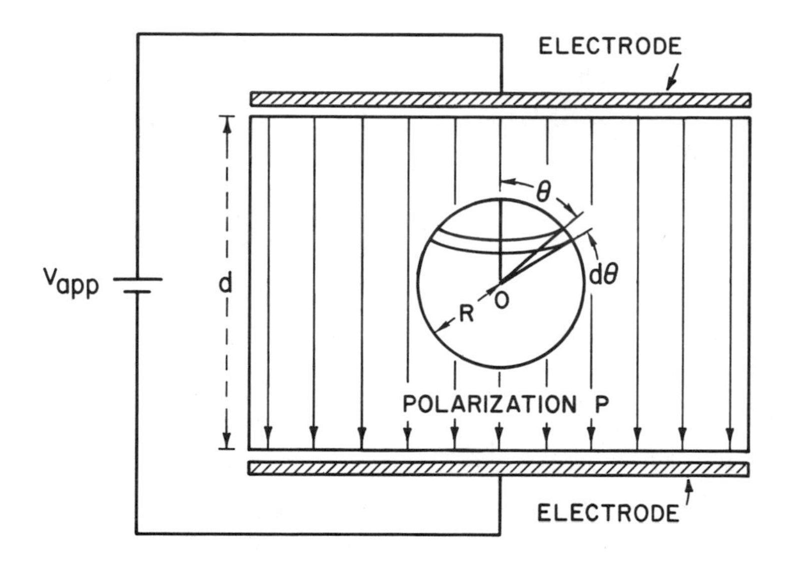

FIG. 4.1. The Lorentz internal field at a point O in a dielectric is calculated by constructing an imaginary sphere of radius R centred on O. The induced dipoles outside the sphere are then treated as a uniformly polarized medium with polarization P, and dipoles inside R are considered separately. For a simple cubic lattice containing the point O the field due to the dipoles inside R vanishes. The field at O due to the charge on the inside surface of the sphere can be found by integrating over the ring-shaped element shown above and has the value $\frac{4}{3}\pi P$.

certain special conditions - e.g. if the environment consists of a cubic lattice of dipoles all oriented in the same direction - $E_{<R}$ vanishes and

$$E_{int}/E_{app} = \frac{1}{3}(\varepsilon_r+2). \qquad (4.7)$$

In the more general case the contribution $E_{<R}$ must also be calculated by summing the fields due to dipoles contained inside the sphere and then added to E_{int} (see next section).

The extension of this argument to the case of an anisotropic dielectric is an obvious one and need not be considered in detail. The imaginary bounding surface is still taken as a sphere, but the polarization $\underline{P}$ is related to $\underline{E}_{\text{app}}$ by the dielectric tensor and is not necessarily parallel to $\underline{E}_{\text{app}}$. The field $\underline{E}_R = \frac{4}{3}\pi\underline{P}$ must therefore be added vectorially to $\underline{E}_{\text{surf}}$ in eqn (4.5). If, however, one of the principal axes of the dielectric ellipsoid is normal to the faces of the slab-shaped sample shown in Fig. 4.1, then $\underline{E}_{\text{app}}$ is parallel to $\underline{P}$ as in the isotropic case, and eqn (4.6) can still be used with ε_r as the appropriate principal value of the relative permittivity.

The internal fields must be expressed as potentials in order to make crystal field calculations. The first-degree potentials $a_1^q r C_1^q(\theta,\phi)$ can be derived from the Cartesian components of E_{int} by means of the relations†

$$a_1^{\pm 1} = (1/\sqrt{2})(E_{x,\text{int}} \pm iE_{y,\text{int}}) ,$$
$$a_1^0 = -E_{z,\text{int}} . \qquad (4.8)$$

The potential due to the Lorentz field is therefore

† The electrostatic potential $\delta V = -\underline{E}\cdot\underline{r}$. The scalar product $\underline{T}\cdot\underline{U}$ of two spherical tensors T_k^q, U_k^q is defined as the sum $\sum_q(-1)^q T_k^q U_k^{-q}$. Hence $\delta V = -r\sum_q(-1)^q E_q^{(1)} C_1^{-q}(\theta,\phi)$, where the $E_q^{(1)}$ are spherical tensor field components (eqn (3.56)) and the $C_1^q(\theta,\phi)$ are first-degree spherical harmonics as in Table A.1 (p.264). Comparing this expression with the first-degree terms from the crystal field expansion (eqn (4.2)) we find that $a_1^q = (-1)^{q+1}E_{-q}^{(1)}$. Substituting from eqn (3.57) we obtain the amplitudes a_1^q in terms of the Cartesian components of the electric field.

$$\delta V_{\text{Lor}} = \frac{1}{3}(\varepsilon_r+2)r\left[+(1/\sqrt{2})E_x\left\{C_1^1(\theta,\phi) - C_1^{-1}(\theta,\phi)\right\}\right.$$

$$\left. - (i/\sqrt{2})E_y\left\{C_1^1(\theta,\phi) + C_1^{-1}(\theta,\phi)\right\} - E_z C_1^0(\theta,\phi)\right] , \qquad (4.9)$$

where E_x, E_y, E_z are the components of the applied electric field. The corresponding spectroscopic crystal field parameters contain the radial integral $\langle r\rangle$ and can be derived from (4.8) by means of eqn (4.3).

4.2. POINT MULTIPOLE POTENTIALS AND THEIR SYMMETRY PROPERTIES

The Lorentz field potential (4.9) is sometimes used as a rough approximation to the internal field even when a contribution $E_{\langle R}$ in (4.5) is physically possible. Such an approximation will, however, exclude effects due to all higher-order harmonics, in particular the effects due to the even harmonics $A_2^q C_2^2(\theta,\phi)$ which play an important part in determining the level splittings for paramagnetic ions in crystals. It is therefore preferable, where possible, to attempt to calculate some of the remaining terms. This is not difficult in simple ionic lattices provided that suitable estimates can be made for the electrostatic moments induced by the applied field. (Some ways of estimating the induced dipole moments are suggested in §4.3) General formulae which describe the interaction between electrostatic multipole moments can then be used to calculate the induced crystal field amplitudes. Since the derivation of these formulae is somewhat lengthy (Carlson and Rushbrooke 1950; Rose 1958; Gray 1968), we shall merely summarize the results here and then specialize to the case of the potential due to a dipole array.

The interaction between the charge cloud on the paramagnetic ion and the charge clouds on its environmental ions can be described in general terms as follows. Let us consider one of the environmental ions situated at a lattice point $\underline{R}$ relative to the centre of the paramagnetic ion and having a charge density $\rho'(\underline{r}')$ where the coordinate $\underline{r}'$ is taken relative to an origin defined by $\underline{R}$ (see Fig. 4.2). The potential at $\underline{r}$ is given by

$$\delta V' = \int \{\rho'(\underline{r}')/|\underline{R}+\underline{r}'-\underline{r}|\}d\underline{r}' ,$$

where $\underline{r}$ defines position relative to the centre of the paramagnetic

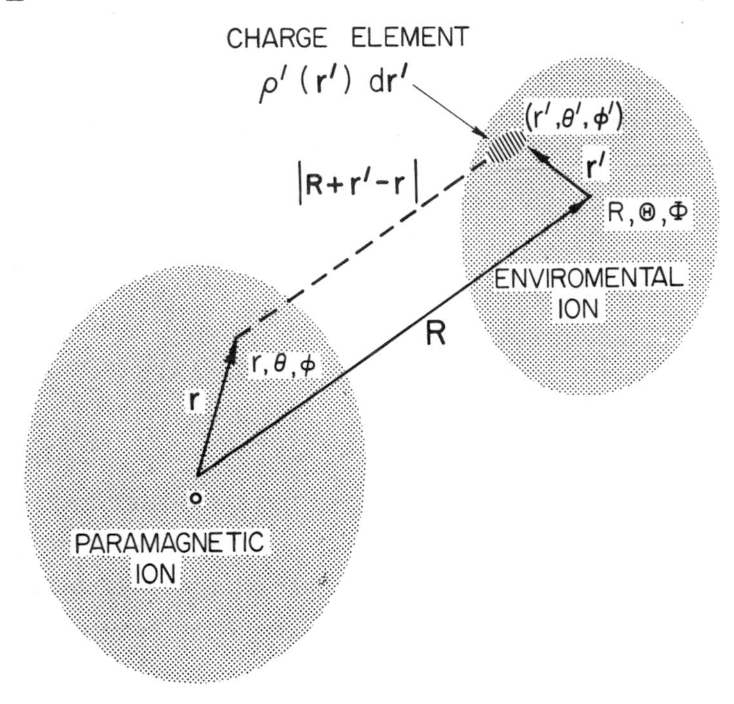

FIG. 4.2. The electrostatic potential at a coordinate $\underline{r} = (r,\theta,\phi)$ of the wavefunction of the paramagnetic electron due to a neighbouring ion centred at $\underline{R} = (R,\Theta,\Phi)$ is obtained by summing the potentials due to all charge elements at $\underline{r}' = (r',\theta',\phi')$. The results can be expressed in terms of the electrostatic multipole moments of the charge on the neighbouring ion. This multipole expansion is only valid provided that the charge distributions defined by $\underline{r}$ and $\underline{r}'$ do not overlap.

ion. The function $|\underline{R}+\underline{r}'-\underline{r}|^{-1}$ can be expanded as a series of spherical harmonics involving the coordinates (R,Θ,Φ), (r',θ',ϕ'), (r,θ,ϕ) of the three vectors. In the references cited earlier it is shown that

$$|\underline{R}+\underline{r}'-\underline{r}|^{-1} = \sum_{k,k'} \sum_{q,q'} (-1)^k \frac{(2K+1)!}{(2k)!(2k')!} \begin{pmatrix} k & k' & K \\ q & q' & -Q \end{pmatrix} \times$$

$$\times \frac{(r)^k (r')^{k'}}{R^{K+1}} C_k^q(\theta,\phi) C_{k'}^{q'}(\theta',\phi') C_K^{-Q}(\Theta,\Phi) , \tag{4.10}$$

where

$$K = k + k', \qquad Q = q + q' . \tag{4.11}$$

It should be noted that in (4.11) the quantities K,k,k' are not vectors and that the conditions are more restrictive than the 'triangular' conditions implied by the 3j symbol (§A.3). Under these special conditions the 3j symbol assumes a simpler form than in the general case (see eqn (A.18)), and eqn (4.10) can be replaced by the equation

$$|\underline{R}+\underline{r}'-\underline{r}|^{-1} = \sum_{k,k'} \sum_{q,q'} (-1)^{k'+Q} \left\{ \frac{(K+Q)!(K-Q)!}{(k+q)!(k-q)!(k'+q')!(k'-q')!} \right\}^{\frac{1}{2}} \times$$

$$\times \frac{(r)^k (r')^{k'}}{R^{K+1}} C_k^q(\theta,\phi) C_{k'}^{q'}(\theta',\phi') C_K^{-Q}(\Theta,\Phi) . \tag{4.12}$$

Substituting (4.12) in the expression for $\delta V'$, we see that the integration involves the multipole moments

$$M_{k'}^{q'} = \int \rho'(\underline{r}')(r')^{k'} C_{k'}^{q'}(\theta',\phi') d\underline{r}' \tag{4.13}$$

of the charge cloud belonging to the environmental ion. Thus

$$\delta V' = \sum_{k,k'} \sum_{q,q'} (-1)^{k'+Q} \left\{ \frac{(K+Q)!(K-Q)!}{(k+q)!(k-q)!(k'+q')!(k'-q')!} \right\}^{\frac{1}{2}} M_{k'}^{q'} \times$$

$$\times \frac{r^k}{R^{K+1}} C_k^q(\theta,\phi) C_K^{-Q}(\Theta,\Phi) . \qquad (4.14)$$

Summing potentials V' due to an array of lattice points $(R,\Theta,\Phi) = (R_j,\theta_j,\phi_j)$, and writing δV for the overall potential we then have

$$\delta V = \sum_{k,q} a_k^q r^k C_k^q(\theta,\phi) , \qquad (4.15)$$

where

$$a_k^q = \sum_j \sum_{k',q'} M_{k',j}^{q'} \eta(k',q',j;k,q) C_K^{-Q}(\theta_j,\phi_j)/R_j^{K+1} \qquad (4.16)$$

and where

$$\eta(k',q',j;k,q) = (-1)^{k'+Q} \left\{ \frac{(K+Q)!(K-Q)!}{(k+q)!(k-q)!(k'+q')!(k'-q')!} \right\}^{\frac{1}{2}} . \qquad (4.17)$$

$M_{k',j}^{q'}$ is a multipole moment associated with the jth environmental ion.

The lowest-order multipole term corresponds to the point charge potential

$$V = \sum_{k,q} A_K^Q r^K C_K^Q(\theta,\phi) ,$$

where

$$A_K^Q = (-1)^Q \sum_j Z_j C_K^{-Q}(\theta_j,\phi_j)/R_j^{K+1} , \qquad (4.18)$$

as may be verified by setting $k' = q' = 0$, $K = k$, $Q = q$ and $M^{q'}_{k',j'} = Z_j$ in eqns (4.15)-(4.17). The next term ($k' = 1$, $K = k + 1$, $Q = q+\mu$) gives the point dipole potential

$$\delta V = \sum_{k,q} a^q_k r^k C^q_k(\theta,\phi) ,$$

where

$$a^q_k = \sum_j \sum_\mu p_{j,\mu}\eta(\mu,k,q)C^{-q-\mu}_{k+1}(\theta_j,\phi_j)/R^{k+2}_j \tag{4.19}$$

and where

$$\eta(\mu,k,q) = (-1)^{1+q+\mu}\left\{\frac{(k+1+q+\mu)!(k+1-q-\mu)!}{(k+q)!(k-q)!(1+\mu)!(1-\mu)!}\right\}^{\frac{1}{2}} \tag{4.20}$$

It should be noted that in (4.19) the dipole moments $p_{j,\mu}$ of the jth environmental ion are the spherical tensor dipole moments which are related to the Cartesian dipole moments by the equations

$$p_{j,\pm 1} = \mp(1/\sqrt{2})(p_{j,x} \pm ip_{j,y});\ p_{j,0} = p_{j,z} , \tag{4.21}$$

or conversely, by

$$p_{j,x} = -(1/\sqrt{2})(p_{j,1}-p_{j,-1});\quad p_{j,y} = (i/\sqrt{2})(p_{j,1}+p_{j,-1});$$

$$p_{j,z} = p_{j,0} . \tag{4.22}$$

In the case of axial dipoles ($\mu = 0$), eqn (4.20) reduces to

$$\eta(0,k,q) = (-1)^{q+1}\{(k+1+q)(k+1-q)\}^{\frac{1}{2}} , \tag{4.23}$$

whilst for transverse dipoles ($\mu = \pm 1$) it becomes

$$\eta(\pm 1,k,q) = (-1)^q (1/\sqrt{2})\{(k+1\pm q)(k+2\pm q)\}^{\frac{1}{2}} . \tag{4.24}$$

Terms due to higher multipole moments can be derived from the same general result if they are needed. For example, the potential δV due to an array of quadrupole moments $M_{2,j}^{p'}$ situated at lattice points R_j is

δV quad =

$$= \sum_j \sum_{q'} \sum_{k,q} M_{2,j}^{q'} \eta_{quad}(q',k,q)(r^k/R_j^{k+3}) C_{k+2}^{-(q+q')}(\theta_j,\phi_j) C_k^q(\theta,\phi), \tag{4.25}$$

where

$$\eta_{quad}(0,k,q) = (-1)^q \tfrac{1}{2}[\{(k+2)^2 - q^2\}\{(k+1)^2 - q^2\}]^{\frac{1}{2}} \tag{4.26}$$

$$\eta_{quad}(\pm 1,k,q) = (-1)^{q+1} \frac{1}{\sqrt{6}}[(k+3\pm q)(k+2\pm q)\{(k+1)^2 - q^2\}]^{\frac{1}{2}} \tag{4.27}$$

$$\eta_{quad}(\pm 2,k,q) = (-1)^q \frac{1}{2\sqrt{6}}[(k+4\pm q)(k+3\pm q)(k+2\pm q)(k+1\pm q)]^{\frac{1}{2}} \tag{4.28}$$

It will generally be found, however, that the additional accuracy obtained by considering these higher-order induced multipoles is more than offset by crudities in other parts of the electric field effect calculation.

Returning to the point dipole case, we now show how to identify the non-vanishing harmonics in δV for any given point symmetry. As in other kinds of EPR calculation this can save a great deal of unnecessary effort. It is well known that for any given point symmetry (except the lowest point symmetry C_1) certain harmonics $C_K^Q(\theta,\phi)$ are excluded from V and that their coefficients $\dot{A}_K^Q$ are zero (see Tables 4.1 and 4.2). This means, of course, that the overall series (4.18) must sum to zero for the K,Q values concerned. But in the case of many crystal lattices this series consists of a number of smaller summations each individually zero

TABLE 4.1

This table gives odd spherical harmonics up to the seventh degree which are permitted in the crystal field potential for each of the twenty-one-odd point groups. The subscript s in $\binom{\pm Q}{K}_s$ denotes that the two harmonics $C_K^{\pm Q}(\theta,\phi)$ appear as a combination $A_K^Q C_K^Q(\theta,\phi) + A_K^{-Q} C_K^{-Q}(\theta,\phi)$ containing the factor $\sin(Q\phi)$ (i.e. $A_K^{-Q} = -(-1)^Q A_K^Q$). The subscript c denotes a combination containing the factor $\cos(Q\phi)$ (i.e. $A_K^{-Q} = (-1)^Q A_K^Q$). Where there is no subscript the combination can be expressed as the sum of sine and cosine terms. The systems of axes used in deriving this table are as shown in Fig. 3.2. The notation $C_2(z)$ indicates that the twofold axis is taken here to be the z-axis.

	Triclinic and monoclinic
C_1	All harmonics
C_s	$\binom{\pm 1}{1}$, $\binom{\pm 1}{3}$, $\binom{\pm 3}{3}$, $\binom{\pm 1}{5}$, $\binom{\pm 3}{5}$, $\binom{\pm 5}{5}$, $\binom{\pm 1}{7}$, $\binom{\pm 3}{7}$, $\binom{\pm 5}{7}$, $\binom{\pm 7}{7}$
	Orthorhombic (vertical twofold)
$C_2(z)$	$\binom{0}{1}$, $\binom{0}{3}$, $\binom{\pm 2}{3}$, $\binom{0}{5}$, $\binom{\pm 2}{5}$, $\binom{\pm 4}{5}$, $\binom{0}{7}$, $\binom{\pm 2}{7}$, $\binom{\pm 4}{7}$, $\binom{\pm 6}{7}$
D_2	$\binom{\pm 2}{3}_s$, $\binom{\pm 2}{5}_s$, $\binom{\pm 4}{5}_s$, $\binom{\pm 2}{7}_s$, $\binom{\pm 4}{7}_s$, $\binom{\pm 6}{7}_s$
C_{2v}	$\binom{0}{1}$, $\binom{0}{3}$, $\binom{\pm 2}{3}_c$, $\binom{0}{5}$, $\binom{\pm 2}{5}_c$, $\binom{\pm 4}{5}_c$, $\binom{0}{7}$, $\binom{\pm 2}{7}_c$, $\binom{\pm 4}{7}_c$, $\binom{\pm 6}{7}_c$
	Trigonal (vertical threefold)
C_3	$\binom{0}{1}$, $\binom{0}{3}$, $\binom{\pm 3}{3}$, $\binom{0}{5}$, $\binom{\pm 3}{5}$, $\binom{0}{7}$, $\binom{\pm 3}{7}$, $\binom{\pm 6}{7}$
D_3	$\binom{\pm 3}{3}_s$, $\binom{\pm 3}{5}_s$, $\binom{\pm 3}{7}_s$, $\binom{\pm 6}{7}_s$
C_{3v}	$\binom{0}{1}$, $\binom{0}{3}$, $\binom{\pm 3}{3}_c$, $\binom{0}{5}$, $\binom{\pm 3}{5}$, $\binom{0}{7}$, $\binom{\pm 3}{7}_c$, $\binom{\pm 6}{7}_c$

TABLE 4.1 (cont.) TABLE 4.1 (cont.)

	Tetragonal (vertical fourfold)
C_4	$\binom{0}{1}$, $\binom{0}{3}$, $\binom{0}{5}$, $\binom{\pm4}{5}$, $\binom{0}{7}$, $\binom{\pm4}{7}$
D_4	$\binom{\pm4}{5}_s$, $\binom{\pm4}{7}_s$
C_{4v}	$\binom{0}{1}$, $\binom{0}{3}$, $\binom{0}{5}$, $\binom{\pm4}{5}_c$, $\binom{0}{7}$, $\binom{\pm4}{7}_c$
S_4	$\binom{\pm2}{3}$, $\binom{\pm2}{5}$, $\binom{\pm2}{7}$, $\binom{\pm6}{7}$
D_{2d}	$\binom{\pm2}{3}_s$, $\binom{\pm2}{5}_s$, $\binom{\pm2}{7}_s$, $\binom{\pm6}{7}_s$
	Hexagonal
C_6	$\binom{0}{1}$, $\binom{0}{3}$, $\binom{0}{5}$, $\binom{0}{7}$, $\binom{\pm6}{7}$
D_6	$\binom{\pm6}{7}_s$
C_{6v}	$\binom{0}{1}$, $\binom{0}{3}$, $\binom{0}{5}$, $\binom{0}{7}$, $\binom{\pm6}{7}_c$
C_{3h}	$\binom{\pm3}{3}$, $\binom{\pm3}{5}$, $\binom{\pm3}{7}$
D_{3h}	$\binom{\pm3}{3}_s$, $\binom{\pm3}{5}_s$, $\binom{\pm3}{7}_s$
	Cubic
T	$\binom{\pm2}{3}_s$
T_d	$\binom{\pm2}{3}_s$
O	No odd harmonics below $\binom{0}{9}$

TABLE 4.2

This table gives even spherical harmonics up to the sixth degree which are permitted in the crystal field potential for each of the twenty-one-odd point groups. The subscript c in $\binom{\pm Q}{K}_c$ denotes that the two harmonics $C_K^{\pm Q}(\theta,\phi)$ appear in a combination containing the factor cos $(Q\phi)$ (i.e. $A_K^{-Q} = (-1)^Q A_K^Q$). Where there is no subscript the combination can be expressed as the sum of the sine and cosine terms. For the point groups T, T_d, and O the harmonics $C_4^{0,\pm 4}$ appear as the combinations $C_4^0 + (\frac{5}{14})^{\frac{1}{2}} (C_4^4 + C_4^{-4})$ and $C_6^0 - (\frac{7}{5})^{\frac{1}{2}} (C_6^4 + C_6^{-4})$ only. The systems of axes used in deriving this table are as shown in Fig. 3.2. The notation $C_2(z)$ indicates that the twofold axis is taken here to be the z-axis. This table can also be used to find the spherical harmonics permitted for each of the eleven centrosymmetric point groups by looking up the equivalent centrosymmetric point group in Table 5.1. (p.141)

	Triclinic and monoclinic
C_1	All harmonics
C_s	$\binom{0}{2}$, $\binom{\pm 2}{2}$, $\binom{0}{4}$, $\binom{\pm 2}{4}$, $\binom{\pm 4}{4}$, $\binom{0}{6}$, $\binom{\pm 2}{6}$, $\binom{\pm 4}{6}$, $\binom{\pm 6}{6}$
	Orthorhombic (vertical twofold)
$C_2(z)$	$\binom{0}{2}$, $\binom{\pm 2}{2}$, $\binom{0}{4}$, $\binom{\pm 2}{4}$, $\binom{\pm 4}{4}$, $\binom{0}{6}$, $\binom{\pm 2}{6}$, $\binom{\pm 4}{6}$, $\binom{\pm 6}{6}$
D_2	$\binom{0}{2}$, $\binom{\pm 2}{2}_c$, $\binom{0}{4}$, $\binom{\pm 2}{4}_c$, $\binom{\pm 4}{4}_c$, $\binom{0}{6}$, $\binom{\pm 2}{6}_c$, $\binom{\pm 4}{6}_c$, $\binom{\pm 6}{6}_c$
C_{2v}	$\binom{0}{2}$, $\binom{\pm 2}{2}_c$, $\binom{0}{4}$, $\binom{\pm 2}{4}_c$, $\binom{\pm 4}{4}_c$, $\binom{0}{6}$, $\binom{\pm 2}{6}_c$, $\binom{\pm 4}{6}_c$, $\binom{\pm 6}{6}_c$

TABLE 4.2 (cont.)

	Trigonal (vertical threefold)
C_3	$\binom{0}{2}$, $\binom{0}{4}$, $\binom{\pm3}{4}$, $\binom{0}{6}$, $\binom{\pm3}{6}$, $\binom{\pm6}{6}$
D_3	$\binom{0}{2}$, $\binom{0}{4}$, $\binom{\pm3}{4}_c$, $\binom{0}{6}$, $\binom{\pm3}{6}_c$, $\binom{\pm6}{6}_c$
C_{3v}	$\binom{0}{2}$, $\binom{0}{4}$, $\binom{\pm3}{4}_c$, $\binom{0}{6}$, $\binom{\pm3}{6}_c$, $\binom{\pm6}{6}_c$
	Tetragonal (vertical fourfold)
C_4	$\binom{0}{2}$, $\binom{0}{4}$, $\binom{\pm4}{4}$, $\binom{0}{6}$, $\binom{\pm4}{6}$
D_4	$\binom{0}{2}$, $\binom{0}{4}$, $\binom{\pm4}{4}$, $\binom{0}{6}$, $\binom{\pm4}{6}$
C_{4v}	$\binom{0}{2}$, $\binom{0}{4}$, $\binom{\pm4}{4}$, $\binom{0}{6}$, $\binom{\pm4}{6}$
S_4	$\binom{0}{2}$, $\binom{0}{4}$, $\binom{\pm4}{4}$, $\binom{0}{6}$, $\binom{\pm4}{6}$
D_{2d}	$\binom{0}{2}$, $\binom{0}{4}$, $\binom{\pm4}{4}_c$, $\binom{0}{6}$, $\binom{\pm4}{6}_c$
	Hexagonal
C_6	$\binom{0}{2}$, $\binom{0}{4}$, $\binom{0}{6}$, $\binom{\pm6}{6}$
D_6	$\binom{0}{2}$, $\binom{0}{4}$, $\binom{0}{6}$, $\binom{\pm6}{6}_c$
C_{6v}	$\binom{0}{2}$, $\binom{0}{4}$, $\binom{0}{6}$, $\binom{\pm6}{6}_c$
C_{3h}	$\binom{0}{2}$, $\binom{0}{4}$, $\binom{0}{6}$, $\binom{\pm6}{6}$
D_{3h}	$\binom{0}{2}$, $\binom{0}{4}$, $\binom{0}{6}$, $\binom{\pm6}{6}_c$

TABLE 4.2 (cont.)

	Cubic
T	$\binom{0}{4}$, $\binom{\pm 4}{4}_c$, $\binom{0}{6}$, $\binom{\pm 4}{6}_c$
T_d	$\binom{0}{4}$, $\binom{\pm 4}{4}_c$, $\binom{0}{6}$, $\binom{\pm 4}{6}_c$
O	$\binom{0}{4}$, $\binom{\pm 4}{4}_c$, $\binom{0}{6}$, $\binom{\pm 4}{6}_c$

since the crystalline environment often consists of many groupings of like ions characterized by a common distance R_j from the paramagnetic centre, each separately obeying the point symmetry operations. Rewriting (4.18) in terms of such groupings we have

$$A_K^Q = (-1)^Q \sum_j Z_j \left\{ \sum_i C_K^{-Q}(\theta_{ij}, \phi_{ij}) \right\} / R_j^{K+1} \; . \tag{4.29}$$

Eqn (4.19) can be similarly rewritten in terms of groupings of like ions in the form

$$a_k^q = \sum_j \sum_\mu \eta(\mu, k, q) p_{j,\mu} \left\{ \sum_i C_{k+1}^{-q-\mu}(\theta_{ij}, \phi_{ij}) \right\} / R_j^{k+2} \; , \tag{4.30}$$

where the parameters $p_{j,\mu}$, $\eta(\mu,k,q)$, R_j are the same within a given grouping. It is easy to see then that if the point symmetry requires that all the sums $\sum_i C_K^{-Q}(\theta_{ij}, \phi_{ij})$ belonging to the term A_K^Q in V should be zero the sums $\sum_i C_{k+1}^{-q-\mu}(\theta_{ij}, \phi_{ij})$ in δV will also be zero when $K = k + 1$ and $Q = q + \mu$. The corresponding harmonic $a_k^q C_k^q(\theta,\phi)$ in δV will therefore be missing. We can sum up the situation by saying that the harmonics C_K^Q and C_k^q which are permitted by symmetry to appear in V and δV respectively are related by modified electric dipole selection rules

$$k = K - 1 ,$$
$$q - Q = -\mu = \pm 1, 0 , \tag{4.31}$$

Q and q will be the same if all the dipole moments in the environment are aligned along the z-axis and will differ by ±1 if the dipoles lie along the x- or y-axes. These selection rules, with the condition $k = K - 1$ (but not $k = K$ and $k = K + 1$), arise from the modified triangular condition (4.11) in the multipole potential formula (4.10). Similar arguments can be used to compare the symmetry conditions which apply to the point charge crystal field potential and to the point quadrupole induced potential (4.25). The selection rules here are

$$k = K - 2 ,$$
$$q - Q = -q' = \pm 2, \pm 1, 0 . \tag{4.32}$$

Tables 4.1 and 4.2 can now be used in conjunction with the modified electric dipole selection rules (4.31) to determine which harmonics are permitted to appear in δV. For example, in S_4 point symmetry the tables show that V contains odd harmonics $C_3^{\pm 2}$, $C_5^{\pm 2}$, $C_7^{\pm 2,\pm 6}$, and even harmonics C_2^0, $C_6^{0,\pm 4}$. Thus, according to the point dipole model, the even harmonics permitted in δV for axial dipoles p_0 will be $C_2^{\pm 2}$, $C_4^{\pm 2}$, $C_6^{\pm 2,\pm 6}$, and the odd harmonics will be C_1^0, C_3^0, $C_5^{0,\pm 4}$ (harmonics up to C_6^q). For non-axial spherical dipoles $p_{\pm 1}$ the harmonics are $C_2^{\pm 1}$, $C_4^{\pm 1,\pm 3}$, $C_6^{\pm 1,\pm 3,\pm 5}$ and $C_1^{\pm 1}$, $C_3^{\pm 1,\pm 3}$, $C_5^{\pm 1,\pm 3,\pm 5}$. Actually it is rarely worth considering any but the lowest-order odd and even harmonics, the lowest-order odd harmonics always being the C_1^q since these terms appear in the long-range Lorentz field (4.9). It should be noted that no even harmonics will be present in δV unless the site is a non-centrosymmetric one.

The summations in eqn (4.19) can be made in a variety of ways, a summation over ions lying within successive spherical shells being fairly easy to compute numerically and affording rapid convergence for all but the first-degree harmonics. In the case of the first-degree harmonics a summation over spherical shells will converge, but it represents only the contribution $E_{<R}$ due to the local atomic environment (see eqn (4.5)) and must be added to the potentials associated with the charge on the electrodes and with non-spherical portions of the remoter environment as represented by the Lorentz field (4.9).

In the present context it is worth noting that a somewhat similar convergence problem is encountered when one attempts to compute the coefficients A_1^q in the normal crystal field V for a material which lacks an overall centre of symmetry (e.g. a piezoelectric or ferroelectric material). These first-degree harmonics are not required in the majority of EPR calculations but are sometimes needed in order to find the linear electric shifts. The calculation can be performed by summing contributions to A_1^q due to point charges lying in successive spherical shells.† Eventually, however, a non-spherical boundary is reached. Remarkably large fields can result from the assumption of certain kinds

---

† Spherical shells lying far enough from the centre to be treated as portions of a uniformly polarized medium make zero contributions to the field at the centre.

of boundary condition - e.g. if the top surface of a parallel-sided sample were to end in a layer of positive ions and the bottom surface in a layer of negative ions. From a practical point of view such boundary conditions are unrealistic however since a surface charge would be neutralized by surface leakage and a long-range bulk field would probably be screened out by charge migration in the dielectric. Some method must therefore be found for eliminating long-range contributions. As a practical expedient one may, for instance, integrate over spherical shells with a hypothetical potential decay factor proportional to $e^{-\lambda R}$.

It might seem from the close relationship existing between the normal and induced potentials that effort could be saved and perhaps a more realistic result obtained by deducing the parameters $a_k^q(s)$ from experimentally measured parameters $A_K^Q(s)$ rather than by means of an ab initio electrostatic calculation. If V and δV were both primarily determined by a single grouping of like ions all lying at the same distance R_j (e.g. the nearest neighbours), this would perhaps be a reasonable approach. By eqns (4.29) and (4.30) we should then obtain the ratio

$$a_{K-1}^{Q+\mu}(s)/A_K^Q(s) = a_{K-1}^{Q+\mu}/A_K^Q = p_{j,\mu}\eta(\mu,K-1,Q+\mu)/Z_j \;, \tag{4.33}$$

the two harmonics being those which are related according to the modified electric dipole selection rules. Considerable caution is needed, however, in making such inferences. The shielding corrections (see references in Abragam and Bleaney 1970 (p. 304) which would be included in the empirical values for the even parameter $A_K^Q(s)$ are not necessarily correct for the related odd-induced parameters $a_{K-1}^{Q+\mu}(s)$, and similar objections could be raised where there are covalency contributions to $A_K^Q(s)$ or $a_{K-1}^{Q+\mu}(s)$. Moreover, even if one assumes the validity of the point charge point dipole model, eqn (4.33) fails in the case when V or δV is determined by more than one grouping of neighbouring ions.

Let us suppose, for example, that contributions to A_K^Q from two groups of neighbouring ions tend to cancel on account of the ions being oppositely charged. No matching cancellation would occur in $a_{K-1}^{Q+\mu}$, since this potential depends on induced dipoles which would most probably have the same sign for both ions.

4.3. THE INDUCED POINT DIPOLES

The applied electric field causes new dipoles p_j to appear at the crystal lattice points surrounding the paramagnetic ion in the following three ways:

(1) by displacing the surrounding ions, each of which carries a charge eZ_j, by an amount $\underline{u}_j$ from their equilibrium position;

(2) by polarizing the charge clouds on the surrounding ions;

(3) by displacing the impurity ion itself.

The polarization of the charge cloud belonging to the paramagnetic ion itself need not be considered here since it is generally allowed for in other ways. The opposite parity mixing mechanism of Chapter 5 allows for the polarization of that part of the electron wavefunction which is responsible for the paramagnetism. Polarization of the rest of electron wavefunction can be allowed for by introducing a shielding correction. It should be noted that although the role of such shielding effects in modifying the even crystal field harmonics has been discussed in the EPR literature (see references in Abragam and Bleaney 1970 (p. 304), no consideration has been given to the shielding of odd harmonics.

The displacements of the impurity ion and of the surrounding ions can both be taken into account by postulating the appearance of ionic dipole moments

$$\underline{p}_{ion,j} = eZ_j(\underline{u}_j-\underline{u}_I) \tag{4.34}$$

at each of the surrounding lattice points (see Fig..4.3). Clearly there will be no contributions from ions which are displaced in

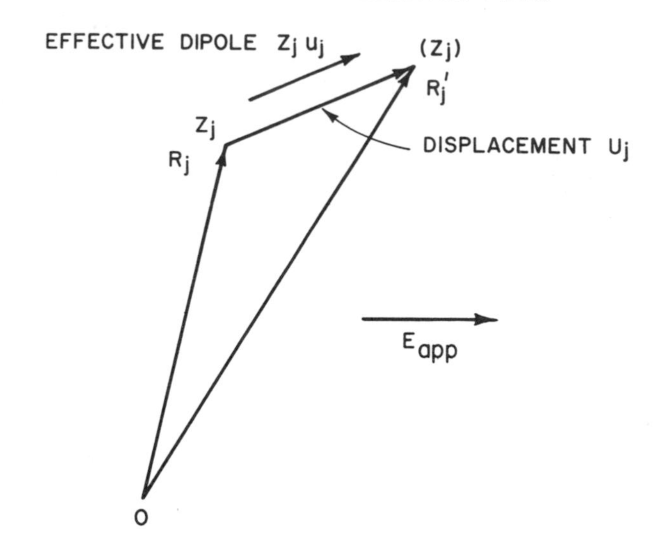

FIG 4.3. An ion which forms part of the environment of a paramagnetic ion centred at O is represented by a point charge Z_j at $\underline{R}_j$. Under the influence of an applied electric field $\underline{E}_{app}$ the ion undergoes a small displacement $\underline{u}_j$ to a new position $\underline{R}'_j$ ($\underline{u}_j$ is not necessarily parallel to $\underline{E}_{app}$.). The electrostatic field due to the charge Z_j at $\underline{R}'_j$ can then be regarded as being made up of two parts: the field due to the charge at its old position $\underline{R}_j$ and the field due to a dipole $\underline{p}_j = Z_j\underline{u}_j$ which in the limit of small displacements can be represented as a point dipole $\underline{p}_j$ at the position $\underline{R}_j$. If the paramagnetic ion is itself displaced by $\underline{u}_I$, the effective dipole $\underline{p}_j = Z_j(\underline{u}_j-\underline{u}_I)$.

---

exactly the same way as the paramagnetic ion. This will only happen in a very limited number of cases, however, since paramagnetic ions often differ in charge or in elastic properties from the ion they replace even when they enter a lattice substitutionally. The actual magnitudes of $\underline{u}_j$ and $\underline{u}_I$ depend on the internal electric field, the ionic charges, and on the interionic forces. Usually a certain amount of guesswork is needed to arrive at suitable values. Interionic forces can sometimes be inferred from the frequency ω_{LO} of the longitudinal optical phonon branch at the zero momentum limit by using the relation

$$\omega_{LO} = 2\pi(k/\mu)^{\frac{1}{2}} \tag{4.35}$$

where μ is a reduced mass and k is the lattice force constant. But it must be remembered here that the electrostatic force which is balanced against the lattice restoring force ku_j is $E_{int}Z_j$, and that the dipole moment

$$p_{j,ion} = \frac{E_{int}Z_j^2}{k} , \tag{4.36}$$

which is calculated in this way will therefore depend on what assumptions are made about the internal field.

As an alternative procedure, in simple lattices it may be possible to estimate values for the ionic dipole moments from the ionic term $\varepsilon_{r,ion}$ in the bulk relative permittivity ε_r. This 'ionic relative permittivity' is obtained by subtracting the free space contribution $\varepsilon_{r,fs} = 1$ and the contribution due to electronic polarization, in order to leave that part of ε_r which can be ascribed to ionic motion only. At optical frequencies the electronic contribution is $\varepsilon_{r,opt}-1$ where $\varepsilon_{r,opt} = n^2$ is the square of the refractive index. The electronic contribution is larger at low frequencies, however, on account of the increase in the internal field $\frac{1}{3}(\varepsilon_r+2)E_{app}$ seen by the atom or ion in question, and it must be replaced by $(\varepsilon_{r,opt}-1)(\varepsilon_r+2)/(\varepsilon_{r,opt}+2)$. Subtracting this low-frequency 'electronic relative permittivity' and $\varepsilon_{r,fs}$ from ε_r we are left with

$$\varepsilon_{r,ion} = 3(\varepsilon_r-\varepsilon_{r,opt})/(\varepsilon_{r,opt}+2) . \tag{4.37}$$

The ionic relative permittivity is related to the ionic dipole moment p_{cell} of each lattice cell by

$$p_{cell} = \varepsilon_{r,ion} E_{app}/4\pi N_{cell} , \qquad (4.38)$$

where N_{cell} is the number of lattice cells per cubic centimetre. Substituting (4.37) in (4.38) we can then obtain the required result. For some purposes this estimate of the ionic dipole moment of a lattice cell is all that is needed.

In certain other calculations (e.g. in the calculation of the 'ionic effect' for a covalently bonded system) it may be necessary to proceed one step further and find the ionic displacement u itself. This can be derived in an NaCl-type lattice by supposing that p_{cell} arises as a result of the displacement u of the negative charge e carried by the Cl^- ion relative to a stationary charge on the Na^+ ion (or the displacement of the Na^+ relative to the Cl^-). Then p_{cell} = eu and

$$eN_0 u = \frac{3(\varepsilon_r - \varepsilon_{r,opt})}{4\pi(\varepsilon_{r,opt} + 2)} E_{app} , \qquad (4.39)$$

where $N_0 = N_{cell}$ is the number of Na^+ or Cl^- ions per cubic centimetre. In a less simple case where there are n ions per cell each having a valency v the same expression can be used with $N_0 = N_{cell} nv$. Thus, for example, in CaF_2 p_{cell} represents the displacement of two monovalent F^- ions (n=2, v=1) with respect to a stationary Ca^{2+} ion, or, alternatively, of one divalent Ca^{2+} ion (n=1, v=2) with respect to two stationary F^- ions. Further refinements can be introduced in (4.39) by considering the possibility of the ions carrying a charge somewhat lower than the integral ionic charge because of covalent bonding effects in the crystal. Szigeti (1949) has suggested that the electronic charge e should be replaced by an effective charge e* = 0·8e. This procedure has subsequently been questioned, however (see Kittel 1956, p. 168), and it is doubtful whether small corrections of this kind are significant in most linear electric field effect calculations.

The electronic polarizabilities of many common ions can be obtained from tables such as those given by Tessman, Kahn, and Shockley (1953) and by Pirenne and Kartheuser (1964). It should be noted that the assumption of a Lorentz internal electric field is already implicit in the values quoted in these tables. The polarizabilities $\alpha = \alpha_{el,j}$ are defined by

$$p_{el,j} = E_{int}\alpha_{el,j} = \frac{1}{3}(\varepsilon_r+2)E_{app}\alpha_{el,j}\,. \tag{4.40}$$

No account is taken of possible anisotropic polarizabilities α (which are, in any case, not to be expected for many of the ions represented in the tables) and in the case of bulk anisotropy the Lorentz factor $\frac{1}{3}(\varepsilon_r+2)$ is approximated by the mean of the Lorentz factors along the three principal dielectric axes. The same approach may therefore be adopted when estimating induced dipole moments for a point dipole calculation although the possibility of α differing according to the orientation of the applied field and of $\underline{p}_{el}$ not being parallel to $\underline{E}_{app}$ should strictly be considered here.

It is also unlikely that the ionic dipole moments $\underline{p}_{ion,j}$ will be parallel to $\underline{E}_{int}$ or to $\underline{E}_{app}$ in any but the simplest lattices, but it is difficult to make a reliable estimate of the anisotropy. The displacements $\underline{u}_j$ are related to the applied force $\underline{E}_{int}Z_j$ by a second-rank tensor $k_{\ell m}$ representing the force constant and consisting of up to 6 parameters depending on the point symmetry of the ionic site. (An ion in a site of axial symmetry would, for example, have two force constants $k_{||}$ and $k_{\perp}$.) Comparatively little is known, however, regarding mechanical properties on the atomic scale, since most physical measurements involve bulk properties and represent averages over different kinds of ion. In most cases the only practical course is to assume an isotropic k.

The same considerations apply to the displacement $\underline{u}_I$ of the paramagnetic ion as to the displacement $\underline{u}_j$ of the ions in its environment, but here the force constants have to some extent been investigated experimentally by comparing the results obtained in a range of similar host lattices. Kiel and Mims (1970, 1971) and Mims and Masuhr (1972) have measured linear electric shifts for a number of paramagnetic ions substituted at the cation site in the scheelite lattices $CaWO_4$, $SrWO_4$, $BaWO_4$. The general pattern of behaviour which emerges is that the linear electric shifts increase, often by considerable factors, when the paramagnetic ion becomes small in relation to the cation which it replaces. Similar results have also been obtained for rare earth ions in some charge-compensated fluoride lattices (Kiel and Mims 1972a, 1973). It seems reasonable to associate this behaviour with the increased value of u_I resulting from a reduction in the restoring force constant, although it should be remembered that other parameters which play a part in determining the magnitude of the shifts will also change with the lattice spacing.

A rudimentary model based on the Born theory of ionic forces Kiel and Mims (1970) gave qualitative agreement with the observed trend but exceptions to the rule can be found. For instance, the small Mn^{2+} ion (ionic radius 0·80 Å) substituted at the Pb^{2+} site in $PbMoO_4$ (Pb^{2+} ionic radius 1·20 Å) gave shifts which were smaller than those observed for Mn in $SrWO_4$ (Sr^{2+} ionic radius 1·12 Å). This result was tentatively attributed to an incipient instability resulting in a situation analogous to that which occurs in the dynamic Jahn-Teller effect (Kiel, Mims, and Masuhr 1973), but in the absence of any independent confirmation this remains little more than a speculation. Further studies of small ions in oversized lattice sites, in particular studies of ions such as Mn^{2+} in BaO which have undergone a spontaneous permanent displacement, (Sochava, Tolparov, and Kovalev 1971; Weightman, Dugdale, and Holroyd 1971) might help in clarifying situations of this kind.

The difficulties which arise when estimating the induced dipoles and ionic displacements required for the point-dipole calculation of δV are relatively simple compared with those encountered when one begins to consider higher-order induced multipoles in the environment of the paramagnetic ion. An applied electric field cannot for symmetry reasons induce a quadrupole moment in a spherical free ion such as F^- or O^{2-}, but quadrupole moments could be induced for ions situated in a crystal lattice. The applied field and odd harmonics present in the local crystal field could in principle combine to induce such a moment in much the same way as they combine to form an 'equivalent even field' for the paramagnetic ion (Chapter 5). Other mechanisms could lead to the same effect. For instance the ionic displacements and electronic polarization of the neighbours surrounding each environmental ion could give rise to quadrupole polarizing fields and thus induce quadrupole moments. Fortunately there is good reason to believe that these induced quadrupole moments are generally small in relation to the induced dipole moments, i.e. $M_{2,j} < p_j r_0$ (where r_0 is the radius of the ion). Moreover, it can be seen from (4.19) and (4.25) that δV_{quad} is smaller than the point dipole potential by a factor $\simeq (M_{2,j}/p_j R_m)$. Under most circumstances one may, therefore, with some justification, neglect the point quadrupole correction to the point-dipole calculation.

Induced even and odd potentials arising from the polarization of nearby ions have been considered by Dreybrodt and Silber (1969) in a study of the linear electric field effect for Mn^{2+} charge-compensated ions in NaCl. A more elaborate analysis of the induced potential in terms of the point dipole model is given for Mn^{2+} in CdS and for Ce^{3+} charge compensated centres in CaF_2 by Kiel and Mims (1972a, 1972b) (see also Chapter 6).

4.4. THE INTERNAL FIELD IN COVALENT-BONDING CALCULATIONS

In the preceding treatment it has been assumed that the paramagnetic electrons are strictly localized on the paramagnetic ion and hence that the factor r/R_j is always less than unity. If this is not true for all values of R_j, as, for instance, when the paramagnetic electron is shared covalently with the surrounding ions, or when it occupies a molecular orbital then the multipole expansion given earlier is no longer valid. In such cases it remains possible in principle to make a multipole expansion (Buehler and Hirschfelder 1951, 1952), but in practice it may be preferable to change the model or to rely on simple ad hoc estimates of the internal field.

To see what is required in order to arrive at a realistic estimate let us consider briefly the nature of the electric field effect calculation for a partially covalent system. Magnetic resonance parameters for covalently bonded ions can be derived by setting up molecular orbitals for the ligand ions (nearest neighbours) and by forming mixed states which involve the ligand wavefunctions and the wavefunctions of the paramagnetic ion. An applied electric field then modifies these parameters in two ways: (1) by polarizing the mixed electron wavefunction (electronic effect) and (2) by displacing the ligand ions relative to the paramagnetic ion thus altering the degree of covalent bonding (ionic effect). The question arises as to what electric field to use in estimating each of these two contribution to the overall effect.

Most authors have chosen to use the Lorentz field $E_{int} = \frac{1}{3}(\varepsilon_r+2)\,E_{app}$ in calculating the electronic effect (Royce and Bloembergen 1963 ; Dreybrodt and Silber 1969; Buch and Gelineau 1971). This seems to be a reasonable guess since the nearest-neighbour ions which generally contribute the largest corrections $E_{<R}$ (see eqn (4.6)) to the Lorentz field are already taken into consideration as part of the covalently bonded complex. But it

can also be argued that since the electrons are partially delocalized electrons a value closer to E_{app} is more appropriate (see §8.3). The internal-field problem is harder to settle for the ionic effect since the field acting on the ligand ions and giving rise to their displacement is partly determined by the polarization of their immediate neighbours. One way of avoiding the problem is to derive the displacement u directly from the bulk relative permittivity via eqn (4.39), a procedure which makes it unnecessary to ask what are the fields actually seen by the ions. This method is of course only strictly applicable in rather simple situations, but it may be used for want of a better one when no specific information regarding the lattice restoring forces acting on individual ions is available.

5. The treatment of odd crystal field potentials

The eigenstates of a free ion have definite odd or even parity. This remains true for ions substituted at centrosymmetric sites in a crystal lattice, but it is no longer the case where the crystal field contains odd harmonics. Let us for example consider the ion Ce^{3+}. Its low lying states consist of a sixfold degenerate $J = \frac{5}{2}$ level and an eightfold degenerate $J = \frac{7}{2}$ level lying 2253 cm^{-1} higher up. These are the eigenstates of the single 4f electron of Ce^{3+}, they have odd parity and they constitute the complete 4f manifold of states. The nearest opposite parity set of states, the 5d manifold, is situated at approximately 50 000 cm^{-1} above the 4f manifold. If the Ce^{3+} ion is now substituted in a crystal lattice at a centrosymmetric site the degeneracy of the $J = \frac{5}{2}$ and $J = \frac{7}{2}$ states will be partially raised and there will be some mixing between these two submanifolds. Analogous changes will occur within the 5d manifold but there will be no 4f-5d coupling and the parity of the states will remain the same as in the free ion. States of mixed parity will only be obtained when the crystal field contains odd harmonics which couple the 4f and 5d manifolds.

The mixing between opposite-parity free-ion states has traditionally been ignored in EPR studies on the grounds that it is often much smaller than state mixing within a manifold of given parity because of the large energy denominators which correspond to the separations between opposite parity manifolds and therefore has little effect on calculations. This approximation is not always justifiable (it fails for many of the divalent rare earths, see Table 5.7 (p. 151)) - but it nevertheless remains possible to give a description of the properties observed in normal EPR experiments in terms of a set of effective even crystal field harmonics. The reason is that the phenomena observed in normal EPR experiments are invariant under reversal of the magnetic fields, i.e. they are invariant under an inversion of coordinates of the probes used to study the system. Although the effective even crystal field harmonics obtained by such a parametrization procedure are not the true even harmonics, the difference is often small and the correction term can sometimes be calculated by perturbation theory as shown later (eqn (5.23)).

The odd harmonics become of primary importance when interpreting the linear electric field effect which offers an almost unique means of studying the deviations from centrosymmetry in the crystal field environment.[†] One mechanism has been discussed in Chapter 4, where it was shown how the polarization of an odd configuration of ions surrounding the paramagnetic ion can result

---

[†] Odd field effects and opposite parity state mixing also play a major role in determining the intensity of some optical transitions. The optical intensities depend on the magnitude of the electric dipole matrix element which is zero if both states concerned in the transition have the same well-defined parity. Transitions occurring within a given manifold (e.g. the 4f manifold) acquire their intensity as a result of opposite parity admixture (e.g. 5d admixture) brought about by odd crystal fields (see e.g. Judd 1962).

in additions to the even crystal field. We now go on to consider a second mechanism which depends explicitly on the odd crystal fields seen by the paramagnetic ion.

5.1. PERTURBATION TREATMENT OF OPPOSITE PARITY STATE MIXING

In order to calculate the state mixing caused by the odd part of the normal crystal field and by the odd part of the induced field, i.e. by V_{odd} and δV_{odd}, we shall require a number of results derived from stationary perturbation theory (Landau and Lifshitz 1958). These results are summarized below.

The first-, second-, and third-order shifts in the energy E_n of an eigenstate ψ_n due to a perturbation V are given by

$$\delta^{(1)}E_n = V_{nn} , \tag{5.1}$$

$$\delta^{(2)}E_n = \sum_{\ell}^{\ell\neq n} \frac{|V_{\ell n}|^2}{E_{n\ell}} , \tag{5.2}$$

$$\delta^{(3)}E_n = \sum_{k}^{k\neq n} \sum_{\ell}^{\ell\neq n} \frac{V_{n\ell}V_{\ell k}V_{kn}}{E_{\ell n}E_{kn}} - V_{nn} \sum_{\ell}^{\ell\neq n} \frac{|V_{n\ell}|^2}{E_{\ell n}^2} , \tag{5.3}$$

where $V_{\ell n} = \langle\psi_\ell|V|\psi_n\rangle$ and $E_{\ell n}$ is the energy interval $E_\ell - E_n$. The first- and second-order changes in the composition of the wavefunction ψ_n are

$$\delta^{(1)}\psi_n = \sum_{\ell}^{\ell\neq n} \frac{V_{\ell n}}{E_{n\ell}} \psi_\ell , \tag{5.4}$$

$$\delta^{(2)}\psi_n = \sum_{\ell}^{\ell\neq n}\sum_{k}^{k\neq n}\frac{V_{\ell k}V_{kn}}{E_{nk}E_{n\ell}}\psi_\ell - V_{nn}\sum_{\ell}^{\ell\neq n}\frac{V_{\ell n}}{E^2_{n\ell}}\psi_\ell -$$

$$-\frac{1}{2}\psi_n\sum_{\ell}^{\ell\neq n}\frac{|V_{\ell n}|^2}{E^2_{\ell n}}, \qquad (5.5)$$

In order to discuss the effects arising from the even part of the crystal field, and to calculate g-shifts (Chapter 6) it is also convenient to have expressions for the first- and second-order changes in the matrix elements $f_{nm} = \langle\psi_n|f|\psi_m\rangle$. These can be derived from eqns (5.4) and (5.5) and are as follows

$$\delta^{(1)}(f_{nm}) = \sum_{\ell}^{\ell\neq n}\frac{V_{n\ell}f_{\ell m}}{E_{n\ell}} + \sum_{\ell}^{\ell\neq m}\frac{V_{\ell m}f_{n\ell}}{E_{m\ell}}, \qquad (5.6)$$

$$\delta^{(2)}(f_{nm}) = \sum_{\ell}^{\ell\neq n}\sum_{k}^{k\neq n}\frac{V_{nk}V_{k\ell}f_{\ell m}}{E_{nk}E_{n\ell}} + \sum_{\ell}^{\ell\neq m}\sum_{k}^{k\neq m}\frac{f_{m\ell}V_{\ell k}V_{km}}{E_{mk}E_{m\ell}} +$$

$$+\sum_{\ell}^{\ell\neq m}\sum_{k}^{k\neq n}\frac{V_{nk}f_{k\ell}V_{\ell m}}{E_{nk}E_{m\ell}} - V_{nn}\sum_{\ell}^{\ell\neq n}\frac{V_{n\ell}f_{\ell m}}{E^2_{n\ell}} -$$

$$-V_{mm}\sum_{\ell}^{\ell\neq m}\frac{f_{n\ell}V_{\ell m}}{E^2_{m\ell}} - \frac{1}{2}f_{nm}\sum_{\ell}^{\ell\neq n}\frac{|V_{n\ell}|^2}{E^2_{n\ell}} -$$

$$-\frac{1}{2}f_{nm}\sum_{\ell}^{\ell\neq m}\frac{|V_{m\ell}|^2}{E^2_{m\ell}}. \qquad (5.7)$$

Let us first consider the perturbation $V = V_{odd}$ where the ψ_n are states of definite parity derived from a Hamiltonian which includes all even crystal fields. The first-order energy perturbation $\delta^{(1)}E_n$ is then zero, but the second-order perturbation $\delta^{(2)}E_n$ contains non-zero terms arising from the summation over wavefunctions ψ_ℓ which are opposite in parity to the ψ_n. Writing ψ_{gj} for the ground-state wavefunctions and ψ_u for the opposite parity manifold† we have

$$\delta E_{gj} = -\sum_u (1/E_{ug}) |\langle\psi_u|V_{odd}|\psi_{gj}\rangle|^2 \quad , \tag{5.8}$$

where $E_{ug} = E(\psi_u) - E(\psi_g)$ (note the change of sign caused by the substitution $E_{ug} = E_{\ell n} = E_{n\ell}$). The third-order perturbation $\delta^{(3)}E_n$ vanishes since at least one of the factors $V_{n\ell}$, $V_{\ell k}$, V_{kn} is zero in the first term of eqn (5.3), whatever the parity of ψ_k, ψ_ℓ, and ψ_{nn} is zero in the second term. The shift in energy due to an odd perturbation only is therefore given by (5.8) up to the third order, although odd and even perturbations together can produce third-order shifts, as we see next.

---

† The subscripts g, u generally stand for <u>gerade</u> (even) and <u>ungerade</u> (odd). Here, however, g stands merely for the ground state and u for an excited state of opposite parity. This will sometimes conflict with conventional usage - e.g. in the case of Ce^{3+} the ground 4f manifold is odd and the excited 5d manifold even - but it avoids confusion in the present discussion.

If we set $V = V_{odd} + V_H$, where V_H represents the Zeeman field perturbation (e.g. $V_H = g\beta(\underline{L}+2\underline{S}).\underline{H}$), we can find energy shifts which depend on the odd field and also on the matrix elements of V_H, these being the shifts described by the parameters T_{ijk} in eqn (3.2)(p.39). In first order the operator V_H, which is even, gives rise to the perturbation $\delta^{(1)}E_n = (V_H)_{nn}$ this being the Zeeman energy. The second-order term,

$$\delta^{(2)}E_n = \sum_{\ell}^{\ell \neq n} (1/E_{n\ell})\{|(V_{odd})_{\ell n}|^2 + (V_{odd})_{\ell n}(V_H)_{n\ell} + $$

$$+ (V_H)_{\ell n}(V_{odd})_{n\ell} + |(V_H)_{\ell n}|^2\} \quad , \tag{5.9}$$

likewise leads to no new results of any significance. The first term has already been considered (eqn 5.8), the two middle terms are zero since one or the other of the matrix elements vanishes for both parities of ψ_ℓ, and the last term constitutes a small quadratic Zeeman shift. It is not until third order that we find terms containing V_{odd} and V_H together. Substituting $V = V_{odd} + V_H$ in (5.3), taking both possible parities for the wavefunctions ψ_k and ψ_ℓ into account, and eliminating zero terms, we can write down the perturbation

$$\delta^{(3)}E_n = \sum_{k}^{k \neq n} \sum_{\ell}^{\ell \neq n} \{(1/E_{\ell n}E_{kn})(V_H)_{n\ell}(V_{odd})_{\ell k}(V_{odd})_{kn}\}_{k(-),\ell(+)} +$$

$$+ \sum_{k}^{k \neq n} \sum_{\ell}^{\ell \neq n} \{(1/E_{\ell n}E_{kn})(V_{odd})_{n\ell}(V_{odd})_{\ell k}(V_H)_{kn}\}_{k(+),\ell(-)} +$$

$$+ \sum_{k}^{k\neq n} \sum_{\ell}^{\ell\neq n} \{(1/E_{\ell n}E_{kn})(V_{odd})_{n\ell}(V_H)_{\ell k}(V_{odd})_{kn}\}_{k(-),\ell(-)} -$$

$$- (V_H)_{nn} \sum_{k}^{k\neq n} \{(1/E_{kn}^2) \mid (V_{odd})_{nk}|^2\}_{k(-)} \qquad (5.10)$$

(plus two terms in higher powers of V_H which can be ignored). The subscript notation k(−), ℓ(+) is used here to indicate that the ψ_k must have opposite parity to the ψ_n and the ψ_ℓ the same parity as the ψ_n for non-vanishing contributions to the sum. This notation is strictly superfluous since the parity conditions are already implicit in the assumption that $(V_{odd})_{k\ell}$ etc are non zero matrix elements, but it will help to focus attention on the main outline of the argument.

Eqn (5.10) can be simplified by taking the relative magnitudes of the energy denominators into account. The first two terms contain the odd-to-even manifold separation only once, whereas in the last two terms this quantity appears as the square. In many instances the odd-to-even interval is much larger (see Tables 5.5–5.7, p.149), than the separation between the ground state and the first few excited states. We can therefore discard these last two terms. By interchanging the subscripts k and ℓ we also see that the second term is the Hermitian conjugate (h.c.) of the first. Making these simplifications and adopting the notation of eqn (5.8), we obtain the result

$$\delta E_{gj,H} = \sum_{u} \sum_{i}^{i\neq j} (1/E_{ug}E_{ij})\{\langle\psi_{gj}|V_H|\psi_{gi}\rangle\langle\psi_{gi}|V_{odd}|\psi_u\rangle\langle\psi_u|V_{odd}|\psi_{gj}\rangle +$$

$$+ \text{h.c.}\} \quad , \qquad (5.11)$$

where the subscript H in $\delta E_{gj,H}$ indicates that the expression accounts for only that part of the energy shift which is associated with the Zeeman field H_0. The total shift is given by the sum of the H_0-independent and H_0-dependent parts in eqns (5.8) and (5.11).

To find the energy shifts associated with the applied electric field, we replace V_{odd} with $V_{odd} + \delta V_{odd}$ in the preceding formulae. Three types of shift can be identified: those involving V_{odd} twice, those involving δV_{odd} twice, and those involving both V_{odd} and δV_{odd}. The first is the correction to the normal crystal field calculation which is obtained by taking the odd harmonics into account. The second is quadratic in the applied field, and the third is the required linear electric effect term. The H_0-independent and H_0-dependent portions derived from (5.8) and (5.11) are

$$\delta E_{gj} =$$

$$-\sum_u (1/E_{ug})\{\langle\psi_{gj}|V_{odd}|\psi_u\rangle\langle\psi_u|\delta V_{odd}|\psi_{gj}\rangle + \text{h.c.}\} , \tag{5.12}$$

$$\delta E_{gj,H} =$$

$$\sum_u \sum_i^{i\neq j} (1/E_{ug}E_{ij})\{\langle\psi_{gj}|V_H|\psi_{gi}\rangle\langle\psi_{gi}|V_{odd}|\psi_u\rangle\langle\psi_u|\delta V_{odd}|\psi_{gj}\rangle +$$

$$+ \langle\psi_{gj}|V_H|\psi_{gi}\rangle\langle\psi_{gi}|\delta V_{odd}|\psi_u\rangle\langle\psi_u|V_{odd}|\psi_{gj}\rangle + \text{h.c.}\}. \tag{5.13}$$

In principle, eqn (5.13) is all that is needed to interpret the result of a frequency-shift experiment. For a Kramers doublet one might, for example, substitute the appropriate operator for V_H, and write

$$\delta g \beta H_0 = 2\delta E^{+}_{g,H} \,, \tag{5.14}$$

where $\delta E^{+}_{g,H}$ is the shift for the upper state. For a low-symmetry site the calculation would have to be repeated at various orientations of H_0, however, and it is usually more convenient to work with general expressions giving the shift in the Zeeman field matrix elements rather than with energy shift expressions such as (5.13). These expressions can be obtained from the perturbation formulae (5.6)-(5.7) by substituting $V = V_{odd}$ and $f = V_H$. It is easily verified that there is no first-order shift $\delta^{(1)}\langle\psi_n|V_H|\psi_m\rangle$ since the matrix elements $(V_{odd})_{n\ell}, (V_{odd})_{\ell m}$ vanish when ψ_ℓ has the same parity to ψ_n, ψ_m whilst $(V_H)_{\ell m}, (V_H)_{n\ell}$ vanish when it has the same parity. The second-order shift $\delta^{(2)}\langle\psi_n|V_H|\psi_m\rangle$ also contains a number of terms which can be discarded at once for parity reasons (i.e. the fourth and fifth terms from eqn (5.7)). We are thus left with the expression

$$\delta^{(2)}\langle\psi_n|V_H|\psi_m\rangle =$$

$$= \sum_{k}^{k\neq n}\sum_{\ell}^{\ell\neq n} \{(1/E_{\ell n}E_{kn})(V_{odd})_{nk}(V_{odd})_{k\ell}(V_H)_{\ell m}\ k(-),\ell(+) \quad +$$

$$+ \sum_{k}^{k\neq m}\sum_{\ell}^{\ell\neq m} \{(1/E_{\ell m}E_{kn})(V_H)_{n\ell}(V_{odd})_{\ell k}(V_{odd})_{km}\ k(-),\ell(+) \quad +$$

$$+ \sum_{k}^{k\neq n}\sum_{\ell}^{\ell\neq m} \{(1/E_{\ell m}E_{kn})(V_{odd})_{nk}(V_H)_{k\ell}(V_{odd})_{\ell m}\}_{k(-),\ell(-)} \quad -$$

$$- \frac{1}{2}\,(V_H)_{nm}\left\{\sum_{k}^{k\neq n}(1/E^2_{kn})\,|(V_{odd})_{kn}|^2\right\}_{k(-)} \quad -$$

$$- \frac{1}{2} (V_H)_{nm} \left\{ \sum_{k}^{k \neq m} (1/E_{km})^2 \, | (V_{odd})_{km} |^2 \right\}_{k(-)} . \qquad (5.15)$$

(the subscripts k(−), ℓ(+), etc. denote the parity of ψ_k, ψ_ℓ as in eqn (5.10)). A further simplification can be made by assuming as was done in deriving eqn (5.11) that the odd-even manifold separation is much larger than separations within the ground manifold. This leads to the elimination of the last three terms in eqn (5.15) and leaves (in the notation of eqns (5.8) and (5.11),) the expression

$$\delta \langle \psi_{gj} | V_H | \psi'_{gj} \rangle$$

$$= \sum_u \sum_i^{i \neq j} \frac{1}{E_{ug} E_{ij}} \langle \psi_{gj} | V_{odd} | \psi_u \rangle \langle \psi_u | V_{odd} | \psi_i \rangle \langle \psi_i | V_H | \psi'_{gj} \rangle \; +$$

$$+ \sum_u \sum_i^{i \neq j'} \frac{1}{E_{ug'} E_{ij'}} \langle \psi_{gj} | V_H | \psi_i \rangle \langle \psi_i | V_{odd} | \psi_u \rangle \langle \psi_u | V_{odd} | \psi'_{gj} \rangle \; , \qquad (5.16)$$

where ψ_{gj}, ψ'_{gj}, and ψ_i belong to the ground manifold, $E_{ij'}$ denotes the interval $E(\psi_i) - E(\psi'_j)$, etc. Eqns (5.10), (5.11) are special cases of (5.15), (5.16), as may be verified by setting m = n and $\psi'_{gj} = \psi_{gj}$.

The linear electric field induced perturbation is found by substituting $V_{odd} + \delta V_{odd}$ for V_{odd} and dropping terms in V^2_{odd}, $(\delta V_{odd})^2$. Thus we have

$$\delta\langle\psi_{gj}|V_H|\psi'_{gj}\rangle$$

$$= \sum_u \sum_i^{i\neq j} \{(1/E_{ug}E_{ij})\langle\psi_{gj}|V_{odd}|\psi_u\rangle\langle\psi_u|\delta V_{odd}|\psi_i\rangle\langle\psi_i|V_H|\psi'_{gj}\rangle +$$

$$+ \langle\psi_{gj}|\delta V_{odd}|\psi_u\rangle\langle\psi_u|V_{odd}|\psi_i\rangle\langle\psi_i|V_H|\psi'_{gj}\rangle\} +$$

$$+ \sum_u \sum_i^{i\neq j'} \{(1/E_{ug}E_{ij'})\langle\psi_{gj}|V_H|\psi_i\rangle\langle\psi_i|V_{odd}|\psi_u\rangle\langle\psi_u|\delta V_{odd}|\psi'_{gj}\rangle +$$

$$+ \langle\psi_{gj}|V_H|\psi_i\rangle\langle\psi_i|\delta V_{odd}|\psi_u\rangle\langle\psi_u|V_{odd}|\psi'_{gj}\rangle\} \quad . \tag{5.17}$$

5.2. THE EQUIVALENT EVEN FIELD

As we have already noted the perturbation expansions for $\delta E_{gj,H}$, etc. can be considerably simplified in those cases when the odd to even energy separation E_{ug} is large in comparison with the separations within the ground manifold. A most useful additional simplification can be made by replacing the distribution of values E_{ug} by a single mean value $\overline{E}_{ug}$ and by taking this factor outside the summation sign. We can then extract from eqns (5.12), (5.13), (5.17) the Hermitian operator

$$\delta V_{EEF} = -\frac{1}{\overline{E}_{ug}} \sum_u \{(V_{odd}|\psi_u\rangle\langle\psi_u|\delta V_{odd}) + (\delta V_{odd}|\psi_u\rangle\langle\psi_u|V_{odd}\} \quad , \tag{5.18}$$

and rewrite the equations in the condensed form

$$\delta E_{gj} = \langle\psi_{gj}|\delta V_{EEF}|\psi_{gj}\rangle \quad , \tag{5.19}$$

$$\delta E_{gj,H} = -\sum_{i}^{i\neq j} \frac{1}{E_{ij}} \{\langle\psi_{gj}|V_H|\psi_{gi}\rangle\langle\psi_{gi}|\delta V_{EEF}|\psi_{gj}\rangle + \text{h.c.}\} \quad , \tag{5.20}$$

$$\delta\langle\psi_{gj}|V_H|\psi'_{gj}\rangle = -\sum_{i}^{i\neq j} \frac{1}{E_{ij}} \langle\psi_{gj}|\delta V_{EEF}|\psi_i\rangle\langle\psi_i|V_H|\psi'_{gj}\rangle -$$

$$-\sum_{i}^{i\neq j'} \frac{1}{E_{ij'}} \langle\psi_{gj}|V_H|\psi_i\rangle\langle\psi_i|\delta V_{EEF}|\psi'_{gj}\rangle \quad . \tag{5.21}$$

The operator δV_{EEF} is an even operator (i.e. one connecting states of the same parity) as shown diagrammatically in Fig. 5.1. It has been termed the 'equivalent even field' (Kiel 1966), and it appears in calculations in the same places as would the induced even potential δV_{ev}. Eqns (5.19)-(5.21) are in fact the same as those we should obtain by taking $V = \delta V_{ev}$ as a perturbation and applying the formulae in §5.1. Thus, from eqn (5.1) we should obtain the first-order perturbation $\delta E_{gj} = \langle\psi_{gj}|\delta V_{ev}|\psi_{gj}\rangle$ (cf. eqn (5.19). Likewise, if we were to set $V = \delta V_{ev} + V_H$ in eqns (5.2) and (5.6) and discard terms in δV_{ev}^2 and V_H^2 we should obtain the formal equivalents of eqns (5.20) and (5.21) (note that $E_{ij} = E_{\ell n} = -E_{n\ell}$). From this similarity between the two types of expression it follows that the total effect of the even and odd induced potentials can be represented by means of an even operator

$$\delta\overline{V}_{ev} = \delta V_{ev} + \delta V_{EEF} \quad , \tag{5.22}$$

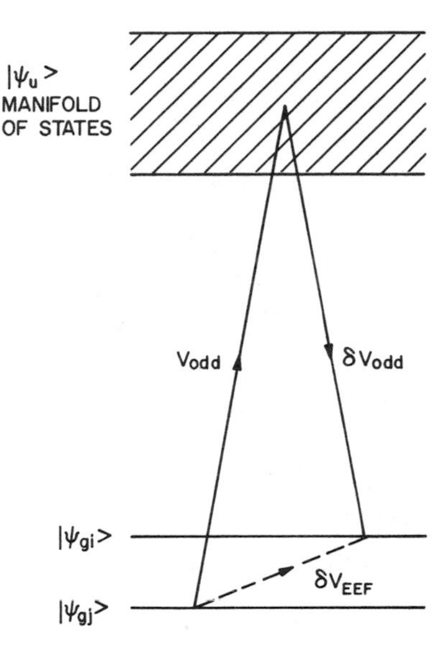

FIG. 5.1. The two odd crystal field potentials V_{odd} and δV_{odd} couple states of opposite parity ψ_u, ψ_g but have no first-order matrix elements within either of the two manifolds. They will couple states ψ_g in second order, however. This second-order perturbation can be reduced to a first-order perturbation, symbolized by an equivalent field operator δV_{EEF}, by summing over all states ψ_u and applying the closure principle.

this operator being used in calculations which involve the ground manifold of states only. The perturbation formulae required in these calculations are one order lower than those required when V_{odd} and δV_{odd} appear explicitly.

Clearly it is possible to write down a similar set of expressions corresponding to the second-order perturbation due to the odd portion of the normal crystal field. Thus

$$V_{EEF} = -\frac{1}{\bar{E}_{ug}} \sum_u V_{odd}|\psi_u\rangle\langle\psi_u|V_{odd} , \tag{5.23}$$

and the operator sum

$$\overline{V}_{ev} = V_{ev} + V_{EEF} \tag{5.24}$$

then represents the even crystal field potential corrected for the second-order effects of the odd harmonics. It should be noted that the harmonics contained in an expansion of the even operator V_{EEF} have the property of being invariant under the symmetry operations of the odd point group and also under inversion. This means that they are the same as the harmonics permitted for the even portion V_{even} of the normal crystal field (see Table 4.2, p.111) and that they are the same as the harmonics permitted in the even point group which is obtained by augmenting the symmetry operations of the odd point group with the inversion operation. The even point groups related to odd point groups in this way are indicated in Table 5.1 and their symmetry operations are shown diagrammatically in Fig. 5.2. Apart from a linear electric field effect experiment there is no EPR method of distinguishing between the point groups in the two columns of Table 5.1 and they are therefore to this extent phenomenologically equivalent.

It remains to find a method of calculating the even operators δV_{EEF}, V_{EEF} as in

$$\langle\psi_{gj}|\delta V_{EEF}|\psi_{gi}\rangle \; - \frac{1}{\overline{E}_{ug}} \sum_{u} \langle\psi_{gj}|V_{odd}|\psi_u\rangle\langle\psi_u|\delta V_{odd}|\psi_{gi}\rangle \; +$$

$$+ \; \langle\psi_{gj}|\delta V_{odd}|\psi_u\rangle\langle\psi_u|V_{odd}|\psi_{gi}\rangle \quad . \tag{5.25}$$

The equivalent even operators can be derived by using a closure method to sum over the complete set of eigenfunctions ψ_u. A simple illustration of the closure principle is provided by the relation

TABLE 5.1

If the symmetry operations of one of the 21 non-centrosymmetric point groups are augmented by inversion we obtain centrosymmetric point groups as below. In EPR experiments which do not involve applied electric fields the non-centrosymmetric point groups and related centrosymmetric point groups are phenomenologically indistinguishable (some alternative notations are shown in brackets).

Non-centrosymmetric point group	Centrosymmetric point group
C_1	$S_2(C_i)$
C_2	C_{2h}
C_3	$S_6(C_{3i})$
C_4	C_{4h}
C_6	C_{6h}
$D_2(V)$	$D_{2h}(V_h)$
D_3	D_{3d}
D_4	D_{4h}
D_6	D_{6h}
C_{2v}	D_{2h}
C_{3v}	D_{3d}
C_{4v}	D_{4h}
$D_{2d}(V_d)$	D_{4h}
C_{6v}	D_{6h}
D_{3h}	D_{6h}
S_4	C_{4h}
$C_s(C_{1h})$	C_{2h}
C_{3h}	C_{6h}
T	T_h
T_d	O_h
O	O_h

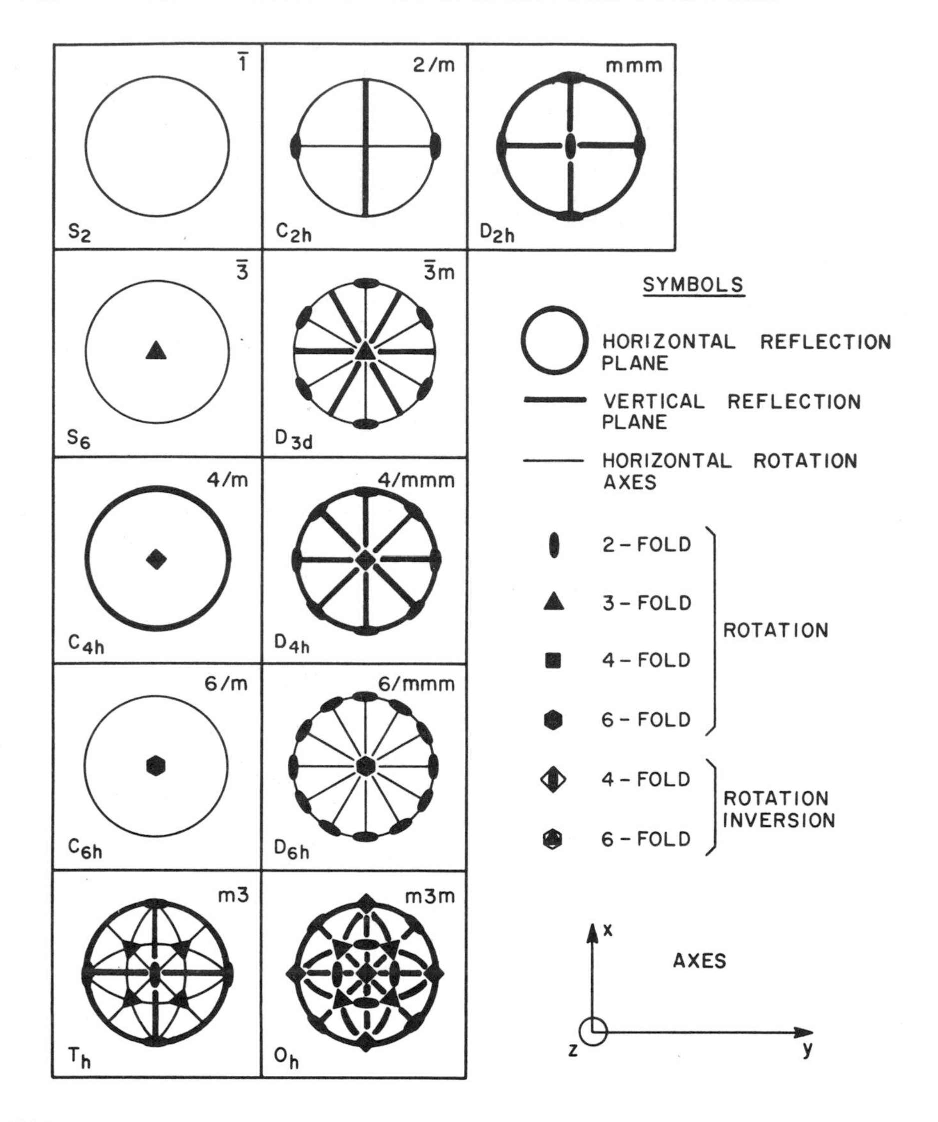

FIG. 5.2. Diagram showing the symmetry elements for the 11 even point groups. EPR phenomena other than the linear electric field effect for the 21 odd point symmetries (see Fig. 3.2) can be described parametrically in terms of an even point group related as in Table 5.1.

$$\langle A|B\rangle = \sum_{C} \langle A|C\rangle\langle C|B\rangle \quad ,$$

where $|A\rangle$, $|B\rangle$ are two eigenfunctions, $\langle A|B\rangle$ is their scalar product, and $\langle A|C\rangle$, $\langle B|C\rangle$ (= $\langle C^*|B^*\rangle$) are the expansion coefficients which give $|A\rangle$, $|B\rangle$ in terms of the complete set of eigenfunctions $|C\rangle$. The operations required in the present instance are somewhat more involved, however, and we therefore merely give the results here, referring reader to original papers by Griffith (1960), Judd (1962), and Kiel (1966) for further details.

Let us suppose that the potentials δV_{EEF}, V_{odd}, δV_{odd} are expressed as a series of spherical harmonics of the form $a_{k'}^{q'}(E)r^{k'}C_{k'}^{q'}(\theta,\phi)$, $A_K^Q r^k C_K^Q(\theta,\phi)$, $a_k^q r^k C_k^q(\theta,\phi)$. We then wish to know which harmonics $C_{k'}^{q'}$ appear in δV_{EEF} for given harmonics C_K^Q, C_k^q, in V_{odd}, δV_{odd} and how the amplitudes $a_{k'}^{q'}(E)$ depend on the amplitudes A_K^Q, a_k^q, on the indices of the spherical harmonics and on the quantum numbers of the wavefunctions in the two manifolds. This relationship is given by the equation[†]

$$a_{k'}^{q'}(E,s) = -\frac{2}{\overline{E}_{ug}}\sum_{K,Q} (-1)^{q'} A_K^Q(s)a_k^q(s)\eta_{EEF}(\ell,\ell',K,k,k') \times \times \begin{pmatrix} K & k & k' \\ Q & q & -q' \end{pmatrix} \quad , \tag{5.26}$$

[†] The factor of 2 in eqn (5.26) appears as a result of adding the two products under the summation sign in (5.25). See Judd (1962) (eqns (9), (14) and the equality above eqn (12)). This factor of 2 does not appear in the corresponding expression for V_{EEF}.

where the crystal field amplitudes A_K^Q, a_k^q have been converted into spectroscopic crystal field parameters as in eqn (4.3) and where

$$\eta_{EEF}(\ell,\ell',K,k,k') = (-1)^{\ell'}(2\ell'+1)(2k'+1)\begin{pmatrix}\ell & \ell' & K\\ 0 & 0 & 0\end{pmatrix}\times$$

$$\times\begin{pmatrix}\ell & \ell' & k\\ 0 & 0 & 0\end{pmatrix}\begin{Bmatrix}\ell & \ell' & k'\\ k & K & \ell\end{Bmatrix}\div\begin{pmatrix}\ell & \ell & k'\\ 0 & 0 & 0\end{pmatrix}, \quad (5.27)$$

The bracketed expressions are the Wigner 3j and 6j symbols. (For 3j symbols see §A.3.) The selection rule

$$q' = Q + q \quad (5.28)$$

and the vector relations (the 'triangular rules')

$$\underline{k}' + \underline{k} + \underline{K} = \underline{\ell} + \underline{\ell}' + \underline{k} = \underline{\ell} + \underline{\ell}' + \underline{k}' = 0 \quad (5.29)$$

are implicit in the 3j symbols and determine the range of values of K,Q (and hence also of k,q) which enter into the summation for any given equivalent even field harmonic. In the present instance K and k are, of course, odd and k' is even.

The quantum numbers ℓ, ℓ' are the angular momentum quantum numbers for the ground manifold and the opposite-parity manifold. It is assumed in deriving eqns (5.26)-(5.27) that the ground-state wavefunctions belong to a configuration $(n\ell)^N$ and the opposite-parity wavefunctions to a configuration $(n\ell)^{N-1}(n'\ell')$, i.e. only one of the electrons has been raised to an excited state to form the opposite-parity manifold. The quantum numbers n, n' determine the magnitude of the radial integrals

$$\langle r^K \rangle = \langle n\ell | r^K | n'\ell' \rangle = \int_0^\infty \mathcal{R}(n\ell)\mathcal{R}(n'\ell') r^{K+2} dr \,,$$
$$\langle r^k \rangle = \langle n\ell | r^k | n'\ell' \rangle = \int_0^\infty \mathcal{R}(n\ell)\mathcal{R}(n'\ell') r^{k+2} dr \,, \tag{5.30}$$

which are needed in order to calculate the spectroscopic crystal field parameters $A_K^Q(s)$, $a_k^q(s)$ for the odd fields (see eqn (4.3)). It should be noted that the spectroscopic crystal field parameter $a_{k'}^{q'}(E,s)$ does not depend on the even radial integral $\langle r^{k'} \rangle$ but on the product of two odd radial integrals. In this respect it differs from the parameters associated with δV_{ev}, all of which contain an even radial integral of the type

$$\langle r^k \rangle = \langle n\ell | r^k | n\ell \rangle = \int_0^\infty \mathcal{R}^2(n\ell) r^{k+2} dr \,. \tag{5.31}$$

Two different types of radial integral are therefore involved when we write

$$\bar{a}_k^q(s) = a_k^q(s) + a_k^q(E,s) \tag{5.32}$$

for the total spectroscopic crystal field parameters due to the induced even potentials and the EEF. Unfortunately there have been very few calculations of the odd radial integrals needed here. Freeman and Watson (1965) give comprehensive tables of even radial integrals (see Tables 5.2 and 5.3 for an excerpt), but an extrapolation of (or interpolation between) these values will not yield the required odd integrals, although such a procedure may be used as a makeshift. A comparison of odd and even radial integrals given by Judd (1962) for some rare-earth ions (see Table 5.4) will indicate the magnitude of the error which can arise from this approximation.

TABLE 5.2

Even radial integrals in Ångströms for some 3d ions, calculated by Freeman and Watson (1965).

Ion	Configuration	$\langle r^2 \rangle$ $(\mathring{A})^2$	$\langle r^4 \rangle$ $(\mathring{A})^4$
Cr^{3+}	$3d^3$	0·405	0·337
Cr^{2+}	$3d^4$	0·499	0·566
Mn^{2+}	$3d^5$	0·434	0·432
Fe^{3+}	$3d^5$	0·322	0·219
Fe^{2+}	$3d^6$	0·390	0·353
Co^{2+}	$3d^7$	0·350	0·287
Ni^{2+}	$3d^8$	0·317	0·236
Cu^{2+}	$3d^9$	0·288	0·196

The summation in eqn (5.26) should, in principle, be extended to cover all of the excited states belonging to opposite-parity manifolds, and should also take account of state mixing due to the excitation of electrons from filled inner shells, but this calculation would be lengthy and hard to make. For an approximate estimate of the EEF one may, therefore, restrict consideration to the nearest excited-state manifold of opposite parity only. Contributions from many of the remaining opposite-parity manifolds are in any case often associated with small radial integrals and large energy separations.† The mean energy separations $\overline{E}_{ug}$ of the ground and nearest opposite-parity excited manifold for some free ions are shown in Tables 5.5, 5.6 and 5.7 together with the

TABLE 5.3

Even radial integrals in Ångströms for some 4f ions, calculated by Freeman and Watson (1965).

Ion	Configuration	$\langle r^2 \rangle$ $(\text{Å})^2$	$\langle r^4 \rangle$ $(\text{Å})^4$	$\langle r^6 \rangle$ $(\text{Å})^6$
Ce^{3+}	$4f^1$	0·336	0·271	0·466
Pr^{3+}	$4f^2$	0·304	0·221	0·345
Nd^{3+}	$4f^3$	0·280	0·188	0·272
Sm^{3+}	$4f^5$	0·247	0·149	0·193
Eu^{3+}	$4f^6$	0·233	0·133	0·163
Gd^{3+}	$4f^7$	0·220	0·119	0·138
Tb^{3+}	$4f^8$	0·211	0·111	0·125
Dy^{3+}	$4f^9$	0·203	0·104	0·112
Ho^{3+}	$4f^{10}$	0·195	0·096	0·099
Er^{3+}	$4f^{11}$	0·187	0·088	0·087
Tm^{3+}	$4f^{12}$	0·181	0·084	0·080
Tm^{2+}	$4f^{13}$	0·204	0·122	0·165
Yb^{3+}	$4f^{13}$	0·172	0·075	0·068

† In the case of some odd point groups mixing with the nearest opposite-parity manifold may not occur, making it necessary to consider more remote manifolds. Thus, for example, 3d ($\ell = 2$) to 4p ($\ell' = 1$) mixing will not occur in D_4 point symmetry since the lowest crystal field harmonic is $C_5^{\pm 4}$ (K = 5) (Table 4.1, p. 109) and the 3j symbol in the numerator of eqn (5.27) vanishes.

TABLE 5.4

Radial integrals in Ångströms $(\text{Å})^k$ given by Judd (1962). The odd integrals connecting 4f and 5d states are the only ones needed in the EEF calculation. The even integrals within the 4f manifold are shown for comparison.

Integral	Pr^{3+}	Nd^{3+}	Er^{3+}	Tm^{3+}
$\langle 4f \mid r \mid 5d \rangle$	0·476	0·460	0·325	0·309
$\langle 4f \mid r^2 \mid 4f \rangle$	0·410	0·390	0·233	0·213
$\langle 4f \mid r^3 \mid 5d \rangle$	0·811	0·766	0·408	0·363
$\langle 4f \mid r^4 \mid 4f \rangle$	0·419	0·389	0·153	0·123
$\langle 4f \mid r^5 \mid 5d \rangle$	2·096	1·955	0·826	0·684
$\langle 4f \mid r^6 \mid 4f \rangle$	0·870	0·799	0·230	0·161

interval $(E_{ug})_{min}$ for the nearest opposite-parity state. The two values $\overline{E}_{ug}$, $(E_{ug})_{min}$ give a rough indication of the energy spread of the manifold. The values for the 3d group were obtained from the tables by Moore (1949, 1952) by averaging over the list of free ion states in these tables (without weighting according to degeneracy). The rare-earth values have been derived from two figures given by Dieke (1968). These values should all perhaps be revised downwards to allow for the fact that the ions are imbedded in a crystal lattice. Little would be gained, however, by expending a great deal of effort on corrections of

TABLE 5.5

Approximate energy separations E_{ug} between the ground state $3d^N$ and the nearest opposite-parity manifold of excited states $3d^{N-1}4p$ for free ions in the iron group (derived from tables by Moore, 1949, 1952). The mean separation for Fe^{3+} is shown in parenthesis since very little data appears for this ion.

Ion	Ground configuration	Opposite-parity configuration	Smallest separation $(E_{ug})_{min}$ ($10^3 cm^{-1}$)	Mean separation $\bar{E}_{ug}$ ($10^3 cm^{-1}$)
Ti^{3+}	$3d$	$4p$	127•9	128•3
Cr^{3+}	$3d^3$	$3d^2 4p$	157•3	167•9
Cr^{2+}	$3d^4$	$3d^3 4p$	93•8	111•1
Mn^{2+}	$3d^5$	$3d^4 4p$	110•0	114•5
Fe^{3+}	$3d^5$	$3d^4 4p$	-	(190•0)
Fe^{2+}	$3d^6$	$3d^5 4p$	89•1	134•6
Co^{2+}	$3d^7$	$3d^6 4p$	103•2	126•3
Ni^{2+}	$3d^8$	$3d^7 4p$	111•9	124•9
Cu^{2+}	$3d^9$	$3d^8 4p$	118•9	135•4

TABLE 5.6

Approximate energy separations E_{ug} between the ground state $4f^N$ and the nearest opposite-parity manifold of excited states $4f^{N-1}5d$ for trivalent rare-earth ions. (Derived from Fig. 17 of Dieke (1968.)

Ion	Ground configuration	Opposite-parity configuration	Smallest separation $(E_{ug})_{min}$ $(10^3 cm^{-1})$	Mean separation $\bar{E}_{ug}$ $(10^3\ cm^{-1})$
Ce^{3+}	$4f$	$5d$	52	53
Pr^{3+}	$4f^2$	$4f5d$	54	62
Nd^{3+}	$4f^3$	$4f^25d$	61	80
Pm^{3+}	$4f^4$	$4f^35d$	60	95
Sm^{3+}	$4f^5$	$4f^45d$	65	111
Eu^{3+}	$4f^6$	$4f^55d$	69	127
Gd^{3+}	$4f^7$	$4f^65d$	92	162
Tb^{3+}	$4f^8$	$4f^75d$	35	137
Dy^{3+}	$4f^9$	$4f^85d$	56	130
Ho^{3+}	$4f^{10}$	$4f^95d$	60	124
Er^{3+}	$4f^{11}$	$4f^{10}5d$	62	117
Tm^{3+}	$4f^{12}$	$4f^{11}5d$	60	104
Yb^{3+}	$4f^{13}$	$4f^{12}5d$	67	95

TABLE 5.7

Approximate energy separations E_{ug} between the ground state and the nearest opposite-parity manifold of excited states for divalent rare-earth ions. (Derived from Fig. 18 of Dieke (1968).

Ion	Ground configuration	Opposite-parity configuration	Smallest separation $(E_{ug})_{min}$ ($10^3 cm^{-1}$)	Mean separation $\bar{E}_{ug}$ ($10^3 cm^{-1}$)
La^{2+}	4f	5d	8	8
Ce^{2+}	$4f^2$	4f5d	7	13
Pr^{2+}	$4f^3$	$4f^2 5d$	11	27
Nd^{2+}	$4f^4$	$4f^3 5d$	13	41
Pm^{2+}	$4f^5$	$4f^4 5d$	17	54
Sm^{2+}	$4f^6$	$4f^5 5d$	21	68
Eu^{2+}	$4f^7$	$4f^6 5d$	42	97
Gd^{2+}	$4f^7 5d$	$4f^8$	5	57
Tb^{2+}	$4f^9$	$4f^8 5d$	3	73
Dy^{2+}	$4f^{10}$	$4f^9 5d$	16	68
Ho^{2+}	$4f^{11}$	$4f^{10} 5d$	18	62
Er^{2+}	$4f^{12}$	$4f^{11} 5d$	18	53
Tm^{2+}	$4f^{13}$	$4f^{12} 5d$	23	46

this kind in view of the approximate nature of the overall calculation and the uncertainties in the values assumed for V_{odd} and δV_{odd}. It should be remembered that crystal field calculations are rarely exact and tend to be more useful for exploring functional relationships between experimental data and various bond and ligand parameters than for providing actual numbers.

The angular-dependent portion of (5.26) consisting of the 3j symbol with arguments Q,q,-q', and the angular-independent portion consisting of the 'reduced matrix element' η_{EEF} are given in Tables 5.8-5.10 for some commonly occurring values of the arguments.[†] Only those combinations which involve the first-degree harmonics in δV_{odd} (k=1) have been taken into consideration, although some additional combinations can be found by interchanging K and k. (This leaves η_{EEF} unaltered; Q and q must of course be interchanged together with K and k.) Table 5.8 gives η_{EEF} for cases in which d-manifolds are mixed with p- or f-manifolds and includes combinations of harmonics C_K^Q, C_k^q which lead to EEFs of the second and fourth degree. Table 5.9 gives η_{EEF} for cases in which f-manifolds are mixed with d- or g-manifolds and includes EEFs of the second, fourth, and sixth degrees. (Sixth-degree harmonics are likely to be quite small but are given here since these harmonics have sometimes been found useful for interpreting the EPR spectra of f-state ions in trigonal crystals.) Table 5.10 gives expressions for the 3j symbols which are required in conjunction with the factors η_{EEF} appearing in Tables 5.8 and 5.9, i.e. those 3j symbols for which $k = 1$, $q = 0,\pm 1$. Combinations involving the third-degree harmonics in δV_{odd} (k=3) have been omitted, mainly to preserve simplicity in the table but can be found in various textbooks (see Appendix A). Such higher order contributions to the equivalent even field are usually small in

---

† These tables were provided by Dr. A. Kiel.

TABLE 5.8

The factor $\eta_{EEF}(\ell,\ell',K,k,k')$ in eqn (5.27) for cases in which d-manifolds (ℓ=2) are mixed with p- (ℓ'=1) or f- (ℓ'=3) manifolds and in which the harmonics in V_{odd} and δV_{odd} give EEFs of the second and fourth degree (k'=2,4). EEFs derived from first-degree harmonics in δV_{odd} (k=1) are the only ones considered in this table. Certain other combinations can be obtained by interchanging K and k, since this leaves η_{EEF} unaltered.

ℓ	ℓ'	K	k	k'	η_{EEF}
2	1	1	1	2	1·28
2	3	1	1	2	0·54
2	1	3	1	2	0·29
2	3	3	1	2	1·17
2	1	3	1	4	-2·04
2	3	3	1	4	-0·23
2	3	5	1	4	2·03

relation to those contributions which arise from the first-degree harmonics in δV_{odd}. This is partly because of the appearance of additional factors $\simeq(r/R_j)^2$ in the third-degree harmonics and partly because the first-degree harmonics contain the long-range Lorentz field E_R (eqns (4.5)-(4.6)) in addition to fields due

TABLE 5.9

The factor $\eta_{EEF}(\ell,\ell',K,k,k')$ in eqn (5.27) for cases in which f-manifolds ($\ell=3$) are mixed with d-($\ell'=2$) or g-($\ell'=4$) manifolds and in which the harmonics in V_{odd} and δV_{odd} give EEFs of the second, fourth, and sixth degree ($k'=2,4,6$). EEFs derived from first-degree harmonics in δV_{odd} ($k=1$) are the only ones considered in this table. Certain other combinations can be obtained by interchanging K and k since this leaves η_{EEF} unaltered.

ℓ	ℓ'	K	k	k'	η_{EEF}
3	2	1	1	2	1·17
3	4	1	1	2	0·65
3	2	3	1	2	-0·42
3	4	3	1	2	-1·05
3	2	3	1	4	1·78
3	4	3	1	4	0·49
3	2	5	1	4	-0·29
3	4	5	1	4	-1·74
3	4	5	1	6	0·19
3	4	7	1	6	-2·47

TABLE 5.10

3j symbols required for use in conjunction with the factors η_{EEF} in Tables 5.8 and 5.9. These tables cover cases for which $k = 1$, $q = 0,\pm 1$ (EEFs derived from first-degree harmonics in δV_{odd}). The necessary 3j symbols therefore have the arguments $k = 1$, $q = 0,\pm 1$; also $k' = K\pm 1$, $q' = Q$ or $q' = Q\pm 1$ as indicated by eqns (5.28) and (5.29). The 3j symbols given here can be derived from the general formula (A.18).

Case $k' = K - 1,\ q' = Q$

$$\begin{pmatrix} K & 1 & K-1 \\ Q & 0 & -Q \end{pmatrix} = (-1)^{K-Q}\left\{\frac{(K+Q)(K-Q)}{(2K+1)K(2K-1)}\right\}^{\frac{1}{2}}$$

Case $k' = K - 1,\ q' = Q \pm 1$

$$\begin{pmatrix} K & 1 & K-1 \\ Q & \pm 1 & -Q\mp 1 \end{pmatrix} = \frac{1}{\sqrt{2}}\,(-1)^{K-Q+1}\left\{\frac{(K\mp Q)(K\mp Q+1)}{(2K+1)K(2K-1)}\right\}^{\frac{1}{2}}$$

Case $k' = K + 1,\ q' = Q$

$$\begin{pmatrix} K & 1 & K+1 \\ Q & 0 & -Q \end{pmatrix} = (-1)^{K-Q+1}\left\{\frac{(K+1+Q)(K+1-Q)}{(2K+3)(K+1)(2K+1)}\right\}^{\frac{1}{2}}$$

Case $k' = K + 1,\ q' = Q \pm 1$

$$\begin{pmatrix} K & 1 & K+1 \\ Q & \pm 1 & -Q\mp 1 \end{pmatrix} = \frac{1}{\sqrt{2}}\,(-1)^{K-Q}\left\{\frac{(K+1\pm Q)(K+2\pm Q)}{(2K+3)(K+1)(2K+1)}\right\}^{\frac{1}{2}}$$

to the neighbouring ions.

In concluding this section it must be stressed once more that the equivalent even field approach to the treatment of odd crystal field potentials is based on the assumption that there is a relatively wide separation between the opposite-parity manifold and any of the other states represented in the perturbation calculation. If this is not so, then we cannot neglect the terms involving E_{ug}^2 in deriving (5.11) from (5.10) and (5.16) from (5.15). In some cases, for instance when calculating the linear electric field effect for divalent rare-earth ions (Table 5.2) or for some valence states of the 3d ions, it may not even be reasonable to begin the calculation with zero-order states of a definite parity. In the La^{2+} free ion, for example, the 4f-5d separation is only ± 8000 cm^{-1}, and the Gd^{2+} ion the lowest $4f^7 5d$ states lie below the 4f state. In cases like this relatively small odd fields will cause extensive state mixing. The linear electric effects have not yet been investigated for these ions but would, presumably, be large. (The optical transitions are strongly enhanced and result in a deep coloration of samples containing divalent rare-earth ions.) In the 3d group the Fe^0 ion, which is characterized by a small even-odd separation has been shown to give large shifts (Ludwig and Woodbury 1961). This case is discussed theoretically by Ham (1961).

The EEF approximation will also fail in many cases where there is strong covalent bonding to the paramagnetic ion. This situation is discussed briefly in the next section.

5.3. ODD FIELDS AND COVALENTLY BONDED SYSTEMS

Covalent bonding and overlap of wavefunctions between the paramagnetic ion and its ligands often plays an important part in determining the values of parameters appearing in the spin Hamiltonian. Covalency effects are relatively small in the rare-earth series where the 4f electrons are partially screened from their surroundings, but they are larger in the 5f series whilst in the 3d and 4d series they may be the dominant factor determining resonance behaviour. There are a number of useful discussions of covalent bonding effects in EPR. See, for example, Owen and Thornley (1967), Abragam and Bleaney (1972), Chapter 20, Simanek and Sroubek (1972).

Although it was realized early that covalent bonding effects were likely to play a major role in determining the magnitude of the linear electric field shifts (see e.g. Royce and Bloembergen 1963) there have been very few detailed theoretical studies based on a covalent model (see however Bates 1968; Buch and Gelineau 1971). Most calculations have followed the established EPR tradition of analysing the problem in terms of the point charge model. It would in any event be difficult to prescribe a general form for a covalent bonding calculation since each case presents special features of its own according to the quantum-mechanical description of the ligands and of the paramagnetic ion concerned, the more so in the case of linear electric field effect calculations since there is the additional problem of allowing for covalency in estimating the electrical polarizability of the ligands. We shall therefore confine ourselves to describing some general features of a covalent calculation and showing how the basic assumptions here are related to the basic assumptions of the point charge/point dipole model described earlier.

The problem of choosing the correct value for the internal field has already been mentioned in §4.4, where it was pointed out that most authors have adopted the Lorentz field approximation (eqn (4.7)) uncorrected for effects due to nearby ions, although some have suggested using a smaller value of the internal field to compensate for the extended nature of the electronic charge distribution. Assuming that some suitable value (or values) can be found for the internal field the linear electric field effect can then be broken down conceptually into two parts, an 'ionic effect' and an 'electronic effect'. The ionic effect is found by calculating the changes in the EPR parameters which results from a relative movement of the paramagnetic ion and its ligands, but without allowing for the polarization of the electronic wavefunction by the internal electric field. The electronic effect is found by calculating the perturbation matrix element $\langle\psi_1|\delta V|\psi_2\rangle$, etc. for the 'covalent' wavefunctions ψ_1,ψ_2 (which belong partly to the paramagnetic ion and partly to its ligands) on the assumption that the centres of the ions remain fixed.

The ionic effect requires an estimate for the displacement of the ligand atoms or molecules in the internal field and also an estimate for the dependence of the EPR parameters concerned on the distances and on the orientations of the ligands. The first can be made by the methods suggested in §4.3. A covalent-type calculation of the normal EPR parameters will yield the second. In the limiting case where covalent bonding tends to zero the ionic effect becomes equivalent to those contributions to δV_{odd} and δV_{even} which, in the point charge/point dipole model, are associated with ionic motion of the nearest neighbours.

In order to calculate the electronic effect it is necessary to set up molecular orbitals or some equivalent approximate wavefunctions for the paramagnetic ion and its ligands. Ground-state wavefunctions, and wavefunctions for the nearer excited states, of the complex will be needed in order to calculate the effects of the electric field. Perturbation theory as in §5.1 can be used to find the energy shifts, etc., since the laboratory field will almost certainly be small compared with the other terms which enter into the covalent calculation. But it may not be a good approximation to begin with zero order states of definite parity and in many cases mixed parity states will have to be constructed at the start of the calculation. (In the limiting case where covalent bonding tends to zero these mixed-parity states are equivalent to the state mixture produced by the point charge potential

V_{odd}, where V'_{odd} is calculated by considering the immediate neighbours only.) The mixed-parity wavefunctions will be coupled by δV_{odd} (e.g. by the Lorentz field) and by δV_{even} thus yielding a shift which is linear in the applied field. The electronic effect in such a covalent treatment is equivalent to the contributions in the point charge/point dipole calculation which arise from the Lorentz field and those portions of δV_{odd}, δV_{even} associated with electronic polarization of the neighbouring ions.

The above discussion shows how, for the purpose of analysing a complex with partial covalent bonding, the physical problem may be resolved into elements in a new way. In the point charge/point dipole case the paramagnetic ion is treated as an isolated quantum-mechanical system interacting with its crystal environment via a configuration of electrostatic fields. The details of the crystal environment are reproduced in the harmonic structure of the electrostatic fields. Here, on the other hand, the paramagnetic ion and its immediate neighbours are treated as the basic entity. Consideration of the internal electrostatic fields is still important, but much of the fine detail can be dispensed with. This new description is perhaps conceptually a simpler one and avoids the seeming paradox of odd applied fields inducing even state mixing (via δV_{even}) in the paramagnetic ion. In practice, however, the calculations tend to be harder to make and, in cases where covalent bonding is fairly weak, it may save trouble to proceed as if the point charge model were correct and then adjust the spectroscopic crystal field parameters semi-empirically to fit the results. A useful rationalisation for this approach is provided by the angular overlap model (Schäffer, 1974).

A glance through the review articles cited at the beginning of this section will show that much useful information regarding covalent bonding has been derived from experimental studies of ligand superhyperfine structure. Studies of electric field induced shifts in the superhyperfine structure might likewise be expected to yield some insight into the role of covalency in linear electric field effects and might possibly provide valuable information regarding the polarizability of different types of bonds. Experiments of this kind have been successfully performed on F-centres in alkali halides, but the technical difficulties are considerable. These experiments are discussed in Chapter 8.

6. g-shifts for Kramers ions: an illustrative calculation

The g- and D-parameters in the spin Hamiltonian are usually calculated by considering the effect of a crystal field consisting of even harmonics only on the ground manifold of free ion states. One mechanism for the electric field induced shift can be understood directly in terms of this picture since, as is shown in Chapter 4, the polarization of a non-centrosymmetric environment by an applied electric field produces new contributions to the even crystal field. But a second mechanism involving the effect of the applied field and the odd crystal fields on the paramagnetic ion itself is often of equal importance. Fortunately this second mechanism can also be represented by increments in the even-field parameters (Chapter 5) and we can simply add the two contributions and continue the analysis by traditional methods, i.e. by evaluating the matrix elements of the perturbing potential within the ground manifold of states.

The exact form taken by this calculation will depend a great deal on the nature of the paramagnetic ion which is being studied, and it is not possible in a short text to review all possible cases. It may prove helpful, however, if we take one particular case and follow the calculation through from beginning to end in order to illustrate how the material given in Chapters 4 and 5 can be used in conjunction with standard crystal field theory. We therefore address ourselves here to the task of calculating the g-shift parameters T_{ijk} for tetragonal Ce^{3+} centres in CaF_2.

As a preliminary we shall derive general formulae for the g-shifts of a rare-earth Kramers doublet ion in terms of an even-field perturbation $\delta\overline{V}_{ev}$. This even perturbation is then estimated for the centre in question and used to find the four T_{ijk} parameters concerned. As will be apparent the CaF_2: Ce^{3+} calculation scarcely requires the elaborate analytical apparatus developed in Chapters 4 and 5. The induced potentials might be obtained more quickly from first principles than from general formulae, and the mixing between the 4f- and 5d-manifold (which contains only an e_g orbital doublet and a t_{2g} orbital triplet) could be treated without introducing the EEF formalism. The treatment from a general standpoint is useful, however, as a means of exemplifying some of the procedures and approximations which can be used in less simple cases.

6.1. THE g-SHIFT PARAMETERS FOR RARE-EARTH KRAMERS DOUBLETS

According to Kramers theorem a system containing an odd number of electrons has at least twofold degeneracy, in the absence of magnetic fields. The pairs of states (the 'Kramers doublets') are time conjugate, one being obtained from the other by means of the time-reversal operator. In the $|J,M\rangle$ representation they can be expanded in the form

$$|\xi\rangle = \sum_{J,M} C_{J,M}|J,M\rangle$$

$$|\overline{\xi}\rangle = \sum_{J,M} C^{*}_{J,M}(-1)^{J-M}|J,-M\rangle\ , \qquad (6.1)$$

where the coefficient $C^{*}_{J,M}$ is the complex conjugate of $C_{J,M}$.

The expansion is not unique, since the linear combination giving two orthogonal time-reversed states can be made in an infinity of ways, but in practice there is usually one combination which recommends itself on the grounds of simplicity and convenience. (For a fuller discussion see e.g. Abragam and Bleaney (1970), pp. 647-53.) For axial and lower point symmetries the pairs of doublets are generally separated by energies which are large compared with the splittings caused by available laboratory magnetic fields, and the composition of the doublet states can be regarded as determined by the crystal field only.

The first-order electric field induced shifts as in eqn (5.19) (p.138) are of no direct concern here. These shifts have the same value for both time-reversed states $\psi^{\pm}_{gj}$ and cannot therefore be observed in a microwave resonance experiment involving transitions between two members of the doublet. The shifts which are observed in such an experiment correspond instead to the second-order perturbation (5.20). Rewriting (5.20) with superscripts ± to denote the two members of the doublet, and generalizing to the crystal field perturbation $\delta\overline{V}_{ev}$ defined in (5.22) we obtain the expression

$$\delta E^{\pm}_{gj,H} =$$

$$-\sum_{i}^{i\neq j}\sum_{+,-}\frac{1}{E_{ij}}\{\langle\psi^{\pm}_{gj}\mid V_H\mid\psi^{+,-}_{gi}\rangle\langle\psi^{+,-}_{gi}\mid\delta\overline{V}_{ev}\mid\psi^{\pm}_{gj}\rangle + \text{h.c.}\}\,, \qquad (6.2)$$

where a common energy separation is assumed for the doublet states $\psi^{\pm}_{gj}$, $\psi^{\pm}_{i}$, and the summation is taken over <u>both</u> states in each of the excited doublets $\psi^{\pm}_{i}$ when calculating shifts for <u>either</u> member of the ground doublet. (The notation $\sum_{+,-}\psi^{+,-}_{gi}$ symbolizes this feature of the summation.) The perturbation pathways implicit in the equivalent even-field portion of $\delta\overline{V}_{ev}$ are illustrated in Fig. 6.1.

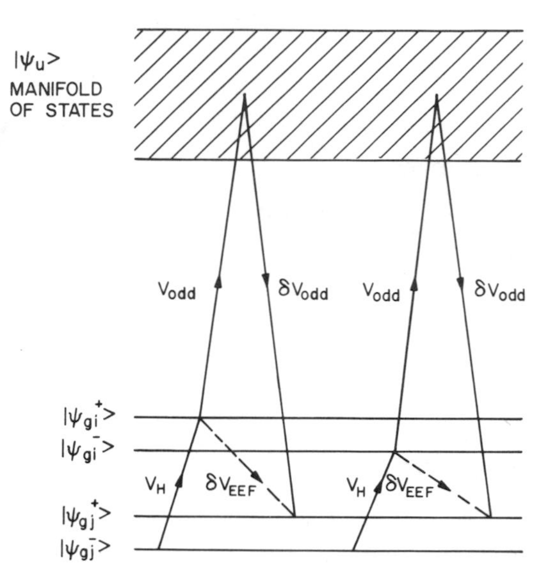

FIG. 6.1. Perturbation pathway involved in the calculation of crystal field matrix elements between Kramers-doublet states $\psi^{\pm}_{gj}$. The third-order perturbation indicated here is reduced to second order when V_{odd} and δV_{odd} are replaced by an equivalent even field, δV_{EEF}, as in eqn (5.18). Even crystal field perturbations δV_{ev} connect the same levels as δV_{EEF}.

As pointed out in Chaper 5 it is more convenient to find the electric field induced shifts in the Zeeman field matrix elements rather than the energy shifts themselves when deriving the g-shift parameters T_{ijk}. The shifts $\delta \langle \psi^{\pm}_{gj} \mid V_H \mid \psi^{\pm}_{gj} \rangle$ in the diagonal elements are already given in eqn (6.2). The shifts in the off diagonal elements are, by eqn (5.21) (p.138),

$$\delta \langle \psi_{gj} \mid V_H \mid \psi^{\mp}_{gj} \rangle =$$

$$- \sum_{i}^{i \neq j} \sum_{+,-} \frac{1}{E_{ij}} \{ \langle \psi^{\pm}_{gj} \mid V_H \mid \psi^{+,-}_{gi} \rangle \langle \psi^{+,-}_{gi} \mid \delta \overline{V}_{ev} \mid \psi^{\mp}_{gj} \rangle +$$

$$+ \langle \psi^{\pm}_{gj} \mid \delta \overline{V}_{ev} \mid \psi^{+,-}_{gi} \rangle \langle \psi^{+,-}_{gi} \mid V_H \mid \psi^{\mp}_{gj} \rangle \} . \qquad (6.3)$$

We can simplify (6.3) further by taking into account the time-reversed nature of the states $\psi^{\pm}_{gj}$, $\psi^{\pm}_{gi}$ and the properties of the two operators $\delta\overline{V}_{ev}$ and V_H under time reversal. Since $\delta\overline{V}_{ev}$ is time even and V_H is time odd, the two terms in (6.3) are equal† and we can write

$$\delta \langle \psi^{\pm}_{gj} \mid V_H \mid \psi^{\mp}_{gj} \rangle$$

$$= -2 \sum_{i}^{i\neq j} \sum_{+,-} \frac{1}{E_{ij}} \langle \psi^{\pm}_{gj} \mid V_H \mid \psi^{+,-}_{gi} \rangle \langle \psi^{+,-}_{gi} \mid \delta\overline{V}_{ev} \mid \psi^{\mp}_{gj} \rangle . \qquad (6.4)$$

Eqn (6.4) will also hold good for time-reversal doublets which do not arise as a result of Kramers degeneracy.

The Zeeman field operator on the right-hand side of eqns (6.1) and (6.3) is given by

$$V_H = \beta g_e \underline{H}_0 \cdot (\underline{L} + 2\underline{S}) \qquad (6.5)$$

where g_e is the free-electron g-value. For simplicity we can also restrict the states ψ_{gi}, ψ_{gj} to a single J-manifold (although the argument can readily be extended to cover the more general case of J-state mixing) thus reducing (6.5) to the form

---

† The proof is the same as that which is used to demonstrate the well known 'Van Vleck cancellation' in the theory of Raman process spin-lattice relaxation. See Abragam and Bleaney (1970), p.649. In that case, however, both operators are crystal field operators, both are time-even, and the second term is opposite in sign to the first.

$$V_H = \beta g_J \underline{H}_0 \cdot \underline{J} \quad , \tag{6.6}$$

where $g_J = \langle J \| \Lambda \| J \rangle$ is the Lande g-value (see Abragam and Bleaney (1970), p. 290, p. 587, also Table 20, p. 874). Eqns (6.2) and (6.4) therefore assume the forms

$$\delta_\eta \langle \psi_{gj}^{\pm} \mid V_H \mid \psi_{gj}^{\pm} \rangle$$

$$= -\beta g_J \sum_\lambda H_\lambda \sum_{i}^{i \neq j} \sum_{+,-} \frac{1}{E_{ij}} \{ \langle \psi_{gj}^{\pm} | J_\lambda | \psi_{gi}^{+,-} \rangle \langle \psi_{gi}^{+,-} | \delta_\eta (\overline{V}_{ev}) | \psi_{gj}^{\pm} \rangle + \text{h.c.} \}, \tag{6.7}$$

$$\delta_\eta \langle \psi_{gj}^{\pm} \mid V_H \mid \psi_{gj}^{\mp} \rangle$$

$$= -2\beta g_J \sum_\lambda H_\lambda \sum_{i}^{i \neq j} \sum_{+,-} \frac{1}{E_{ij}} \langle \psi_{gj}^{\pm} | J_\lambda | \psi_{gi}^{+,-} \rangle \langle \psi_{gi}^{+,-} | \delta_\eta (\overline{V}_{ev}) | \psi_{gj}^{\mp} \rangle \quad . \tag{6.8}$$

In eqns (6.7)-(6.8) H_λ, J_λ (λ = x,y,z) are the Cartesian components of $\underline{H}_0, \underline{J}$. $\delta_\eta(\overline{V}_{ev})$ (η = x,y,z) is the total even crystal field potential (5.22)(p.138) induced by an applied electric field component E_η, and $\delta_\eta \langle \psi_{gj}^{\pm} \mid V_H \mid \psi_{gj}^{\pm} \rangle$, $\delta_\eta \langle \psi_{gj}^{\pm} \mid V_H \mid \psi_{gj}^{\mp} \rangle$ are the corresponding shifts in the Zeeman field matrix elements.† J operates on the wavefunctions on the right-hand side of eqns (6.7) and (6.8) as in

† The subscripts η,λ,ρ are used in place of i,j,k in the subsequent analysis to avoid confusion with the subscripts in ψ_{gi}, ψ_{gj}.

$$J_+ \mid J,M\rangle = \hbar\{(J-M)(J+M+1)\}^{\frac{1}{2}}\{\mid J,M+1\rangle\} ,$$

$$J_- \mid J,M\rangle = \hbar\{(J+M)(J-M+1)\}^{\frac{1}{2}}\{\mid J,M-1\rangle\} ,$$

$$J_z \mid J,M\rangle = \hbar M\{\mid J,M\rangle\} , \tag{6.9}$$

$$J_\pm = J_x \pm iJ_y ,$$

The matrix elements on the left-hand side of eqns (6.7)-(6.8) can be defined in terms of a two-state manifold with effective spin $S' = \frac{1}{2}$ since they involve only the ground doublet states $\psi^\pm_{gj}$. V_H is in this case replaced by the effective Hamiltonian operator

$$V_H = \beta \underline{H}_0 \cdot \underline{g} \cdot \underline{S}$$

in which the components of $\underline{S}$ can be represented by the Pauli spin matrices (3.14), and g is the 'g-tensor' (§3.4). The shifts $\delta_\eta\langle\psi^\pm_{gj} \mid V_H \mid \psi^\pm_{gj}\rangle$, $\delta_\eta\langle\psi^\pm_{gj} \mid V_H \mid \psi^\mp_{gj}\rangle$ are then given by the first-order matrix elements $\langle\psi^\pm_{gj} \mid \delta_\eta(V_H) \mid \psi^\pm_{gj}\rangle$, $\langle\psi^\pm_{gj} \mid \delta_\eta(V_H) \mid \psi^\mp_{gj}\rangle$, where the operators $\delta_\eta(V_H)$ stand for the g-shift operators in the electric field effect spin Hamiltonian (3.2). Thus

$$\delta_\eta(V_H) = \beta\sum_{\lambda\rho} T_{\eta\lambda\rho}E_\eta H_\lambda S_\rho , \tag{6.11}$$

whence we obtain

$$\delta_\eta\langle\psi^\pm \mid V_H \mid \psi^\pm\rangle = \pm(E_\eta\beta/2)(H_x T_{xz} + H_y T_{\eta yz} + H_z T_{\eta zz}) \tag{6.12}$$

and

$$\delta_\eta\langle\psi^{\pm}|V_H|\psi^{\mp}\rangle$$

$$=\frac{E_\eta\beta}{2}\{(H_xT_{\eta xx}+H_yT_{\eta yx}+H_zT_{\eta zx})\mp i(H_xT_{\eta xy}+H_yT_{\eta yy}+H_zT_{\eta zy})\}. \qquad (6.13)$$

The coefficients $T_{\eta\lambda\rho}$ can be obtained in terms of $\delta_\eta(\overline{V}_{ev})$ etc., by comparing the right-hand sides of (6.12) and (6.13) with the right-hand sides of (6.7) and (6.8) and by equating the coefficients of H_x, H_y, H_z. This yields nine relations of the form

$$T_{\eta\lambda\rho} =$$

$$4g_J\sum_i\sum_{+,-}\{\text{Re or Im}\ \langle\psi|J\ |\psi_{gi}^{+,-}\rangle\langle\psi_{gi}^{+,-}\ |(\delta_\eta(\overline{V}_{ev})/E_\eta)|\psi'\rangle\}, \qquad (6.14)$$

where ψ, ψ' are states belonging to the doublet ψ_{gj}. The results are given in full in Table 6.1. The components $g_{\lambda\rho}$ of the g-tensor can be obtained by a similar procedure, i.e. by comparing the matrix elements of the operator (6.6) between states $\psi_{gj}^{\pm}$ expressed as in (6.1) with matrix elements of the operator (6.10) in the effective spin $S'=\frac{1}{2}$ manifold. They are given in Table 6.2.

Slightly different, though equivalent forms in the right-hand columns of Tables 6.1 and 6.2 can be obtained by equating different elements (6.12), (6.7), and (6.13), (6.8). For instance, we can obtain the result

$$T_{\eta xy} = +4g_J\sum_i\frac{1}{E_{ij}}\text{Im}\{\langle\psi^-|J_x|\psi_i\rangle\langle\psi_i|\delta V_\eta|\psi^+\rangle\}$$

in place of that appearing in Table 6.1. In the general case we shall however find that $T_{\eta\lambda\rho}\neq T_{\eta\rho\lambda}$ and that $g_{\lambda\rho}\neq g_{\rho\lambda}$. The form of $T_{\eta\lambda\rho}$ or of $g_{\lambda\rho}$ depends on the way in which the Kramers doublet

TABLE 6.1

The coefficients of the g-shift tensor $T_{\eta\lambda\rho}$ (η = x,y,z; likewise λ,ρ) in terms of matrix elements of the angular-momentum operator J_μ within a single J-manifold of a Kramers doublet ion. $\psi^\pm$ are the states of the ground doublet $\psi^\pm_{gj}$, ψ_i the states of excited doublets $\psi^\pm_{gi}$, $E_{ij} = E(\psi_i) - E(\psi_j)$ is the energy separation between ground and excited doublets. The sum $\sum_i$ must be taken over both members of each excited doublet. δV_η is the total value $(\delta\overline{V}_{ev})_\eta$ of the even crystal field perturbation due to the electric field component E_η divided by E_η. For values of the constant g_J, see Abragam and Bleaney (1970), Table 20, p. 874.

g-shift coefficient	Perturbation formula
$T_{\eta xx}$	$4g_J \sum_i (1/E_{ij})\mathrm{Re}\{\langle\psi^+\lvert J_x\rvert\psi_i\rangle\langle\psi_i\lvert\delta V_\eta\rvert\psi^-\rangle\}$
$T_{\eta yy}$	$-4g_J \sum_i (1/E_{ij})\mathrm{Im}\{\langle\psi^+\lvert J_y\rvert\psi_i\rangle\langle\psi_i\lvert\delta V_\eta\rvert\psi^-\rangle\}$
$T_{\eta zz}$	$4g_J \sum_i (1/E_{ij})\mathrm{Re}\{\langle\psi^+\lvert J_z\rvert\psi_i\rangle\langle\psi_i\lvert\delta V_\eta\rvert\psi^+\rangle\}$
$T_{\eta yz}$	$4g_J \sum_i (1/E_{ij})\mathrm{Re}\{\langle\psi^+\lvert J_y\rvert\psi_i\rangle\langle\psi_i\lvert\delta V_\eta\rvert\psi^+\rangle\}$
$T_{\eta zy}$	$-4g_J \sum_i (1/E_{ij})\mathrm{Im}\{\langle\psi^+\lvert J_z\rvert\psi_i\rangle\langle\psi_i\lvert\delta V_\eta\rvert\psi^-\rangle\}$
$T_{\eta zx}$	$4g_J \sum_i (1/E_{ij})\mathrm{Re}\{\langle\psi^+\lvert J_z\rvert\psi_i\rangle\langle\psi_i\lvert\delta V_\eta\rvert\psi^-\rangle\}$
$T_{\eta xz}$	$4g_J \sum_i (1/E_{ij})\mathrm{Re}\{\langle\psi^+\lvert J_x\rvert\psi_i\rangle\langle\psi_i\lvert\delta V_\eta\rvert\psi^+\rangle\}$
$T_{\eta xy}$	$-4g_J \sum_i (1/E_{ij})\mathrm{Im}\{\langle\psi^+\lvert J_x\rvert\psi_i\rangle\langle\psi_i\lvert\delta V_\eta\rvert\psi^-\rangle\}$
$T_{\eta yx}$	$4g_J \sum_i (1/E_{ij})\mathrm{Re}\{\langle\psi^+\lvert J_y\rvert\psi_i\rangle\langle\psi_i\lvert\delta V_\eta\rvert\psi^-\rangle\}$

TABLE 6.2

The coefficients of the g-tensor in the effective spin $S' = \frac{1}{2}$ Hamiltonian $\mathcal{H} = \beta\, \underline{H}.\underline{g}.\underline{S}$ as matrix elements of the operators J_x, J_y, J_z, connecting the two states $\psi^{\pm}$ of a Kramers doublet. For values of the constant g_J, see Abragam and Bleaney (1970), Table 20, p. 874.

g-coefficient	Matrix element
g_{xx}	$2g_J\{\mathrm{Re}\langle\psi^+ \mid J_x \mid \psi^-\rangle\}$
g_{yy}	$2g_J\{-\mathrm{Im}\langle\psi^+ \mid J_y \mid \psi^-\rangle\}$
g_{zz}	$2g_J\langle\psi^+ \mid J_z \mid \psi^+\rangle$
g_{yz}	$2g_J\langle\psi^+ \mid J_y \mid \psi^+\rangle$
g_{zy}	$2g_J\{-\mathrm{Im}\langle\psi^+ \mid J_z \mid \psi^-\rangle\}$
g_{zx}	$2g_J\{\mathrm{Re}\langle\psi^+ \mid J_z \mid \psi^-\rangle\}$
g_{xz}	$2g_J\langle\psi^+ \mid J_x \mid \psi^+\rangle$
g_{xy}	$2g_J\{-\mathrm{Im}\langle\psi^+ \mid J_x \mid \psi^-\rangle\}$
g_{yx}	$2g_J\{\mathrm{Re}\langle\psi^+ \mid J_y \mid \psi^-\rangle\}$

is expanded in terms of the magnetic eigenstates of the J-manifold. If, as is often convenient, we adopt an expansion of $\psi^{\pm}_{gj}$ which makes the g-matrix symmetric, this will generally mean that $T_{\eta\lambda\rho} \neq T_{\eta\rho\lambda}$ (see §3.4). It is perhaps fortunate that this lack of symmetry in $g_{\lambda\rho}$ and $T_{\eta\lambda\rho}$ does not reveal itself in experimental determinations of resonance frequencies or of the electric field induced frequency shifts although it can be investigated in other ways (§10.6). The resonance frequencies depend on an intrinsically symmetric matrix which describes the quantity g^2, and the shifts depend on a tensor $B_{\eta\lambda\rho}$ for which $B_{\eta\lambda\rho} = B_{\eta\rho\lambda}$ under all circumstances (see §3.5). Theoretical values for the g-shifts $T_{\eta\lambda\rho}$ can be compared with experiment by first converting them to 'g^2-shift' parameters $B_{\eta\lambda\rho}$ as in eqn (3.32).

6.2. g-SHIFTS FOR TETRAGONAL CENTRES IN CaF_2:Ce

When Ce^{3+} ions (or other trivalent rare-earth ions) are substituted for Ca^{2+} in CaF_2, the extra positive charge is sometimes balanced by an F^- ion in an interstitial site lying along one of the six equivalent (001) directions in the cubic lattice (see Fig. 6.2). The resulting paramagnetic centre provides one of the simplest systems in which odd-field effects can be studied since the odd crystal field is due almost entirely to the F^- interstitial. (It is entirely due to it if we ignore indirect effects arising out of small distortions of the lattice.) The calculation of the induced crystal field terms and the g-shifts for this centre follows the lines of one made by Kiel and Mims (1972a, 1974)). The relevant physical parameters are summarized in Table 6.3 and a flow chart for the calculation itself is shown in Fig. 6.3.

6.2.1. NORMAL AND INDUCED CRYSTAL FIELD POTENTIALS.

Let us first consider the components occurring in the harmonic expansion of the normal crystal field V. The point symmetry of the site is C_{4v}. Thus, from Tables 4.1 and 4.2 (p. 109-113) we see that the

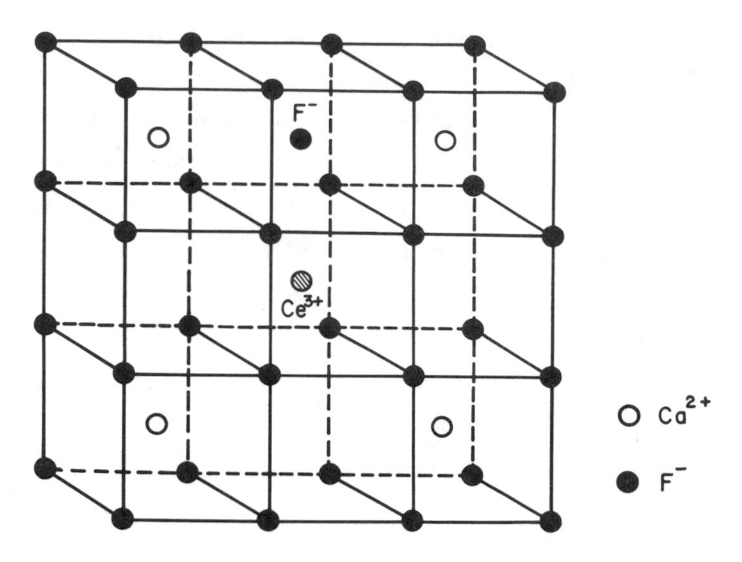

FIG. 6.2. Ce^{3+} tetragonal site in a CaF_2 lattice. Ce^{3+} substitutes for Ca^{2+} the charge balance being preserved by an F^- interstitial ion situated along one of the cubic axes. Six such arrangements can occur; F^- ions situated on opposite sides of the Ce correspond to inversion image sites. There is in actual fact some distortion of the lattice and the Ce^{3+} ion and the F^- interstitial are not located exactly at the centre of cubes of F^- ions, as shown in the figure.

allowed odd field harmonics (up to C_7^q) are C_1^0, C_3^0, C_5^0, $C_5^4 + C_5^{-4}$, C_7^0, $C_7^4 + C_7^{-4}$ and the allowed even field harmonics are C_2^0, C_4^0, $C_4^4 + C_4^{-4}$, C_6^0, $C_6^4 + C_6^{-4}$. If there were no interstitial F^- ion the harmonics would be C_4^0, $C_4^4 + C_4^{-4}$, C_6^0, $C_6^4 + C_6^{-4}$ and they would obey the cubic field relationships as indicated in the caption to Table 4.2. The remaining harmonics are associated with the F^- ion and with lattice distortions to which it gives rise.

In order to calculate the equivalent even field we shall begin by considering the two lowest-order odd harmonics A_1^0, A_3^0 in the normal crystal field (although as we show later the

TABLE 6.3

Values assumed in the $CaF_2{:}Ce^{3+}$ calculation. See also the energy-level diagram of Fig. 6.3 and the g-values in Table 6.6.

Ce-F^- (interstitial) distance	R_F	2·73 Å
Ce^{3+} radial integral	$\langle r \rangle$	0·50 Å
Ce^{3+} radial integral	$\langle r^3 \rangle$	0·86 Å
electronic polarizability of F^-	$\alpha_{e\ell}(F^-)$	$0{\cdot}64 \times 10^{-24} cm^3$
d.c. relative permittivity of CaF_2	ε_r	7·36
ionic part of relative permittivity	$\varepsilon_{r,ion}$	3·92
CaF_2 units per cm^3	n_{CaF_2}	$2{\cdot}45 \times 10^{22}$

contribution due to A_3^0 is a relatively small one). Ignoring lattice distortions and substituting $R_j = R_F = 2{\cdot}73$ A for the separation of Ce^{3+} and F^- in eqn (4.18), we obtain the point charge values

$$A_1^0 = -2{\cdot}15 \ \ Cm^{-2} \ , \quad A_3^0 = -2{\cdot}89 \times 10^{19} \ Cm^{-4} \qquad (6.15)$$

(In actual fact the Ce^{3+} ion may move towards the F^- ion under the influence of Coulomb attraction, resulting in a slightly reduced value of R.) These coefficients can be converted into spectroscopic crystal field parameters $A_K^Q(s) = eA_K^Q \langle r^K \rangle$ by using

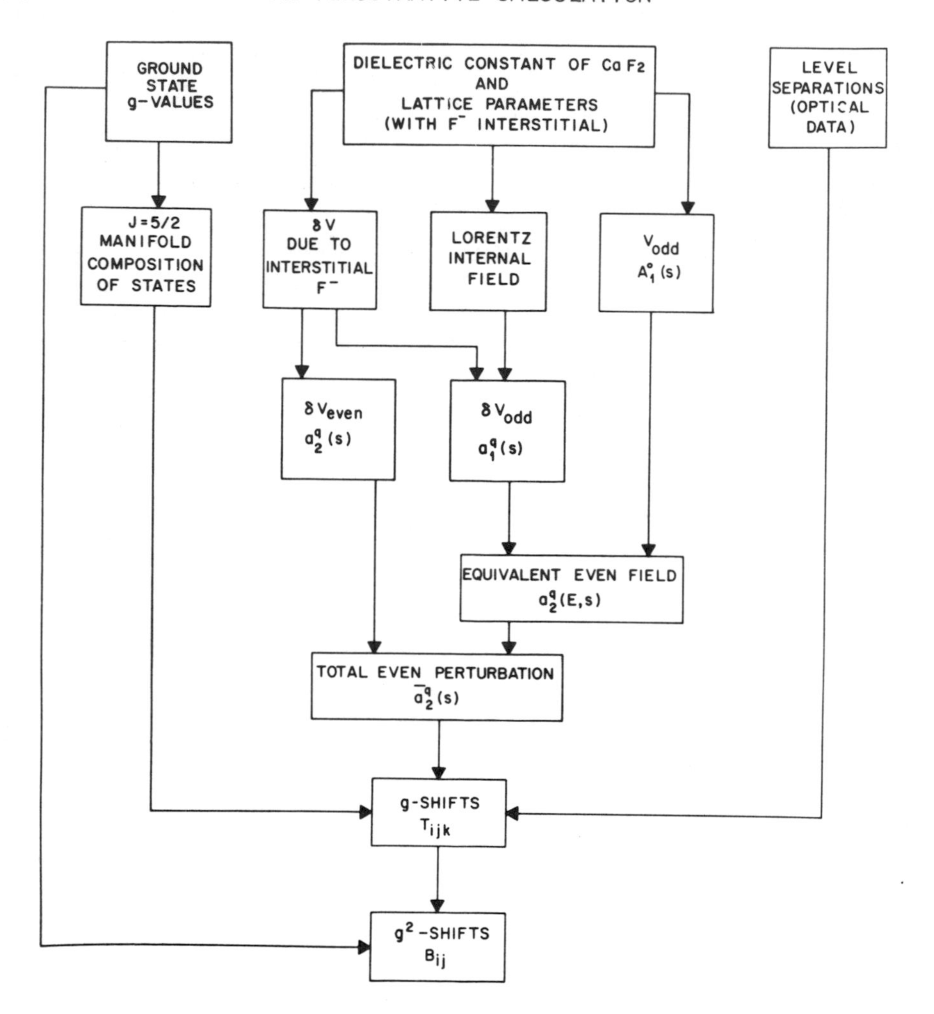

FIG. 6.3. Flow chart for the calculation of g-shifts for tetragonal Ce^{3+} sites in CaF_2.

the radial integrals†

$$\langle r \rangle = 0{\cdot}50\ \text{Å}, \quad \langle r^3 \rangle = 0{\cdot}86\ \text{Å}^3 \qquad (6.16)$$

† These values for the radial integrals $\langle 4f \mid r^k \mid 5d \rangle$ have been extrapolated from values given for Pr^{3+} and other rare-earth ions by Judd (1962); see Table 5.4 (p.148).)

We thus obtain the spectroscopic crystal field parameters

$$A_1^0(s) = 7790 \text{ cm}^{-1}, \; A_3^0(s) = 1800 \text{ cm}^{-1} \; . \tag{6.17}$$

The higher-order odd harmonics A_5^0, A_7^0 generated by the F^- ion, and the odd harmonics $A_5^{\pm 4}$, $A_5^{\pm 7}$ associated with distortions of the lattice can be ignored since they result in contributions which are yet smaller than those due to A_3^0. The even harmonics likewise need not be calculated since the required properties which depend on them (the energy separations and the state compositions) can be inferred directly from experiments without relying on the point charge model.

Next, let us consider the potential δV due to the applied field. We can, without loss of generality, assume this field to lie in the xz-plane, since the shifts calculated for E_x, E_z involve all three independent parameters in the C_{4v} third-rank tensor (see Fig. 3.1 p.46). The resulting induced potential consists of a long-range component associated with the classical Lorentz field and of components arising from the polarization of nearby lattice ions. Since the Lorentz factor $\frac{1}{3}(\varepsilon_r+2)$ for CaF_2 is 3.12; by eqn (4.9), the Lorentz field potential is

$$\delta V_{Lor} = 2{\cdot}21 \; rE_x\{C_1^1(\theta,\phi) - C_1^{-1}(\theta,\phi)\} - 3{\cdot}12 \; rE_z C_1^0(\theta,\phi). \tag{6.18}$$

Turning next to that portion of the induced potential which is associated with ions in the immediate neighbourhood of the Ce^{3+} ion we assume, as in Chapter 4, that it arises from an array of point dipoles which are situated at the lattice sites and are proportional in magnitude to the applied field. The crystal field harmonics arising from this dipole array are related to those which occur in the normal crystal field potential (see Tables 4.1 and 4.2, p.109-113) by the modified dipole selection rules (4.31). Thus, in the present case of C_{4v} point symmetry, induced dipoles p_0, polarized along the z-axis, give rise to even harmonics C_2^0, C_4^0, $C_4^4 + C_4^{-4}$, C_6^0, $C_6^4 + C_6^{-4}$ and to odd harmonics C_1^0, C_3^0, C_5^0. Induced dipoles $p_{\pm 1}$ (see eqns (4.21)-(4.22), corresponding to polarization in the xy-plane, give rise to even harmonics $C_2^{\pm 1}$, $C_4^{\pm 1}$, $C_4^{\pm 3}$, $C_6^{\pm 1}$, $C_6^{\pm 3}$, $C_6^{\pm 5}$, and to odd harmonics $C_1^{\pm 1}$, $C_3^{\pm 1}$, $C_3^{\pm 3}$, $C_5^{\pm 1}$, $C_5^{\pm 3}$, $C_5^{\pm 5}$. Examining the situation more closely we see that only the harmonics $C_k^{0,\pm 1}$ are directly associated with the interstitial fluorine. The harmonics $C_3^{0,\pm 1,\pm 3}$, $C_5^{0,\pm 1,\pm 3}$ are due to dipoles situated on the cubic lattice points, and the remaining harmonics only enter when distortions of the lattice are taken into account. In a simple calculation of the shifts it is usually sufficient to take the lowest odd and even terms C_1^q, C_2^q and ignore the rest. Here this means that we shall ignore the polarization of the CaF_2 lattice except in so far as it contributes to the long-range Lorentz field, and base our estimate of the induced potential on fields generated by the induced dipole at the F^- interstitial site only.

The electronic contribution to the F^- dipole moment can be obtained from tables of electronic polarizabilities given by Tessman, Kahn, and Shockley (1953). These tables yield the value $\alpha_{e\ell}(F^-) = 0{\cdot}64 \times 10^{-24}\,cm^{-3}$, it being assumed in the tables that the field seen by the ion is the Lorentz internal field. If we make the same assumption in the present case, we have†

† The assumption of a Lorentz field is convenient but possibly inaccurate in the present instance. The electronic polarizabilities in the Tessman, Kahn, and Shockley study were deduced from dielectric measurements in cubic crystals and in other highly symmetric crystals, for which the Lorentz field can be expected to give a good approximation to the internal field. Here, on the other hand, the F^- interstitial is in a highly asymmetric environment with a Ca^{2+} ion on one side and a Ce^{3+} on the other.

$$p_{e\ell} = \frac{1}{3}(\varepsilon_r+2)E_{app}\alpha_{e\ell}(F^-) = 2\cdot00 \times 10^{-24}\,E_{app} \qquad (6.19)$$

(where $p_{e\ell}$ and E_{app} are in the same system of units). Since ε_r is isotropic for a cubic lattice the Lorentz field assumption implies that $\underline{p}_{e\ell}$ is parallel to $\underline{E}_{app}$ and the same constant of proportionality $\frac{1}{3}(\varepsilon_r+2)$ can be used for all orientations of the dipole.

The ionic polarizability of the F^- interstitial (i.e. the displacement u_F-u_I with respect to the Ce^{3+} ion per unit applied field) has not been measured, but it can be estimated by one of the methods suggested in Chapter 4. For the present purpose we shall assume that the ionic dipole arising from the displacement of the F^- interstitial relative to the Ce^{3+} ion is the same as the ionic dipole associated with the displacement of one F^- lattice ion relative to a Ca^{2+} ion.† Substituting $\varepsilon_{r,ion} = 3\cdot92$ and $n_{CaF_2} = 2\cdot45 \times 10^{-22}$ in eqn (4.38) and dividing by two for the number of dipoles in each CaF_2 cell, we have

$$p_{ion} = 6\cdot36 \times 10^{24}\,E_{app}\ \text{cm}^{-3} \qquad (6.20)$$

Adding electronic and ionic dipole moments together, we thus obtain

$$p_{tot} = 8\cdot36 \times 10^{-24}\,E_{app}\ , \qquad (6.21)$$

---

† It might be argued that we should assume a larger relative displacement for Ce^{3+} and F^- than for Ca^{2+} and F^- since Ce^{3+} has an extra charge and will be acted on more strongly by the applied field. But Ce^{3+} has a larger ionic radius than Ca^{2+} and may therefore be subject to stronger elastic restoring forces. For simplicity we leave the estimate as it stands.

whence, substituting $p_x = 8{\cdot}36 \times 10^{-24} E_x$, $p_z = 8{\cdot}36 \times 10^{-24} E_z$ in eqn (4.21) (p.107), we derive the spherical tensor dipole components

$$p_1 = -p_{-1} = -p_x/\sqrt{2} = -5{\cdot}91 \times 10^{-24} E_x \, ,$$

$$p_0 = p_z = 8{\cdot}36 \times 10^{-24} E_z \qquad (6.22)$$

($p_y = 0$ since we have assumed that E_{app} is in the xz-plane.)

The induced crystal field potentials can now be obtained by using eqn (4.19). Since we are only considering a single environmental ion at coordinates $(R_j, \theta_j, \phi_j) = (R_F, \theta_F, \phi_F)$, where $\theta_F = 0$, this equation reduces to

$$a_k^q = \sum_{\mu} p_\mu \eta(\mu,k,q) C_{k+1}^{-q-\mu}(\theta_F=0) R_F^{k+2} \quad .$$

A further simplification can be made by noting that $C_{k+1}^{-q-\mu}(\theta=0) = 1$ when $q = -\mu$ and is otherwise zero (Table A.1 p.264) thus leaving the single term

$$a_k^q = p_\mu \eta(\mu,k,q=-\mu)/R_F^{k+2} \quad . \qquad (6.23)$$

The essentials of the calculation for the lowest-order odd and even harmonics associated with the polarization of the F^- ion are summarized in Table 6.4. Adding the results in the last column to the Lorentz field (eqn (6.18)), we obtain[†]

[†] It will be noted that the field due to the polarization of the F^- interstitial adds to the long-range Lorentz field when $\underline{E}_{app}$ is along the z-axis but subtracts from it when $\underline{E}_{app}$ is in the x-direction. One might of course have arrived at this conclusion at once by noting that for E_z the induced dipole is in the end-on position, and for E_x it is in the broadside-on position.

TABLE 6.4

Quantities entering into the calculation of the amplitudes a_1^q, a_2^q of the induced crystal field potentials due to the polarization of the F^- interstitial ion along the z-axis from the Ce^{3+} site in CaF_2. The applied field is assumed to be in the xz-plane. The amplitudes a_k^q are calculated by means of eqn (6.23) and are in the same system of electrical units as the applied field. The parameters $\eta(\mu,k,q)$ are defined in eqns (4.20), (4.23), and (4.24).

μ	p_μ (10^{-24} cm^3)	k	q	$\eta(\mu,k,q)$	R_F^{k+2} (cm^{k+2})	a_k^q (cm^{1-k})
0	$8{\cdot}35\ E_z$	1	0	-2	$20{\cdot}3 \times 10^{-24}$	$-0{\cdot}82\ E_z$
1	$-5{\cdot}82\ E_x$	1	-1	-1	$20{\cdot}3 \times 10^{-24}$	$-0{\cdot}29\ E_x$
-1	$5{\cdot}82\ E_x$	1	1	-1	$20{\cdot}3 \times 10^{-24}$	$0{\cdot}29\ E_x$
0	$8{\cdot}35\ E_z$	2	0	-3	$55{\cdot}6 \times 10^{-32}$	$-0{\cdot}45 \times 10^8\ E_z$
1	$-5{\cdot}82\ E_x$	2	-1	$-\sqrt{3}$	$55{\cdot}6 \times 10^{-32}$	$0{\cdot}18 \times 10^8\ E_x$
-1	$5{\cdot}82\ E_x$	2	1	$-\sqrt{3}$	$55{\cdot}6 \times 10^{-32}$	$-0{\cdot}18 \times 10^8\ E_x$.

$$a_1^0 = -3 \cdot 94\ E_z,\ a_1^{\pm 1} = \pm 1 \cdot 92\ E_x\ ,$$

$$a_2^0 = -0 \cdot 45 \times 10^8\ E_z,\ a_2^{\pm 1} = \pm 0 \cdot 18 \times 10^8\ E_x\ .$$

The spectroscopic crystal field parameters $a_k^q(s) = e \langle r^k \rangle a_k^q$ are derived from these amplitudes by substituting the radial integrals $\langle r \rangle = 0 \cdot 50 \times 10^{-8}$ cm (eqn (6.16)) and $\langle r^2 \rangle = 0 \cdot 34 \times 10^{-16}$ cm^2 (Table 5.3, p.147) and changing to cm^{-1} energy units. We thus obtain the values

$$\begin{aligned} a_1^0(s) &= 1 \cdot 59 \times 10^{-4}\ E_z\ cm^{-1};\ a_1^{\pm 1}(s) = \mp 0 \cdot 78 \times 10^{-4}\ E_x\ cm^{-1}; \\ a_2^0(s) &= 1 \cdot 24 \times 10^{-5}\ E_z\ cm^{-1};\ a_2^{\pm 1}(s) = \pm 0 \cdot 50 \times 10^{-5}\ E_x\ cm^{-1} \end{aligned} \tag{6.24}$$

where E_x, E_z are in volts per centimetre.

The even harmonics in (6.24) can be used at once in the perturbation formulae in Table 6.1, but the odd harmonics must first be combined with the odd harmonics in V (Eqn (6.17)) to form an equivalent even field. According to the composition rules (5.28)-(5.29) $A_1^0(s)$ and $A_3^0(s)$ both combine with $a_1^0(s)$, $a_1^{\pm 1}(s)$ to form harmonics $a_2^0(E,s)$, $a_2^{\pm 1}(E,s)$, the equivalent even field amplitudes being calculated by the equation (eqn (5.26))

$$a_{k'}^{q'}(E,s) = -\frac{2}{\bar{E}_{ug}} \sum_{K,Q} (-1)^{q'} A_K^Q(s) a_k^q(s) \eta_{EEF} \times \begin{pmatrix} K & k & k' \\ Q & q & -q' \end{pmatrix} .$$

Limiting consideration to state mixing between the 4f ground manifold (ℓ=3) and the 5d excited manifold (ℓ'=2) we can now proceed with the EEF calculation whose details are summarized in Table 6.5. It can be seen that the combinations with $A_3^0(s)$ have little effect on the overall result and are likely to be

TABLE 6.5

Calculation of equivalent even field harmonics arising from the coupling between 4f- and 5d-manifolds for Ce^{3+} in tetragonal sites in CaF_2 according to eqn (5.26). For $A_K^Q(s)$ see eqn (6.17), for $a_k^q(s)$ eqn (6.24), for $\overline{E}_{ug}$ Fig 6.4, for η_{EEF} Table 5.9, and for the 3j symbols Table 5.10. The result $a_{k'}^{q'}(E,s)$ is in cm^{-1} energy units. The fields E_x, E_z are in volts per centimetre.

$A_K^Q(s)$ (cm^{-1})	$a_k^q(s)$ (10^{-4} cm^{-1})	$\overline{E}_{ug}$ (cm^{-1})	η_{EEF}	$\begin{pmatrix} K & k & k' \\ Q & q & -q' \end{pmatrix}$	$a_{k'}^{q'}(E,s)$ (10^{-4} cm^{-1})
$A_1^0(s) = 7790$	$a_1^0(s) = 1{\cdot}59E_z$	43 340	0·80	$\sqrt{\frac{2}{15}}$	$a_2^0(E,s) = -0{\cdot}271\ E_z$
$A_1^0(s) = 7790$	$a_1^{\pm 1}(s) = \mp 0{\cdot}77\ E_x$	43 340	0·80	$-\sqrt{\frac{1}{10}}$	$a_2^{\pm 1}(E,s) = \pm 0{\cdot}116\ E_x$
$A_3^0(s) = 1800$	$a_1^0(s) = 1{\cdot}59\ E_z$	43 340	-0·29	$-\sqrt{\frac{3}{35}}$	$a_2^0(E,s) = -0{\cdot}018\ E_z$
$A_3^0(s) = 1800$	$a_1^{\pm 1}(s) = \mp 0{\cdot}77\ E_x$	43 340	-0·29	$\sqrt{\frac{2}{35}}$	$a_2^{\pm 1}(E,s) = \pm 0{\cdot}007\ E_x$

of the same order as the errors in our basic assumptions. Ignoring these and other small contributions to the EEF† we are left with the EEF parameters

$$a_2^0(E,s) = -2{\cdot}44 \times 10^{-5}\ E_z\ \text{cm}^{-1};\ a_2^{\pm 1}(E,s) = \pm 1{\cdot}03 \times 10^{-5}\ E_x\ \text{cm}^{-1} \tag{6.25}$$

It may at first sight seem surprising that the perturbation δV_{even} should turn out to be smaller than the perturbation δV_{EEF} arising from δV_{odd}, especially in view of the large energy denominator entering into the latter. This happens partly because the terms in C_1^q belonging to $E_{<R}$ (eqn (4.6)) are larger than terms in C_2^q by a factor $\simeq R_F/r$ (where r is the radius of the Ce^{3+} wavefunction) and partly also because the lowest-order odd harmonics contain the long-range Lorentz field (eqn (4.9)) in addition to the fields due to the polarization of the F^- interstitial. Simple point charge/point dipole calculations such as the above cannot settle the question of whether the odd fields or induced even fields are primarily responsible for the shift, however. The amplitudes A_1^q and a_2^q entering into $a_2^q(E,s)$ and the amplitudes $a_2^q(s)$ in the induced field were calculated without taking lattice screening or screening due to the outer electrons of the Ce^{3+} ion into account, and it is not easy to estimate what the corrected amplitudes might be. Lacking any more specific information we merely add $a_2^q(s)$ and $a_2^q(E,s)$, as in eqn (5.32), to give the resultant even-field parameters

† Combinations between $A_3^0(s)$ and $a_1^q(s)$ giving $a_4^0(E,s)$ and $a_4^q(E,s)$ are also allowed by the composition rules. In addition to this it is possible to form combinations between $A_1^0(s)$ and induced field components $a_3^q(s)$.

$$\bar{a}_2^0(s) = -1{\cdot}20 \times 10^{-5}\ E_z\ \text{cm}^{-1};\ \bar{a}_2^{\pm 1}(s) = \pm 1{\cdot}53 \times 10^{-5}\ E_x\ \text{cm}^{-1}. \quad (6.26)$$

where E_x, E_z are in volts per centimetre.

6.2.2. THE g-SHIFTS AND g^2-SHIFTS. To calculate the g-shifts from the even field perturbations in eqn 6.26 we need the matrix elements of the perturbation operations $\bar{a}_2^0(s)\ C_2^0(\theta,\psi), \bar{a}_2^{\pm 1}\ C_2^{\pm 1}(\theta,\psi)$ and of the operators J_x, J_z between wavefunctions corresponding to the 4f-manifold of levels. The crystal field splits the six states of the $J=\frac{5}{2}$ manifold into three Kramers doublets, as shown in Fig. 6.4. If we ignore state mixing between $J=\frac{7}{2}$ and $J=\frac{5}{2}$

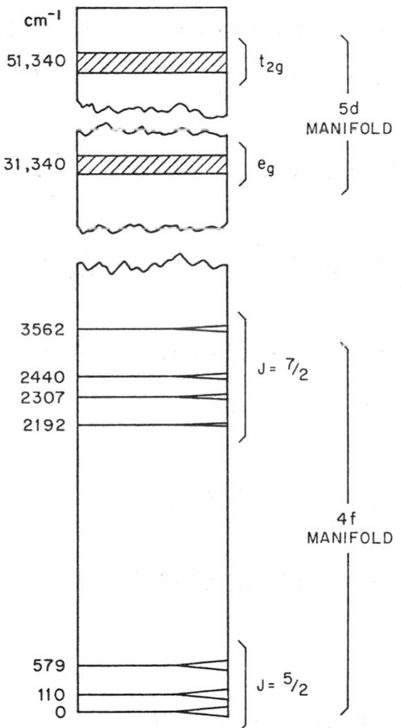

FIG. 6.4. Energy levels for the C_{4v} Ce^{3+} site in CaF_2 according to Manthey (1973). The mean value $\bar{E}_{ug}$ for the separation between the ground state and the states in the 5d-manifold, allowing for the degeneracies in the latter, is 43 340 cm^{-1}.

manifolds these doublets have the composition

$$\psi_1^{\pm} = b\left|\tfrac{5}{2},\pm\tfrac{5}{2}\right\rangle - a\left|\tfrac{5}{2},\mp\tfrac{3}{2}\right\rangle ,$$

$$\psi_2^{\pm} = \left|\tfrac{5}{2},\pm\tfrac{1}{2}\right\rangle \quad , \qquad (6.27)$$

$$\psi_3^{\pm} = a\left|\tfrac{5}{2},\pm\tfrac{5}{2}\right\rangle + b\left|\tfrac{5}{2},\mp\tfrac{3}{2}\right\rangle ,$$

where $|a|^2 + |b|^2 = 1$ (cf. Abragam and Bleaney (1970), p.285 et seq.). According to Manthey (1973) the $\left|\tfrac{5}{2},\pm\tfrac{1}{2}\right\rangle$ doublet is the middle doublet. The parameters a, b which determine state mixing in the remaining doublets can be derived by fitting experimental g-values (Table 6.6) to the expressions in Table 6.2 as evaluated for the wavefunctions $\psi_3^{\pm}$ in eqn (6.27). Thus from

$$g_{xx} = g_{\perp} = 2g_J\{\mathrm{Re}\langle\psi_{gj}^{+} \mid J_x \mid \psi_{gj}^{-}\rangle \quad ,$$

$$g_{zz} = g_{||} = 2g_J\langle\psi_{gj}^{+} \mid J_z \mid \psi_{gj}^{+}\rangle \quad , \qquad (6.28)$$

where $g_J = \langle J||\Lambda||J\rangle = \frac{6}{7}$ (see e.g. Abragam and Bleaney (1970), Table 20) we conclude that

$$g_{\perp} = (12\sqrt{5}/7)ab,$$

$$g_{||} = (6/7)(5a^2-3b^2) \quad , \qquad (6.29)$$

whence

$$a = 0{\cdot}912;\ b = 0{\cdot}410 \ . \qquad (6.30)$$

The fit is not an exact one, most probably because the $J = \frac{5}{2}$ manifold of states is partially mixed with the $J = \frac{7}{2}$ manifold which lies $\simeq 2600\ \mathrm{cm}^{-1}$ above it.

From Table 6.1 we select the g-shift formulae

TABLE 6.6

g-values and the parameters B_{ij} for Ce^{3+} in tetragonal sites in CaF_2. The B_{ij} denote shifts in g^2 as described in §3.5. They are given in units of 10^{-9} V^{-1}cm. The calculated values are based on the assumption that the ground doublet has the form $0{\cdot}912|\frac{5}{2}, \pm\frac{5}{2}\rangle + 0{\cdot}410|\frac{5}{2}, \mp\frac{3}{2}\rangle$. The state-mixing parameters are obtained by making a best fit to the experimental g-values.

	$g_{\parallel}$	$g_{\perp}$	B_{33}	B_{31}	B_{15}
Experimental	3•038	1•396	68	-16	5•5
	±0•003	±0•002	±10	±3	±1
Calculated	3•13	1•43	83	-19	55

$$T_{zxx} = T_{311} = 4g_J \sum_i \frac{1}{E_i} \mathrm{Re}\{\langle\psi_3^+ \mid J_x \mid \psi_i\rangle\langle\psi_i \mid \delta V_z \mid \psi_3^-\rangle\} ,$$

$$T_{zzz} = T_{333} = 4g_J \sum_i \frac{1}{E_i} \mathrm{Re}\{\langle\psi_3^+ \mid J_z \mid \psi_i\rangle\langle\psi_i \mid \delta V_z \mid \psi_3^+\rangle\} ,$$

$$T_{xxz} = T_{113} = 4g_J \sum_i \frac{1}{E_i} \mathrm{Re}\{\langle\psi_3^+ \mid J_x \mid \psi_i\rangle\langle\psi_i \mid \delta V_x \mid \psi_3^+\rangle\} , \tag{6.31}$$

$$T_{xzx} = T_{131} = 4g_J \sum_i \frac{1}{E_i} \mathrm{Re}\{\langle\psi_3^+ \mid J_z \mid \psi_i\rangle\langle\psi_i \mid \delta V_x \mid \psi_3^-\rangle\} ,$$

and substitute the crystal field operators

$$\delta V_z = (\bar{a}_2^0(s)/E_z)C_2^0(\theta,\phi) = -1{\cdot}20 \times 10^{-5}\, C_2^0(\theta,\phi) ,$$

$$\delta V_x = \left\{\bar{a}_2^1(s)/E_x\right\}\left\{C_2^1(\theta,\phi) - C_2^{-1}(\theta,\phi)\right\} \tag{6.32}$$

$$= 1{\cdot}53 \times 10^{-5}\left\{C_2^1(\theta,\phi) - C_2^{-1}(\theta,\phi)\right\}$$

from eqn (6.26). The summation $\sum_i$ need only be taken over the states $\psi_i = \psi_3^\pm$ for T_{zxx}, T_{zzz}, since δV_z has no matrix elements between $\psi_2^\pm$ and $\psi_1^\pm$, but it will include both excited doublets in the case of T_{xxz}, T_{xzx}.

The matrix elements $\langle M_J \mid J_\lambda \mid M_J'\rangle$ connecting states within $J = \frac{5}{2}$ manifold are

$$\langle\pm \tfrac{5}{2} \mid J_x \mid \pm \tfrac{3}{2}\rangle = \langle\pm \tfrac{3}{2} \mid J_x \mid \pm \tfrac{5}{2}\rangle = \frac{\sqrt{5}}{2} ,$$

$$\langle\pm \tfrac{3}{2} \mid J_x \mid \pm \tfrac{1}{2}\rangle = \langle\pm \tfrac{1}{2} \mid J_x \mid \pm \tfrac{3}{2}\rangle = \sqrt{2} , \tag{6.33}$$

$$\langle \pm \tfrac{5}{2} \mid J_z \mid \pm \tfrac{5}{2} \rangle = \pm \tfrac{5}{2}; \quad \langle \pm \tfrac{3}{2} \mid J_z \mid \pm \tfrac{3}{2} \rangle = \pm \tfrac{3}{2} \ ,$$

The crystal field matrix elements can be derived from matrix elements of the normalized operator equivalents† $\tilde{O}_k^q$ by using the relation

$$\langle M_J \mid C_k^q(\theta,\phi) \mid M_J' \rangle = \langle J \| f(k) \| J \rangle \langle M_J \mid \tilde{O}_k^q \mid M_J' \rangle \qquad (6.34)$$

in which the $\langle J \| f(k) \| J \rangle$ are 'reduced matrix elements' commonly written as $\langle J \| \alpha \| J \rangle$, $\langle J \| \beta \| J \rangle$, $\langle J \| \gamma \| J \rangle$ for the cases $k = 2,4,6$ respectively (see Abragam and Bleaney (1970), Table 20, p. 874). Here we only need $\langle J \| \alpha \| J \rangle$. The required $\tilde{O}_k^q$ are expressed in terms of the angular-momentum operators by

$$\tilde{O}_2^{\pm 1} = \mp \tfrac{1}{4} \sqrt{6}\ (J_z J_\pm + J_\pm J_z) \ ,$$

$$\tilde{O}_2^{0} = \tfrac{1}{2}(3J_z^2 - J(J+1)) \ ,$$

and the corresponding matrix elements in a $J = \frac{5}{2}$ manifold are

$$\langle J \| \alpha \| J \rangle = -\tfrac{2}{35} \ ,$$

$$\langle \pm \tfrac{5}{2} \mid \tilde{O}_2^0 \mid \pm \tfrac{5}{2} \rangle = 5; \quad \langle \pm \tfrac{3}{2} \mid \tilde{O}_2^0 \mid \pm \tfrac{3}{2} \rangle = -1 \ ,$$

$$\langle \pm \tfrac{5}{2} \mid \tilde{O}_2^{\pm 1} \mid \pm \tfrac{3}{2} \rangle = -\langle \pm \tfrac{3}{2} \mid \tilde{O}_2^{\mp 1} \mid \pm \tfrac{5}{2} \rangle = -\sqrt{30} \ , \qquad (6.35)$$

$$\langle \pm \tfrac{3}{2} \mid \tilde{O}_2^{\pm 1} \mid \pm \tfrac{1}{2} \rangle = -\langle \pm \tfrac{1}{2} \mid \tilde{O}_2^{\mp 1} \mid \pm \tfrac{3}{2} \rangle = -2\sqrt{3}$$

---

† A different form of operator equivalents O_k^q is often used in tabulations (see Appendix A.2). Here $\tilde{O}_2^{\pm 1} = \mp \frac{1}{2}\sqrt{6}\ O_2^1$, $\tilde{O}_2^0 = \frac{1}{2} O_2^0$.

(see Abragam and Bleaney (1970), Table 17, p. 864; also see tables given by Buckmaster (1962)).

The energy separations E_{13}, E_{23} are

$$E_{13} = 579 \text{ cm}^{-1}; \; E_{23} = 110 \text{ cm}^{-1} \tag{6.36}$$

(Manthey 1973; see Fig. 6.4). Substituting these values in eqns (6.27), (6.29)-(6.35), we obtain the g-shift parameters

$$\begin{aligned} T_{zxx} &= -6{\cdot}8 \times 10^{-9}, \quad T_{zzz} = 13{\cdot}6 \times 10^{-9} \\ T_{xxz} &= -1{\cdot}4 \times 10^{-9}, \quad T_{xzx} = 42{\cdot}4 \times 10^{-9}. \end{aligned} \tag{6.37}$$

The 'g^2-shift' parameters can be calculated from the g-shift parameters by means of eqns (3.32) (p.66), which in the case of C_{4v} symmetry reduce to $B_{31} = 2g_{\|}T_{zxx}$; $B_{33} = 2g_{\perp}T_{zzz}$; $B_{15} = g_{\|}T_{xzx} + g_{\perp}T_{xxz}$. Substituting the g-values from Table 6.3 we have

$$B_{31} = -19 \times 10^{-9}; \; B_{33} = 83 \times 10^{-9}; \; B_{15} = 55 \times 10^{-9}. \tag{6.38}$$

It will be noted that in (6.37) the parameters T_{xxz} and T_{xzx} are not equal. The values depend, as pointed out earlier, on the basis states chosen to represent the three Kramers doublets, and would be different if a new basis, e.g. a set of eigenstates quantized with respect to an axis other than the z-axis, had been chosen instead of the one used here. The representation (6.27) is convenient since it yields a symmetric g-tensor. If, however, the representation were changed in order to make T_{xxz} and T_{xzx} equal the g-tensor would become asymmetric and the expression for B_{15} would assume a more complicated form. This element of arbitrariness has, as shown in Chapter 3, no effect on the

g^2-tensor G_{jk}, derived from g_{jk} by eqn (3.24)(p. 60) which continues to be diagonal with elements $g_\perp^2$, $g_\perp^2$, $g_\parallel^2$, nor on the g^2-shift tensor B_{ij}, derived from g_{jk} and T_{ijk} by (3.32), which is independent of the representation chosen in order to calculate the result.

Substitution of the parameters a,b in eqn (6.28) gives positive g-values $g_\perp$ and $g_\parallel$. It has not been experimentally shown however that $g_\parallel$ and $g_\perp$ have the same sign here, and it is conceivable that the signs might be opposite (see e.g. Blume, Geschwind, and Yafet 1969). If so, the data could be fitted by changing the sign of a or b. Such a change of sign would have no effect on the calculated values for B_{33}, B_{31}, B_{15}, but would reverse the sign of T_{zxx}, T_{xzx}.

The experimental parameters are shown for comparison in Table 6.6. B_{33} and B_{31} agree surprisingly well with the theoretical values, but B_{15} is wrong by a factor of 10. There are, of course, a number of places in the calculation where arbitrary assumptions have been made, and the close agreement for B_{33} and B_{31} should be regarded as partly fortuitous. We have, for instance, ignored mixing with the $J = \frac{7}{2}$ 4f-manifold, excluded all opposite-parity states but the 5d-states, and failed to make any allowance for screening effects when estimating the crystal field potentials. Yet another source of error may be in the value taken for the interval E_{12}. According to Manthey (1973) this interval was inferred indirectly from optical data and was not observed in fluorescence, as was the interval E_{13}. The analysis shows that E_{12} has a critical effect on B_{15} but no effect at all on the other two parameters. This outcome is not untypical of linear electric field effect calculations. Although the right order of magnitude can often be obtained for one or two of the larger coefficients the relative values of the coefficients remain hard to interpret.

7. Paraelectric resonance

Transitions can be excited by the microwave electric field as well as by the microwave magnetic field for paramagnetic ions at non-centrosymmetric lattice sites. This possibility is implicit in the form of the linear electric field effect spin Hamiltonian $\mathcal{H}_{elec}$, as one can see, for example, by comparing the terms $\beta T_{ijk}E_iH_jS_k$ and $\beta g_{jk}H_jS_k$ in eqns (3.2) and (3.1)(pp.38-39). An oscillating electric field $E_i = E_{io}\cos\omega_{12}t$ and an oscillating magnetic field $H_j = H_{jo}\cos\omega_{12}t$ can both induce transitions between states ψ_1 and ψ_2 separated by an interval $\hbar\omega_{12}$, the transition matrix elements being $\beta T_{ijk}H_j\langle\psi_1|S_k|\psi_2\rangle$ in the first case and $\beta g_{jk}\langle\psi_1|S_k|\psi_2\rangle$ in the second. (H_j is the static Zeeman field component in the first case.) Electric field induced, or 'paraelectric', resonance transitions may also be associated with other terms in $\mathcal{H}_{elec}$, e.g. the term $E_iR_{ijk}S_jS_k$ for which the transition matrix elements are of the form $R_{ijk}\langle\psi_1|S_jS_k|\psi_2\rangle$. Transitions which are forbidden in normal magnetic resonance may be induced in this way. It is furthermore interesting to note that parameters such as T_{ijk} and T_{ikj}, which are represented by the single parameter B_{ijk} in frequency-shift experiments (§3.5), correspond to two different matrix elements $\beta T_{ijk}H_j\langle\psi_1|S_k|\psi_2\rangle$ and $\beta T_{ikj}H_k\langle\psi_1|S_j|\psi_2\rangle$, which can be determined separately in electric resonance experiment by aligning the Zeeman field along either the j- or k-axes (see e.g. Jones and Moore 1969). The values of the parameters T_{ijk} are, of course, determined only in relation to a particular representation of the spin operators (§3.4), this generally being the representation which makes the g-matrix symmetric.

Paraelectric resonance transitions result from coupling between the microwave electric field and electric dipole transition moments associated with the resonance states. These moments may be due directly to the odd symmetry component of the crystal field as in the case of the $R_{ijk}\langle\psi_1|S_jS_k|\psi_2\rangle$ transition moment, or may arise from the odd crystal field and the Zeeman field acting in conjunction. The physical origins of such electric moments are explored in more detail in the next section.

It should be noted that the term 'paraelectric resonance' is also applied to phenomena which do not involve magnetic fields and which have no connection with the kinds of transition studied in EPR. For example, the centres formed by OH^- molecular ions in KCl possess electric dipole moments and a microwave electric field can induce transitions between the corresponding energy levels (see e.g. Feher, Shepherd, and Shore (1966), Bron and Dreyfus 1967). These resonance transitions will not be discussed here. They are more closely related to the resonance phenomena observed in the microwave spectroscopy of gases than to those associated with paramagnetic ions in solids.

7.1. ELECTRIC DIPOLE MOMENTS ASSOCIATED WITH EPR STATES

The electric dipole moment can be defined by the matrix element

$$\underline{p}_{nm} = \langle\psi_n \mid e\underline{r} \mid \psi_m\rangle \ , \qquad (7.1)$$

where e is the electronic charge. If $n \neq m$, the definition applies to the transition dipole moment between states ψ_n and ψ_m, otherwise eqn (7.1) defines the static electric dipole moment

$$\underline{p}_n = \langle \psi_n \mid e\underline{r} \mid \psi_n \rangle \quad . \tag{7.2}$$

If both states have well-defined parity and belong to the same manifold, e.g. if ψ_n, ψ_m are the two states ψ_{gj} $\psi_{gj'}$ of Chapter 5, then $\underline{p}_{nm} = \underline{p}_{jj'} = 0$. Small finite values of $\underline{p}_{nm}$ can, however, occur when the states are mixed by odd crystal fields as in the case of ions at non-centrosymmetric sites. The dipole moments can then be calculated by means of the perturbation formulae given in Chapter 5.1. According to eqn (5.6) the first-order value of $\underline{p}_{nm}$ due to the odd perturbation V is

$$\delta^{(1)}\underline{p}_{nm} = \sum_{\substack{\ell \\ \ell \neq m \\ \ell \neq n}} \{V_{n\ell}\underline{p}_{\ell m}/E_{n\ell}) + (V_{\ell m}\underline{p}_{n\ell}/E_{m\ell})\} \quad , \tag{7.3}$$

or, in the notation employed later on in Chapter 5,

$$\delta^{(1)}\underline{p}_{jj'} = -\sum_{u}\frac{1}{E_{ug}}\{\langle \psi_{gj} \mid V_{odd} \mid \psi_u\rangle\langle \psi_u \mid e\underline{r} \mid \psi_{gj'}\rangle + \langle \psi_{gj} \mid e\underline{r} \mid \psi_u\rangle\langle \psi_u \mid V_{odd} \mid \psi_{gj'}\rangle\}. \tag{7.4}$$

This equation gives the transition dipole moment between the two zero-order states ψ_{gj}, $\psi_{gj'}$. The static dipole moment corresponding to (7.4) is

$$\delta^{(1)}\underline{p}_j = -\sum_{u}\frac{1}{E_{ug}}\{\langle \psi_{gj} \mid V_{odd} \mid \psi_u\rangle\langle \psi_u \mid e\underline{r} \mid \psi_{gj}\rangle + \text{h.c.}\} \, . \tag{7.5}$$

(As in Chapter 5, we have approximated by setting

$E_u - E_{gj'} \simeq E_u - E_{gj} \simeq E_{ug}$.)

A higher order contribution to the electric dipole moment involving the Zeeman field as well as the odd crystal field can be obtained by setting $V = V_{odd} + V_H$ in eqn (5.7), V_H being the Zeeman field operator. The summations are taken over states ψ_u in the opposite-parity manifold and ψ_i in the ground manifold, and the result is simplified by eliminating terms with an energy denominator $\simeq E_{ug}^2$ (on the grounds that they are usually an order of magnitude smaller than terms with the denominator $E_{ug}E_{ij}$). In this way one can derive the transition dipole moment

$$\delta^{(2)}\underline{p}_{jj'} =$$

$$\sum_u \sum_i^{i\neq j} \frac{1}{E_{ug}E_{ij}} \{ \langle\psi_{gj} \mid V_H \mid \psi_{gi}\rangle\langle\psi_{gi} \mid V_{odd} \mid \psi_u\rangle\langle\psi_u \mid e\underline{r} \mid \psi_{gj'}\rangle +$$

$$+ \langle\psi_{gj} \mid V_H \mid \psi_{gi}\rangle\langle\psi_{gi} \mid e\underline{r} \mid \psi_u\rangle\langle\psi_u \mid V_{odd} \mid \psi_{gj'}\rangle +$$

$$+ \sum_u \sum_i^{i\neq j'} \frac{1}{E_{ug}E_{ij'}} \{ \langle\psi_{gj}|e\underline{r}|\psi_u\rangle\langle\psi_u|V_{odd}|\psi_{gi}\rangle\langle\psi_{gi}|V_H|\psi_{gj'}\rangle +$$

$$+ \langle\psi_{gj} \mid V_{odd} \mid \psi_u\rangle\langle\psi_u \mid e\underline{r} \mid \psi_{gi}\rangle\langle\psi_{gi} \mid V_H \mid \psi_{gj'}\rangle \quad . \tag{7.6}$$

and the static dipole moment

$$\delta^{(2)}\underline{p}_j =$$

$$\sum_{u}\sum_{i}^{i\neq j}\frac{1}{E_{ug}E_{ij}}\{\langle\psi_{gj}\mid V_{H}\mid\psi_{gi}\rangle\langle\psi_{gi}\mid V_{odd}\mid\psi_{u}\rangle\langle\psi_{u}\mid e\underline{r}\mid\psi_{gj}\rangle +$$

$$+\langle\psi_{gj}\mid V_{H}\mid\psi_{gi}\rangle\langle\psi_{gi}\mid e\underline{r}\mid\psi_{u}\rangle\langle\psi_{u}\mid V_{odd}\mid\psi_{gj}\rangle + \text{h.c.}\}\,, \quad (7.7)$$

both moments depending on the magnitude of the Zeeman field. A further simplification occurs when the experimental observations are confined to the two states of a Kramers doublet (see eqn (6.1)). Only the higher-order dipole moments $\delta^{(2)}\underline{p}_{jj'}$, $\delta^{(2)}\underline{p}_{j}$ need then be considered since the static dipole moment $\delta^{(1)}\underline{p}_{j} = \delta^{(1)}\underline{p}_{j'}$ is the same for both members of the doublet and there is no first-order transition moment $\delta^{(1)}\underline{p}_{jj'}$. In this case eqn (7.6) can be reduced to the form,

$$\delta^{(2)}\underline{p}_{jj'} =$$

$$2\sum_{u}\sum_{i}^{i\neq j}\sum_{+,-}\frac{1}{E_{ug}E_{ij}}\{\langle\psi_{gj}|V_{H}|\psi_{gi}^{+,-}\rangle\langle\psi_{gi}^{+,-}|V_{odd}|\psi_{u}\rangle\langle\psi_{u}|e\underline{r}|\psi_{gj'}\rangle +$$

$$+\langle\psi_{gj}|V_{H}|\psi_{gi}^{+,-}\rangle\langle\psi_{gi}^{+,-}|e\underline{r}|\psi_{u}\rangle\langle\psi_{u}|V_{odd}|\psi_{gj'}\rangle\}\,, \quad (7.8)$$

by taking advantage of the properties under time reversal of the operators V_H, V_{odd}, $e\underline{r}$, and approximating $E_{ij} \simeq E_{ij'}$ (cf. §6.1 where the notation $\sum_{+,-}$ is defined).

It will be apparent here that we are more or less duplicating the arguments of §5.1. If we write $\underline{E}\cdot\delta^{(1)}\underline{p}_{j}$ or $\underline{E}\cdot\delta^{(2)}\underline{p}_{j}$ for the energies of the dipoles in an electric field, we obtain expressions very similar to the expressions for the electric field induced energy shifts given in eqns (5.12) and (5.13). But there is an important difference. The shifts calculated in Chapter 5 were obtained by combining V_{odd} with the induced potential δV_{odd} and not merely with the potential $e\underline{E}\cdot\underline{r}$. An induced even potential δV_{even} which couples with quadrupole and higher even moments of the paramagnetic ion was also taken into account. These extra terms represent the energy of interaction of the external electric field with the electrostatic polarization induced by the paramagnetic ion in its crystal lattice environment. The dipole moment associated with this polarisation can be deduced by equating the scalar product $\underline{E}\cdot\underline{p}_{eff}$ to the linear shift (or to the transition matrix element) calculated by taking all internal field contributions into account as in Chapter 4. The effective dipole moment $\underline{p}_{eff}$ then consists of two parts

$$\underline{p}_{eff} = \underline{p} + \underline{p}_{\Delta} \quad , \tag{7.9}$$

where $\underline{p}_{\Delta}$ is the lattice contribution.

The physical origins of $\underline{p}_{\Delta}$ can be traced by considering the situation in more detail. First let us take the case of a dipole moment $\underline{p}$ placed at the centre of a sphere hollowed out from a homogeneous dielectric. By classical electrostatics it can then be shown that a moment $\underline{p}_{\Delta,\mathrm{dielec}} = \frac{1}{3}(\varepsilon_r - 1)\underline{p}$ is induced in the surroundings. The two moments $\underline{p}$ and $\underline{p}_{\Delta,\mathrm{dielec}}$ together have an energy of interaction $\frac{1}{3}(\varepsilon_r + 2)\underline{p}\cdot\underline{E}_{app}$ with the applied electric field and correspond to the shift which one would calculate by taking the Lorentz field (eqn (4.7),p.101) as the field interacting with the dipole.

If we examine the interaction between the paramagnetic ion and its near environment more carefully, we find that there can be a number of other contributions to $\underline{p}_{eff}$, i.e. polarizations of the near environment depending on the quantum state of the paramagnetic ion. A full consideration of the general case would essentially amount to a rehearsal of the discussion given in Chapter 4, so we shall use a single example for the purpose of illustration. Let us suppose that the ionic charge distribution possesses an electric quadrupole moment. This moment generates short range electrostatic fields (falling off $\propto 1/R^4$) and induces dipole moments in the atoms in the immediate neighbourhood. The net effect depends on the geometry of the environment. If the environment contains equivalent pairs of atoms lying on opposite sides of the paramagnetic ion (i.e. if the paramagnetic ion is at a centrosymmetric site) then there is no net contribution to $\underline{p}_\Delta$ since the induced dipoles are oppositely oriented and cancel one another. If, however, the surrounding ions do not subtend inversion symmetry at the paramagnetic centre, then the induced moments in the environment will sum vectorially to give a resultant electric dipole moment $\underline{p}_\Delta$. (Electronic polarization and ionic motion of the surroundings may of course both contribute to this induced lattice moment.†) The lattice dipole moment arising in the manner described above corresponds to the shift associated with the second-degree term in the induced even potential δV_{even}. Other terms in δV_{even} and δV_{odd} correspond to polarization of the lattice environment by dipole, quadrupole, and higher moments of the paramagnetic ion.

It should be noted that permanent electric dipole moments do not occur for ions at sites with D_3, D_4, S_4, D_{2d}, D_6, C_{3h}, D_{3h}, T, T_d point symmetry, although they may be induced by the action of the Zeeman field. This characteristic is associated

---

†The polarization of the environment associated with ionic movements attains equilibrium in times which are short compared with the period of a microwave resonance field. It is reasonable therefore to use static values for the induced potentials, and include the effects of ionic motion, when deriving effective values for the electric dipole transition moments.

with the absence of the lowest-order odd harmonics $C_l^q(\theta,\phi)$ in the crystal field (Table 4.1,p.109). It can also be inferred from the fact that, barring the case of non-Kramers degeneracy, the tensor parameters (Fig. 3.3,p.52) yield no first-order frequency shift in zero magnetic field. Transition dipole moments can occur however as may be seen by writing out the linear electric field effect spin Hamiltonian for these point symmetries.

7.2. PARAELECTRIC RESONANCE EXPERIMENTS

Experiments are most conveniently considered from the phenomenological standpoint. Brief consideration of the conditions of a typical experiment, and a glance at the experimental values for T_{ijk}, R_{ijk}, will show that electric field resonance is usually relatively weak, and that one can only expect to observe it under special circumstances. A cavity arrangement for observing electric resonance is shown schematically in Fig. 7.1. The sample is first located in position A where the microwave magnetic field is at its maximum. It is then moved to position B where the magnetic field is at a minimum and the electric field at a maximum. Resonance signals are measured in both locations and are compared with a standard signal (e.g. from a sample of DPPH) which remains in position C throughout. For an empty TE_{101} cavity the peak electric field (in volts) is ≃ 300 times the peak magnetic field (in Gauss). Ignoring for the moment the reduction of the electric field which tends to occur in the sample, we therefore estimate that the transition probabilities associated with the spin operator S_k for a Kramers doublet sample placed in the two positions will roughly be in the ratio

$$W_B/W_A = (300\, T_{ijk}H_j/g_{j'k})^2 , \qquad (7.10)$$

where the subscript i denotes the axis of the microwave $\underline{E}$ field

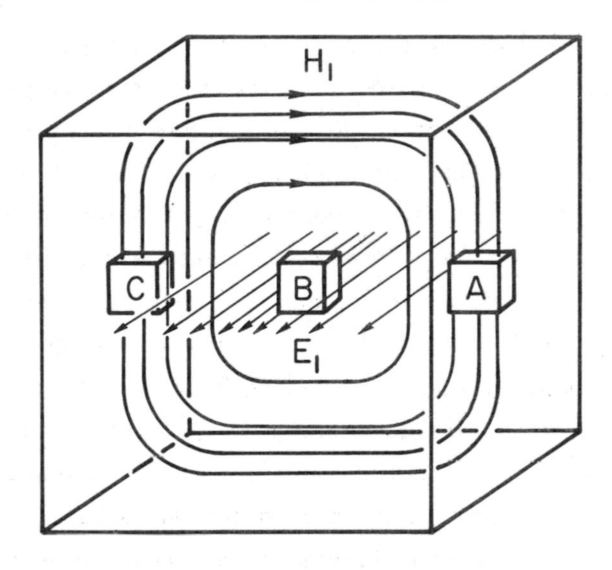

FIG. 7.1. Microwave electric and magnetic fields in a TE_{101} cavity. In a typical paraelectric resonance experiment the sample is placed at position B. Comparison with the magnetic resonance signal can be made by moving the sample to position A. A standard magnetic resonance sample (e.g. DPPH) located at position C throughout the experiment is useful for facilitating comparisons between signals obtained with the test sample at positions A and B.

vector, j' the axis of the microwave H field vector, and j (perpendicular to E and H) the axis of the Zeeman field.

Even in a favourable case, this ratio is quite small. Suppose we take $g \simeq 2$, $H_{j'} \simeq 3500$ G (frequency $\simeq$ 10 GHz) and $T \simeq 10^{-7}$ (see tables of experimental values in Chapter 10). We then obtain the ratio $W_B/W_A = 2{\cdot}8 \times 10^{-2}$. A paraelectric resonance effect which is as small as this in relation to the magnetic resonance effect is hard to demonstrate experimentally since any finite sized sample will extend partly into a region of microwave magnetic field even when placed at position B. By working with larger values of the Zeeman field and using cavities designed specifically to concentrate the electric field in the sample, it might, however, be possible to make the detection of electric resonance somewhat easier. It should also be noted that the detection of paraelectric resonance in a Kramers doublet becomes easier at higher operating frequencies. The ratio (7.10) would be ≃ 0·34 for the case just discussed if the experiment were performed at 35 GHz.

Demonstrations of the electric resonance effect have for the most part been based on the transition matrix element $R_{ijk}\langle\psi_1 \mid S_jS_k \mid \psi_2\rangle$ or on matrix elements occurring in the special type of Hamiltonian discussed in §3.10, since cases can be found in which these are quite large whilst the corresponding magnetic transitions are forbidden or only weakly allowed. The experiments of Ludwig and Ham (1962) on the Mn^+ substitutional site in silicon afford a good illustration since the spin Hamiltonians are simple and the relevant parameters are known from a d.c. frequency shift experiment.

The Mn^+ ion occupies a site with T_d symmetry. The electron configuration is $(3d)^6$ and there are two manifolds of states which can be observed in EPR of which only the $J = 1$ manifold need concern us here. The normal spin Hamiltonian contains an isotropic g-value and no D-term and the electric effect Hamiltonian is

$$\mathcal{H}_{\text{elec}} =$$

$$\beta T_{14}\{E_x(H_yS_z+H_zS_y) + E_y(H_xS_z+H_zS_x) + E_z(H_xS_y+H_yS_x)\} +$$

$$+ R_{14}\{E_x(S_yS_z+S_zS_y) + E_y(S_xS_z+S_zS_x) + E_z(S_xS_y+S_yS_z)\}\,, \qquad (7.11)$$

with $T_{14} = 850 \times 10^{-9}\ V^{-1}$ cm and $R_{14} = 7{\cdot}5 \times 10^4$ Hz V^{-1} cm
The g-shift portion of (7.11) is expressed in terms of an equivalent symmetrical parameter T_{14} but this need not concern us here since the experiments are based on the R_{14} term.

The form of the Hamiltonian makes it possible to test for

electric resonance by merely rotating the Zeeman field, as well as by actually moving the sample. Thus if $\underline{H}_0$ and $\underline{E}$ are both along the z-axis, the levels are eigenstates of S_z and the term $R_{14}E_z(S_xS_y+S_yS_x)$ can induce $\Delta M_J = 2$ transitions between the $M_J = \pm 1$ states, whilst if $\underline{H}_0$ is along the z-axis and $\underline{E}$ along the x-axis (in practice $\underline{H}_0$ is rotated relative to $\underline{E}$) the relevant term is $R_{14}E_x(S_yS_z+S_zS_y)$ which cannot induce $\Delta M_J = 2$ transitions. The cavity used in these experiments was cylindrical rather than rectangular, as in Fig. 7.1, with position A on the cylindrical axis (where H_1 is at a maximum in the TE_{011} mode). In sample-moving experiments position B was displaced radially towards the cavity wall.

The tests showed the paraelectric resonance effect clearly but at the same time they illustrated some of the difficulties encountered in performing such experiments. Rotation of $\underline{H}_0$ with the sample in position B resulted in a virtual disappearance of the signal when $\underline{E}$ was perpendicular to $\underline{H}_0$. On the other hand, a displacement of the sample towards position A increased the signal strength in spite of the fact that the E field tends to zero here and the $\Delta M_J = 2$ transition is magnetically forbidden. This anomaly was explained by pointing out that random strains in the sample weaken the $\Delta M_J = 2$ selection rule. Even so, supposing the selection rule to be entirely inoperative, it is perhaps surprising to find that the signal is actually stronger in position A. We should however remember that our rough estimates have taken no account of the sample depolarizing factor[†] which further reduces the electric resonance signal without affecting magnetic resonance. In the present instance this factor is especially large on account of the high relative permittivity of silicon.

Some similar experiments have been performed by Culvahouse, Schinke, and Foster (1967) on Pr^{3+} in lanthanum zinc double nitrate, by Williams (1967) on Pr^{3+} in yttrium ethyl sulphate, and by Christensen (1969) in Co^{2+} in CdTe. In the first two cases the symmetry is trigonal and the ground state consists of a non-Kramers doublet describable by the spin Hamiltonians of eqn (3.74) (p.92). Systems with this type of spin Hamiltonian tend to be good ones for demonstrating the electric resonance effect since the electric effects are usually large while the interaction with the microwave magnetic field is weak and would vanish altogether in the absence of distortions and crystal strains. The microwave magnetic field transition probability for Pr^{3+} in the two lattices noted above is $W_A = \frac{1}{4} G(\omega)\hbar^{-2}\left(g_z \beta H_1 \bar{\Delta}/\hbar\omega_{12}\right)^2$, where $\bar{\Delta}^2 = \bar{\Delta}_x^2 + \bar{\Delta}_y^2$ is the r.m.s. value of the distortion parameters and $\hbar\omega_{12}$ is the resonance interval. The electric effect Hamiltonian is given by eqn (3.80) and the electric resonance transition probability $W_B = \frac{1}{4} G(\omega)\hbar^{-2}(E_x\delta)^2$. The electric field shift was experimentally estimated to be of the order of 10^4 Hz V^{-1} cm in both cases. A figure comparing the resonance signals obtained by placing the sample at the electric field and magnetic field maxima in a rectangular cavity is given by Williams and clearly demonstrates the paraelectric resonance effect. (The figure is reproduced in Abragam and Bleaney (1970), p.216.)

The results obtained for Pr^{3+} in trigonal non-centrosymmetric lattices show that it can sometimes be better to place the sample in the microwave electric field rather than in the magnetic field, especially when magnetic resonance signals are weak because of symmetry and selection rules. Further investigations of this type

---

† The Hamiltonian $\mathcal{H}_{elec}$ is defined in terms of the bulk fields E_i in the sample. In parallel-plate geometry the field inside the sample and normal to the surface is ε_r times smaller than the field just outside (e.g. the cavity field). The sample will, of course, distort the cavity field and the actual relationship between the E_i and the microwave power level has to be computed with regard to the geometry of sample and cavity.

have been made by Moore, Bates, and Al Sharbati (1973), who use a novel thermal method to detect resonance.

The Pr^{3+} results also suggest that the electric resonance effect may sometimes afford the simplest and most convenient way of measuring the electric field shift parameters themselves. This is probably true for a limited number of cases where the shift is large and where measurement by another method would pose special difficulties. For example, in the case of Pr^{3+} in trigonal crystals the line is very broad and the directly observed shifts are proportional to the random strain parameter Δ (eqn (3.83),p.96). This parameter would have to be determined separately in order to extract δ from the measurements. In a paraelectric resonance experiment, on the other hand, the result depends on δ alone as it appears in the transition matrix element. (Comparison would have to be made with a standard sample and not with the magnetic resonance signal from the Pr^{3+} ions to avoid re-introducing Δ into the ratio.)

Electric resonance experiments might also prove useful in cases where it is desirable to distinguish between the parameters T_{ijk} and T_{ikj}, since these cannot be separated from one another in frequency-shift experiments (see §10.6). Accurate determinations would most probably require the design of special cavity structures both in order to maximize the electric field strength in the sample and to provide a geometry in which the electric resonance field could be calculated reliably.

7.3. MAGNETOELECTRIC EFFECTS IN PARAMAGNETISM

The static electric dipole moments associated with the resonance states can, under the appropriate circumstances, sum to give a bulk electrostatic polarization of the sample which is detectable by its dependence on the Zeeman field or by changes associated with resonance transitions between the states. To form some idea of the orders of magnitude concerned, let us estimate the electrostatic dipole moment for a single 'paramagnetic' ion in debye units (1 debye unit = 10^{-18} e.s.u. cm = $3{\cdot}33 \times 10^{-30}$ Cm). In the case of an ion having an electric field induced D-shift we can write

$$\underline{E}{\cdot}\underline{p}_{eff} = h\delta\nu = hE\overline{R}\ , \tag{7.12}$$

where $\overline{R}$ is the shift in hertz per unit electric field ($\overline{R} \sim R_{ij}$), $\delta\nu$ is the frequency shift, and h is Planck's constant. Expressing p_{eff} in debye units and taking E in volts per centimetre we find that

$$p_{eff} = 1{\cdot}8 \times 10^{-6}\ \overline{R}\ . \tag{7.13}$$

If, on the other hand, the electric dipole moment is associated with the g-shift parameters it will be proportional to the Zeeman field. For one level of a doublet, we have

$$\underline{E}{\cdot}\underline{p}_{eff} = \frac{1}{2}\ \delta g\beta H_0 = E(\overline{B}/4g^2)g\beta H_0\ , \tag{7.14}$$

where

$$E\overline{B} = \delta(g^2),\quad (\overline{B} \simeq B_{ij})\ .$$

Substituting $g\beta H_0 = \frac{1}{3}\ cm^{-1}$ (as for resonance experiments in the X-band region) and expressing p_{eff} in debye units, we have

$$p_{eff} = 0{\cdot}5 \times 10^4\ \overline{B}/g^2\ . \tag{7.15}$$

Taking $\overline{R}$ = 100 Hz V^{-1} cm and $\overline{B} = 10^{-7}\ V^{-1}$ cm as typical values for the shift parameters and setting g = 2, in eqns (7.14)-(7.15) we thus obtain the dipole moments

$p_{eff} \simeq 1{\cdot}8 \times 10^{-4}$ debye units due to the D-shift,

$p_{eff} \simeq 1{\cdot}25 \times 10^{-4}$ debye units due to the g-shift.

The resulting bulk polarization in a sample containing only one kind of site, and at very low temperatures where all the spins occupied the same quantum state, would be appreciable. For instance in a dilute paramagnetic sample with 10^{19} spins per cm^3 the bulk polarization $\simeq 10^{-3}$ e.s.u. cm^{-2} ($3{\cdot}3 \times 10^{-9}$ Cm^{-2}) and the field at a surface normal to the polarization vector $\simeq 30$ mV cm^{-1}. But in a typical situation the bulk polarization is likely to be considerably smaller than this since the spins are distributed between two or more levels and may also occupy different kinds of sites giving rise to dipoles with different orientations. Further knowledge of the system concerned is needed in order to estimate how much the bulk polarization is reduced on account of the multiplicity of different sites. The bulk polarization will of course disappear altogether if the host lattice contains similarly populated inversion image sites, since in this case equivalent energy levels correspond to oppositely oriented electric dipoles.

From the experimental point of view the means used to demonstrate the existence of a bulk polarization can be as significant a consideration as the magnitude of the polarization itself. Since a d.c. polarization tends to be neutralized by the migration of surface charges, it is necessary to induce some kind of change as, for instance, by altering the populations of the levels. A magnetic resonance method might perhaps be suitable here, although it does not appear to have been tried. As an alternative the level populations can be changed thermodynamically by raising or lowering the Zeeman field. The change, of course, will generally amount to only a fraction of the total population, and the effects will be correspondingly smaller than those estimated above.

An experiment of this type has been reported by Hou and Bloembergen (1965) using a 100 per cent concentrated sample of $NiSO_4.6H_2O$. There are four types of site in this material related by 90° rotations about the crystal c-axis and arranged in such a way that the induced dipoles only partially cancel. Both D-shifts and g-shifts can occur in Ni^{2+} (S=1) the former being quite large ($\overline{R} \simeq 10^3$ Hz V^{-1} cm. The magnetoelectric effects were observed non-resonantly by connecting an electrometer amplifier with lock-in to the sample and applying a modulating field ≃ 90 G in conjunction with a d.c. field of several kilogauss.

The magnetic modulating field causes changes in the bulk electrostatic polarization in two ways. It changes the value of the individual electric dipoles and can also cause a redistribution of the Boltzmann populations. Thus in the simple case of a Kramers doublet where $p \propto H$, and the population difference $\propto H$, the bulk polarization, which is the product of these two factors $\propto H^2$. Writing $H = H_0+H_{mod}$ (where H_{mod} is the amplitude of the modulating field) we see that the modulated component of polarization is proportional to the product H_0H_{mod}. (If the modulating period is shorter than the spin lattice relaxation time the modulated component is due only to changes in p and has half its full value.) The dipoles $\underline{p}_{eff}$ associated with the D-shift can also give rise to changes in the bulk electrostatic polarization when the magnetic field is modulated. Here again population changes and changes in the state composition both contribute to the overall effect which is proportional to $H_0{}^2$ (or $\propto H_0H_{mod}$).

In thermodynamic equilibrium the bulk changes in the material due to the above mechanisms can be represented by writing down a thermodynamic potential

$$F(\text{magnetoelectric}) = -\xi_{ijk}E_iH_jH_k \quad , \qquad (7.16)$$

where ξ_{ijk} is a third-rank tensor. The elements of this tensor are restricted according to the point symmetry of the crystal lattice and not the point symmetry of the paramagnetic site. For instance, in $NiSO_4.6H_2O$ the point symmetry at each Ni^{2+} site is C_2, allowing for eight coefficients T_{ijk} (seven coefficients R_{ijk}), but the lattice symmetry is D_4, and there is therefore only one coefficient ξ_{ijk} (see Fig. 3.1, p.46). From a microscopic point of view this simplification is a consequence of summing the contributions from the different dipoles $\underline{p}_{eff}$ at four sites in the crystal.

Magnetoelectric effects can also be observed by measuring changes in the equilibrium magnetization when electric fields are applied to the sample. This is implicit in the form of the thermodynamic potential (7.16) and is also easily understood from a microscopic point of view. For instance, in a Kramers doublet the electric field induced frequency shift $\delta\nu$ can be thought of as being associated with small changes $\pm\delta\mu$ in the magnetic moments of the two states, these changes being caused by electric field induced modifications of the crystal field and of the state compositions. Since $|\delta\mu|$ is proportional to E, and the population difference between the two states is proportional to H_0, the change equilibrium bulk magnetization is proportional to EH_0. The D-shift can likewise change the bulk magnetization by an amount which is proportional to E and to H_0, the effect here being due to the small redistribution of populations which occurs when the levels are shifted by the applied electric field. This electrically induced bulk magnetization was also observed by Hou and Bloembergen in $NiSO_4.6H_2O$, but proved to be more difficult to detect than the inverse effect.

The interest in these experiments in paramagnetic materials derives largely from their resemblance to magnetoelectric effects observed in ferromagnetic and antiferromagnetic crystals (Astrov 1959; Folen, Rado, and Stalder 1961; Rado 1964). Such effects are much larger than those in paramagnetic materials and do not require helium temperatures for their observation. Attempts have been made to interpret them microscopically in terms of D- and g-shifts (Rado 1961), but it appears that electric field induced shifts in the exchange coupling parameters must also be considered (Date, Kanamori, and Tachiki 1961). The effects are, of course, true bulk effects involving a cooperative phenomenon and do not merely represent the summation of effects due to an assembly of individual non-interacting centres. Some useful insights could perhaps be gained, however, by making linear electric field effect measurements in dilute materials, especially if shifts were to be measured for coupled pairs of ions (see §8.2).

8. Electric field effects in endor and for coupled pairs

8.1. ELECTRIC FIELD EFFECTS IN ENDOR

The parameter A_{jk} belonging to the electron-nuclear term $A_{jk}S_jI_k$ in the spin Hamiltonian (eqn (3.1),p.38) can, when large enough, be measured by observing the fine structure separation of the EPR lines in a microwave resonance spectrum. But the accuracy of the measurement is limited by the inhomogeneous broadening of the EPR lines (widths are typically $\gtrsim$ 10 MHz). A more precise measurement can often be made by using a variable radio-frequency ω_{RF} in conjunction with the microwave resonance apparatus to induce resonance transitions between the nuclear hyperfine levels. Such transitions are indicated by changes in the microwave resonance transitions between the nuclear hyperfine levels. Such transitions are indicated by changes in the microwave resonance conditions (usually in the degree of saturation) which appear when the radio-frequency is swept through the appropriate values.

This technique is known as electron-nuclear double resonance (ENDOR) and is described in detail elsewhere (see e.g. Abragam and Bleaney (1970), Chapter 4). The ENDOR linewidth (i.e. the range of values of ω_{RF} over which a double resonance effect can be observed) is usually two or more orders of magnitude less than the EPR linewidth, thus making it possible not only to increase the accuracy but also to measure very small couplings such as those which are associated with the interaction between electron spins and nuclei in their immediate environment. Line-splittings due to these couplings tend otherwise to be concealed by the inhomogeneous broadening of the electron resonance line.

The parameters F_{ijk} in the electric field shift terms $F_{ijk}E_iS_jI_k$ (eqn (3.2)) can also sometimes be measured in microwave resonance experiments by finding the difference between electric field shifts associated with different hyperfine lines in the EPR spectrum (see Table 10.5, p.251). But the accuracy is poor and double resonance methods must generally be used. Reichert and Pershan (1965) and Usmani and Reichert (1969, 1970) have performed a series of such experiments in which the electric field shifts were measured for the superhyperfine coupling between F-centres and the neighbouring nuclei in alkali halides. Some similar experiments have also been reported by Baran, Grachev, Ishchenko, and Chernenko (1973).

The method used was analogous to the 'direct method' described in §2.3. ENDOR resonance lines were observed by the usual microwave saturation technique, a comparison being made between the spectra obtained with and without the application of a d.c. electric field (see Fig. 8.1). As may be imagined, a number of technical difficulties, associated with the simultaneous application of d.c. and r.f. fields to a sample in the microwave cavity, must be faced when performing experiments of this kind (for cavity see Fig. 2.7, p.23). An additional problem is also sometimes encountered in F-centre experiments because of the low dielectric strength of the samples resulting from the X-irradiation of the material. Dielectric breakdown limited the applied field to values < 60 kV cm^{-1} in the work reported by Reichert and Pershan and by Usmani and Reichert. Baran et al (1973),however, were able to reach fields as high as 700 kV cm^{-1} for F-centres in LiF.

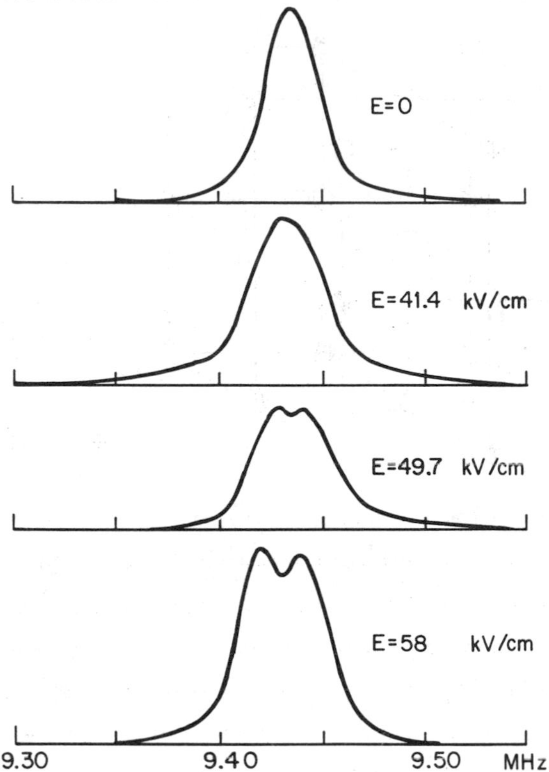

FIG. 8.1. Electric field induced splitting of the ENDOR line associated with the $M_{\perp} = \frac{3}{2} \rightleftarrows \frac{1}{2}$ transition of the second shell of ^{35}Cl ^{37}-Cl nuclei coupled with the F-centre in NaCl. (Usmani and Reichert 1969.)

8.1.1. DATA REDUCTION FOR ENDOR FREQUENCY SHIFTS. The analysis of data obtained in this case of simple lattices is often complicated by the fact that there are a number of like nuclei coupled to the electron spin. The problem of extracting the required parameters for a system of this kind is illustrated by the case of F-centres in halides studied by Usmani and Reichert, whose work is used as the basis for the following discussion. The resonance properties of the system of one electron spin and six nearest-neighbour nuclei, as shown in Fig. 8.2, can be described by the spin Hamiltonians

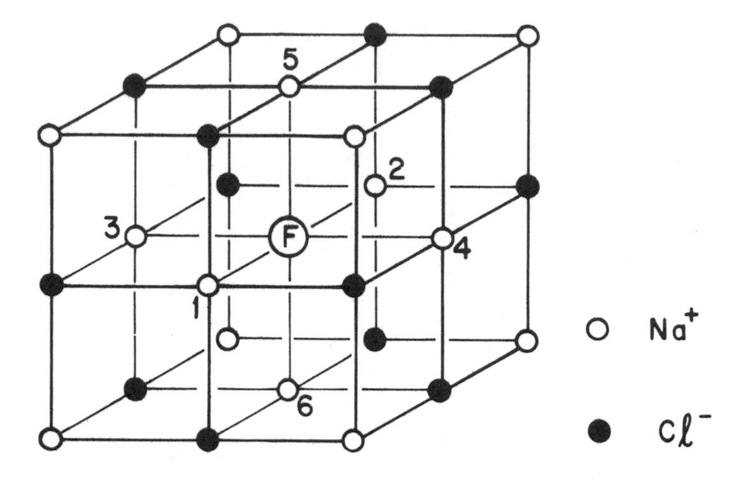

FIG. 8.2. F-centre in NaCl lattice. The electric field induced shift in the contact interaction parameter between the F-centre and the nearest-neighbour ^{23}Na nuclei is obtained by measuring shifts in the corresponding ENDOR lines. The experiment is performed by orienting $\underline{H}_0$ and $\underline{E}_{app}$ along one of the crystalline axes, e.g. the line joining nuclei 5 and 6, and observing the ENDOR resonance due to these two nuclei only.

$$\mathcal{H} = g\beta\underline{H}.\underline{S} + \sum_{\nu=1}^{6} \{A_{jk\nu}S_j I_{k\nu} + \gamma_{N\nu}\underline{H}.\underline{I}_\nu + Q_{jk\nu}I_{j\nu}I_{k\nu}\} \tag{8.1}$$

and

$$\mathcal{H}_{elec} = \sum_{\nu=1}^{6} F_{ijk\nu}E_i S_j I_{k\nu} \quad , \tag{8.2}$$

where a summation over i,j,k is implied by the repeated subscripts as in eqns (3.1) and (3.2). The description has been specialized to the case in which $S = \frac{1}{2}$, g is isotropic, and the g-shift term in $\mathcal{H}_{elec}$ vanishes as is appropriate for an F-centre electron at a centrosymmetric site. The shifts in the nuclear quadrupole term have been omitted in eqn (8.2), since it appears that these shifts are unimportant for the system in question.

ENDOR experiments in the halide systems were performed with $\underline{E}_{app}$ and $\underline{H}_0$ lying along a line joining the F-centre with two nuclei situated on opposite sides of it. Thus, for measurements involving the nearest-neighbour nuclei $\underline{E}_{app}$ and $\underline{H}_0$ were oriented along the (001) direction joining nuclei 5 and 6 in Fig. 8.2, this direction being defined as the z-axis. Provided that there is no mixing of eigenstates between these two nuclei and the rest† we can then work with the simplified Hamiltonians

$$\mathcal{H} = g\beta H_z S_z +$$

$$+ \sum_{\nu=5,6} \{a_\nu \underline{S}\cdot\underline{I}_\nu + b_\nu(3S_z I_{z\nu} - \underline{S}\cdot\underline{I}_\nu) + Q_\nu(I_{z\nu}^2 - \tfrac{1}{3} I_\nu(I_\nu+1))\} \quad , \tag{8.3}$$

$$\mathcal{H}_{elec} = \sum_{\nu=5,6}{}' F_{33\nu} E_z S_z I_{z\nu} + F_{31\nu} E_z S_z (I_{x\nu} + I_{y\nu}). \tag{8.4}$$

Eqns (8.3)-(8.4) correspond to the case where the point symmetry at the nuclear sites is C_{4v} (as for nuclei 5,6) or C_{3v} (as for certain remoter nuclei), and would assume a some what more complicated form for some outer-shell nuclei. In the experimental work discussed here it is however argued that electric field induced shifts in the anisotropic electron nuclei coupling terms will be small compared with shifts in the isotropic term $a\underline{S}\cdot\underline{I}$. Hence,

---

† The criterion here is that differences in the energies of the superhyperfine levels due to the quadrupole term and to the anisotropy in the electron nuclear term should be large compared with any indirect coupling between nuclei 5,6 and the remaining nuclei. This will become clear from the subsequent discussion.

only the first term in eqn (8.4) need be retained as in

$$\mathcal{H}_{elec} = \sum_{\nu=1,2} F_{33\nu} E_z S_z I_{z\nu}, \tag{8.5}$$

$$F_{33\nu} = \pm\ \partial a / \partial E_{app} \tag{8.6}$$

this form of Hamiltonian being adequate to describe all pairs of neighbouring nuclei (denoted henceforth as 1,2) for which observations can be made. The shift parameters are opposite in sign for the nuclei on opposite sides of the F-centre, the two nuclear sites being inversion images of one another.

Before discussing the situation defined by the Hamiltonians (8.3)-(8.4) let us consider some simplified cases. First let us suppose that one of the two nuclei has a spin $I = \frac{1}{2}$ but that the other nucleus consists of a different species for which $I = 0$. The shifts for the states $|M_S, M_I\rangle = |\frac{1}{2}, \pm\frac{1}{2}\rangle$ are then $\pm\frac{1}{4} F_{33}E_z$, and the shift in the $M_S = \frac{1}{2}$ ENDOR line is $-\frac{1}{2} F_{33}E_z$.

The situation is essentially no different when there are two nuclei with $I = \frac{1}{2}$ with negligible coupling between them. We can then construct four wavefunctions $|M_S, M_{I_1}, M_{I_2}\rangle = |\frac{1}{2}, \frac{1}{2}, \frac{1}{2}\rangle$, $|\frac{1}{2}, \frac{1}{2}, -\frac{1}{2}\rangle$, $|\frac{1}{2}, -\frac{1}{2}, \frac{1}{2}\rangle$, $|\frac{1}{2}, -\frac{1}{2}, -\frac{1}{2}\rangle$ for the $M_S = \frac{1}{2}$ manifold of shfs states, the middle two being degenerate. This degeneracy is raised in <u>first order</u> by the applied electric field as it is, for example, in the case of the linear Stark effect of hydrogen, giving shifts $0, \frac{1}{2} F_{33}E_z, -\frac{1}{2} F_{33}E_z, 0$ for the four levels (see Fig. 8.3(a)). The shifts for the $M_S = -\frac{1}{2}$ manifold of states are similar but opposite in sign. For this reason, and also because the shift reverses sign when one interchanges M_{I_1} and M_{I_2}, the ENDOR line will be observed to split just as it does for inversion image sites in electron resonance. Physically we can regard the shifts associated with the nuclei I_1 and

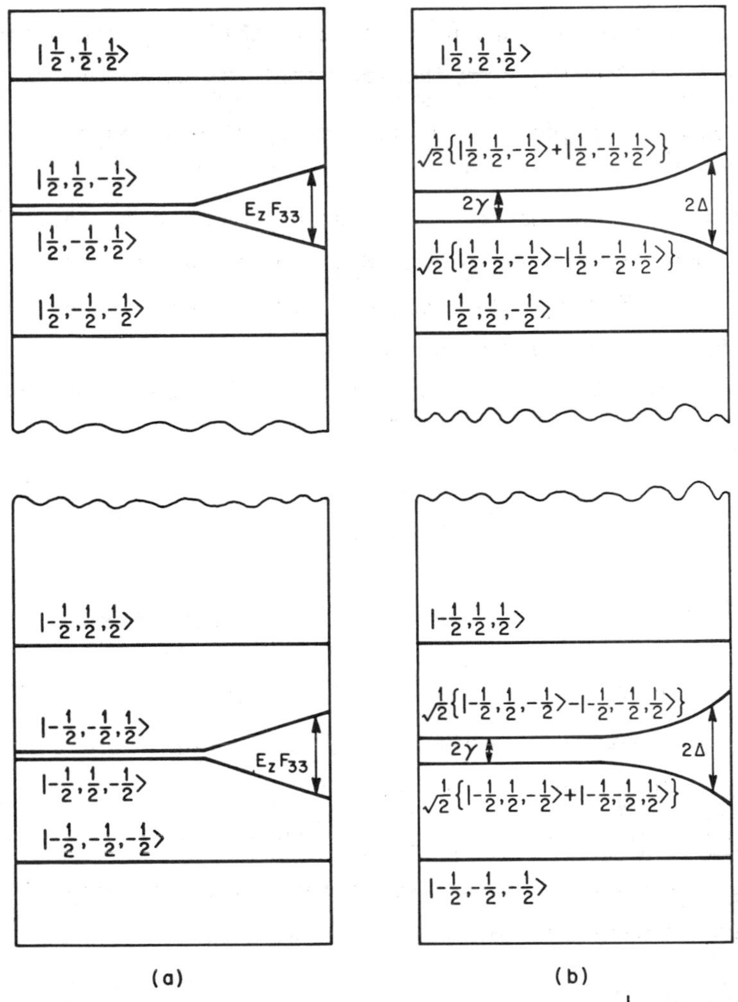

FIG. 8.3. Level schemes for an electron spin ($S = \frac{1}{2}$) coupled to two nuclei ($I_1 = I_2 = \frac{1}{2}$) at positions 5,6 in Fig. 8.2 showing the shifts due to the electric field effect term $F_{33}E_zS_z(I_{1z} + I_{2z})$. State functions are written in the form $|M_S, M_{I_1}, M_{I_2}\rangle$.

(a) No coupling between I_1 and I_2. The shift is linear in E_z.

(b) I_1 and I_2 coupled by a flip-flop term $\gamma(I_{1+}I_{2-} + I_{1-}I_{2+})$. The splitting between the middle pairs of levels is 2Δ, where $\Delta = \{\gamma^2 + (\frac{1}{2}E_zF_{33})^2\}^{\frac{1}{2}}$. The electric field shift is quadratic for small values of E_z and becomes linear when $E_zF_{33} \gg \gamma$.

I_2 as independent of one another, the zero shift for the states with $M_{I_1} = M_{I_2}$ following from the fact that the coefficients F_{ijk} have opposite signs for nuclei on opposite sides of the F-centre.

Next let us consider coupling between the two nuclei. This does not appear explicitly in eqn (8.3) but arises as a result of common coupling of the nuclei to the electron spin via the terms in a_ν and b_ν. It can be represented formally by introducing a 'flip-flop' term $\gamma(I_{1+}I_{2-} + I_{2+}I_{1-})$ into the nuclear Hamiltonian, the constant

$$\gamma = (a-b)^2/4g\beta H_0 \tag{8.7}$$

being derived by contracting the second-order perturbation terms $\langle\frac{1}{2}, \frac{1}{2}, -\frac{1}{2}|A_{jk}S_jI_{k2}| -\frac{1}{2}, \frac{1}{2}, \frac{1}{2}\rangle\langle -\frac{1}{2}, \frac{1}{2}, \frac{1}{2}| A_{jk}S_jI_{k1}|\frac{1}{2}, -\frac{1}{2}, \frac{1}{2}\rangle/g\beta H_0$, which couple eigenstates $|M_S, M_{I1}, M_{I2}\rangle$ of the full Hamiltonian and replacing them with first-order terms $\gamma\langle\frac{1}{2}, -\frac{1}{2}|I_{1+}I_{2-}+I_{2+}I_{1-}| -\frac{1}{2}, \frac{1}{2}\rangle$ in the nuclear Hamiltonian. For the $M_S = \frac{1}{2}$ manifold of superhyperfine states the effective nuclear Hamiltonians then assume the forms

$$\mathcal{H}^{(N)} = \alpha(I_{1z}+I_{2z}) + \gamma(I_{1+}I_{2-} + I_{1-}I_{2+}) \quad , \tag{8.8}$$

$$\mathcal{H}^{(N)}_{elec} = \frac{1}{2}\,\delta(I_{1z}-I_{2z}) \quad , \tag{8.9}$$

where

$$\alpha = \gamma_N H_0 + \frac{1}{2}a+b-\gamma \quad ,$$

$$\delta = E_z F_{33} \quad .$$

The flip-flop coupling term breaks the degeneracy of the states $|\frac{1}{2}, \frac{1}{2}, -\frac{1}{2}\rangle$, $|\frac{1}{2}, -\frac{1}{2}, \frac{1}{2}\rangle$, giving two new states $1/\sqrt{2}\ \{|\frac{1}{2}, \frac{1}{2}, -\frac{1}{2}\rangle \pm |\frac{1}{2}, -\frac{1}{2}, \frac{1}{2}\rangle\}$ separated by an interval 2γ. (see Fig. 8.3(b)). Each of these states has a definite parity, the sum state being even and the difference state odd, and neither state will be perturbed in first order by an electric field. An exact diagonalization of the energy matrix yields the energies $\Delta = \pm\ \{\gamma^2 + (\frac{1}{2}\ E_zF_{33})^2\}^{\frac{1}{2}}$ indicating that the shift only becomes linear when $E_zF_{33} >> \gamma$ thus breaking the flip-flop coupling. For $E_zF_{33} \stackrel{\sim}{<} \gamma$ there is a transition between a low-field region of quadratic shifts and a high-field region of linear shifts analogous to the Zeeman-Paschen Back effects in atomic spectroscopy.

The generalization to the case of $I_1 = I_2 > \frac{1}{2}$ to anisotropic A_{ij}, to other geometrical arrangements, or to more than two nuclei complicates the problem, for example by introducing terms of the form $\beta(I_{1z}^{\ 2} + I_{2z}^{\ 2} - \frac{5}{2})$, $(\beta = Q-\gamma)$ into the nuclear Hamiltonian $\mathcal{H}^{(N)}$, but it leaves the basic features the same as in the above example. The relationship between the magnitudes of the flip-flop coupling and of the parameters which break the degeneracy of the superhyperfine states in the absence of this term remains the essential criterion. In the F-centre experiments in alkali halides degeneracy may be broken by the nuclear quadrupole coupling since the surrounding nuclei K^{39}, Br^{81}, Cl^{35}, Na^{23}, etc., have spin $I = \frac{3}{2}$. The nuclei on opposite sides of the F-centre may also belong to two different species as for example when one nucleus is ^{35}Cl (25 per cent abundant) and the other is ^{37}Cl (75 per cent abundant). There are then two distinct ENDOR lines for each M_S-state, and the shifts are the same as they would be for single nuclei interacting with the electron.

It should also be remembered that the two nuclei may be effectively independent of one another even when they belong to the same species, if they are in quantum states which are not coupled by the flip-flop term. Thus for two identical $I = \frac{3}{2}$ nuclei we have the following possibilities. The six states $|\frac{3}{2},-\frac{1}{2}$, $|-\frac{1}{2},\frac{3}{2}$, $|\frac{3}{2},-\frac{3}{2}$, $|-\frac{3}{2},\frac{3}{2}$, $|\frac{1}{2},-\frac{3}{2}$, $|-\frac{3}{2},\frac{1}{2}$ are not coupled by the flip-flop term and have linear shifts which can be found by summing the shifts associated with M_{I_1} and M_{I_2}. (For example, the state $|\frac{3}{2},-\frac{1}{2}$ has a shift $\frac{3}{4}\delta + \frac{1}{4}\delta = \delta$.) The six states coupled by the flip-flop term give combinations which have (in zero electric field) the composition $\{|\frac{1}{2},\frac{3}{2} \pm |\frac{3}{2},\frac{1}{2}\}$, $\{|-\frac{1}{2},\frac{1}{2} \pm |\frac{1}{2},-\frac{1}{2}\}$, $\{|-\frac{3}{2},-\frac{1}{2} \pm |-\frac{1}{2},-\frac{3}{2}\}$. Their field dependence is quadratic when $\delta \quad \gamma$ and linear when $\delta \quad \gamma$. Between these two limits the shifts will be $\pm\{(\frac{1}{2}\delta)^2 + (4\gamma)^2\}^{\frac{1}{2}}$ for the states $\{|-\frac{1}{2},\frac{1}{2} \pm |\frac{1}{2},-\frac{1}{2}\}$ and $\pm\{(\frac{1}{2}\delta)^2 + (3\gamma)^2\}^{\frac{1}{2}}$ for each of the remaining pairs of states. (The parameter γ is relatively small for F-centres in all but the LiF lattice, and it is generally possible with laboratory fields to pass through Paschen Back regime and observe effects which are linear in spite of the presence of flip-flop coupling.) The energies of the four remaining states $|\frac{3}{2},\frac{3}{2}$, $|-\frac{3}{2},-\frac{3}{2}$, $|\frac{1}{2},\frac{1}{2}$, $|-\frac{1}{2},-\frac{1}{2}$ are unaffected by the electric field since the shifts associated with M_{I_1} and M_{I_2} are equal and opposite and cancel out.

In the above classification of the superhyperfine states it has been assumed that $Q \quad \gamma$ and that the flip-flop coupling mechanism can therefore be ignored for many combinations of nuclear states. However if the quadrupole term is small compared with the flip-flop coupling term the resultant nuclear spin $\underline{I} = \underline{I}_1 + \underline{I}_2$ becomes the appropriate spin operator and I, M, I_1, I_2, and P (parity) are good quantum numbers of the system. Parity is even for $I = 3,1$ and odd for $I = 2,0$. No linear electric effects would be observable for any of the resulting states except in the limit $\delta \quad \gamma$ when the $\underline{I}_1 \cdot \underline{I}_2$ coupling would be broken by the applied electric field.

8.1.2. THEORETICAL CALCULATION OF SUPERHYPERFINE SHIFTS FOR HALIDE F-CENTRE. The shift parameter $\partial a/\partial E = F_{33}$ and the fractional shift parameter $(1/a)\ \partial a/\partial E$ obtained for various F-centre couplings by Usmani and Reichert are shown in Table 8.1. We can picture

TABLE 8.1

Linear electric field shifts in the contact interaction $a\underline{S}\cdot\underline{I}$ between F-centres and surrounding nuclei in halide lattices. The quantity $\partial a/\partial E$ is approximately the same as the parameter F_{33} as defined for a z-axis in the direction of the nucleus concerned. The fractional changes $(1/a)\ \partial a/\partial E$ have been calculated from the table given by Usmani and Reichert (1969).

Crystal	Shell	Direction	Nucleus	$\partial a/\partial E$ ($H_z\ V^{-1}$ cm)	$(\frac{1}{a})\ \partial a/\partial E$ (V $cm^{-1} \times 10^9$)
KBr	I	100	^{39}K	1·0±0·05	55·0
	II	110	^{81}Br	2·0±0·05	47·4
	IV	200	^{81}Br	0·33±0·02	57·5
KCl	I	100	^{39}K	0·9±0·05	43·7
	II	110	^{35}Cl	0·25±0·03	36·2
	IV	200	^{35}Cl	0·05±0·005	47·2
NaCl	I	100	^{23}Na	2·0±0·5	32·5
	II	110	^{35}Cl	0·5±0·05	40·0

these shifts as being caused in two ways: (1) by the physical movement of the ion containing the $I = \frac{1}{2}$ nucleus relative to the electron spin (ionic effect) and (2) by the polarization of the electronic charge cloud (electronic effect). Both mechanisms would cause changes in the term $a\underline{S}\cdot\underline{I}$.

The calculation resembles the calculation of g- and D-shifts for paramagnetic ions, but is in some respects simpler since the induced fields need not be treated in such detail and only one opposite-parity state need be considered instead of an entire manifold of excited states. The contact interaction constant a is given by the expression

$$a = \langle \psi_g | \mathcal{H}_a | \psi_g \rangle , \tag{8.10}$$

where ψ_g is the ground-state wavefunction of the F-centre and

$$\mathcal{H}_a = \frac{8\pi}{3} g \, g_N \mu_B \mu_N \delta(\underline{r}-\underline{R}_N) , \tag{8.11}$$

$\underline{R}_N$ being the coordinate of the neighbouring nucleus concerned. The odd field mixes an opposite-parity wavefunction ψ_u belonging to the F-centre into ψ_g, thus modifying the ground-state wavefunction to ψ_g' where

$$\psi_g' = \psi_g - \frac{1}{E_{ug}} \langle \psi_u | \delta V_{odd} | \psi_g \rangle \psi_u , \tag{8.12}$$

and giving a new contact interaction constant $a + \Delta a = \langle \psi_g' | \mathcal{H}_a | \psi_g' \rangle$. The quantities g, g_N, etc. can then be eliminated from the result by expressing it in the form $\Delta a/a$, and we are left with the fractional shift

$$\frac{\Delta a(\text{electronic})}{a} = \frac{\langle \psi_g | \delta V_{odd} | \psi_u \rangle \langle \psi_u | \delta(\underline{r}-\underline{R}_N) | \psi_g \rangle}{E_{ug} \langle \psi_g | \delta(\underline{r}-\underline{R}_N) | \psi_g \rangle} . \tag{8.13}$$

The ground state ψ_g is a hydrogen-like 1S-state. The state ψ_u is the hydrogen-like 2P state which has been shown by theoretical calculation to be the only state of opposite parity lying between the valence and conduction bands (Kubler and Friauf 1965).

The calculation of the internal field acting on the F-centre wavefunction is relatively simple. Since the centre has inversion symmetry, there is no induced even potential δV_{even}. Moreover, since the site is cubic, the lowest harmonics in V are $C_4^{0,\pm4}$ and hence by eqn (4.31)(p.114) the lowest harmonics in δV arising from polarization of the nearby atoms are the C_3^q. These harmonics cannot mix the hydrogen-like states ψ_g(1S), ψ_u(2P), and, according to the arguments given in Chapter 4, the internal field should therefore be adequately given by the Lorentz field $\frac{1}{3}(\varepsilon_r+2)\underline{E}_{app}$. The use of the Lorentz field here can be criticised however on the grounds that the F-centre wavefunction extends beyond the charges on the neighbouring ions and cannot be thought of as being contained inside a hollowed-out sphere in the dielectric. Part of the dielectric medium lies within the radius of the wavefunction. It has been suggested (Mott and Gurney 1940) that in such situations the applied field without the Lorentz correction factor $\frac{1}{3}(\varepsilon_r+2)$ may give a better approximation to the true internal field. According to this viewpoint (which is the one adopted by Usmani and Reichert) $\delta V_{odd} = e\underline{E}_{app}\cdot\underline{r}$ should be used in eqn (8.13). The spherical harmonic form of this potential corresponds to eqn (4.9) with $\frac{1}{3}(\varepsilon_r+2)$ deleted.

The ionic displacement ΔR_N due to the applied field required for the calculation of the ionic effect can be estimated from relative-permittivity data by means of eqn (4.39). The fractional change in the parameter a resulting from this mechanism is

$$\frac{\Delta a(\text{ionic})}{a} = \frac{\langle\psi_g \mid \delta(r-R_N-\Delta R_N) \mid \psi_g\rangle - \langle\psi_g \mid \delta(r-R_N) \mid \psi_g\rangle}{\langle\psi_g \mid \delta(r-R_N) \mid \psi_g\rangle}$$

$$= \frac{|\psi_g(R_N+\Delta R_N)|^2 - |\psi_g(R_N)|^2}{|\psi_g(R_N)|^2} \quad . \qquad (8.14)$$

The electronic and ionic effects were evaluated by substituting hydrogen-like wavefunctions as calculated by Gourary and Adrian (1957) in eqns (8.13) and (8.14). An alternative calculation with molecular-orbitals gave similar results, the theoretical values being within a factor 2 of the experimental measurements in both cases. The matrix elements $\langle \psi_g | \delta(r-R_N) | \psi_g \rangle$ and $\langle \psi_u | \delta(r-R_N) | \psi_g \rangle$ are of course very sensitive to the form of the F-centre wavefunction in the vicinity of the ionic core and differ by a large factor according to which kind of wavefunction is used, but fortunately the errors tend to cancel when taking the ratio $\Delta a/a$.

Some further experiments were made by Usmani and Reichert (1970) to find the electric field induced shift in the contact term for F-centres in LiF. These experiments proved more difficult since the quadrupole splitting of the ENDOR lines is unresolved, and the flip-flop coefficient γ is considerably larger than it is for F-centres in the other halides thus making it difficult to pass through the Paschen Back region into the region of linear shifts. The problem was overcome by enriching the sample in Li so that it contained a high proportion of centres having different nuclei at the two positions on opposite sides of the F-centre (e.g. positions 5,6 in Fig. 8.2). The electric effect is linear for coupled systems of this kind since the shifts due to ^{6}Li, ^{7}Li do not cancel, and the two nuclei are not coupled by a flip-flop term. The experimental result $\partial a/\partial E = 0{\cdot}36 \pm 0{\cdot}03$ Hz V^{-1} cm for the contact interaction with ^{6}Li nearest neighbours was again in good agreement with the result calculated by using simple hydrogen-like wavefunctions for the F-centre.

The Li-F centre system using unenriched LiF has been studied by Baran et al. (1973) with electric fields ≃ 700 kV cm^{-1}. (A diagram of the sample mounting arrangement, though not of the cavity, is given in the reference.) They obtain values $\partial a/\partial E = 0{\cdot}94 \pm 0{\cdot}01$ Hz V^{-1} cm for the shift in the interaction constant of the nearest-neighbour ^{7}Li nucleus with the F-centre electron and $\partial a/\partial E = 1{\cdot}21 \pm 0{\cdot}02$ Hz V^{-1} cm for the shift in the interaction constant of the nearest ^{19}F nucleus. Theoretical calculations are given by Baran et al. (1973) and by Deigen and Roitsin (1970) and give results which are, like those of Usmani and Reichert, in fair accord with experiments. ENDOR shift measurements have also been reported for the F_A(Li)-centre in KCl (Fedotov, Grachev, and Bagmut 1973). The shift in the isotropic coupling parameter for the F_A-centre and the Li nucleus is given by $|\, da/dE \,| = 0{\cdot}67 \pm 0{\cdot}05$ Hz V^{-1} cm.

The good agreement between theory and experiment obtained in the F-centre studies suggests that the measurement of electric field induced shifts in superhyperfine lines affords a reasonably reliable method for investigating the covalency of the bonds between paramagnetic ions and their ligands. Such measurements might also be used to estimate the strength of the mechanical restoring forces acting on ions in crystals. (The F_A-centre measurement reported above has been interpreted as showing that an Li^+ ion is displaced eight times as easily as a K^+ ion in KCl.) The experimental technique is not an easy one, but it appears that with data accumulation methods (as used by Usmani and Reichert) and possibly with larger fields (as used by Baran et al.) sufficiently accurate results could be obtained. Some of the difficulties encountered due to the presence of equivalent nuclei on opposite sides of the paramagnetic centre are, of course, peculiar to very regular lattices such as the halides and would not arise for sites with lower point symmetry, thus greatly simplifying the task of interpreting the data.

8.2. ELECTRIC FIELD EFFECTS FOR COUPLED PAIRS OF IONS

When two paramagnetic ions are situated close enough together for the exchange interaction $J\underline{S}_1 \cdot \underline{S}_2$ to be comparable with the other terms in the spin Hamiltonian, new sets of EPR lines corresponding to the coupled pair of ions can be observed in the resonance spectrum. (For a review of pair spectra see Owen and Harris (1972). See also Abragam and Bleaney (1970), pp. 502-14, pp. 529-35.) The question arises as to what electric field induced shifts, if any, will be seen in these resonance lines.

The situation has many points in common with that considered in the previous section. Thus two similar $S = \frac{1}{2}$ ions at inversion image sites coupled by an exchange term $J\underline{S}_1 \cdot \underline{S}_2$ will show no linear shift since the overall system is centrosymmetric and is characterized by eigenstates of well-defined parity. The shift will be quadratic unless the electric field induced perturbation is sufficient to overpower the exchange coupling. If $S > \frac{1}{2}$, however, the D-term in the spin Hamiltonian may serve to differentiate the coupled spins in the same way as the nuclear quadrupole terms in the earlier example, the relevant criterion being that the D-splitting should exceed the exchange coupling.

The case of Cr^{3+}-Cr^{3+} pairs in Al_2O_3 affords an illustration which is both convenient and has the advantage that some of the predictions have been verified experimentally. Fig. 8.4 shows the Al_2O_3 lattice. Cr^{3+} ions substitute for Al^{3+} ions in any one of the four distinct sites a, b, c, d. Sites a and b and sites c and d are related to one another by a small rotation of the oxygen nearest neighbours about the crystal c-axis. Experiments have been performed with electric and magnetic fields both parallel to the c-axis. In this case isolated Cr^{3+} ions ($S = \frac{3}{2}$) can be described by magnetic quantum states $|\pm\frac{3}{2}\rangle$, $|\pm\frac{1}{2}\rangle$, the zero field splitting ($= 2|D|$) between the $|\pm\frac{3}{2}\rangle$ states and the $|\pm\frac{1}{2}\rangle$ states being 11.454 GHz. No distinction need be made between

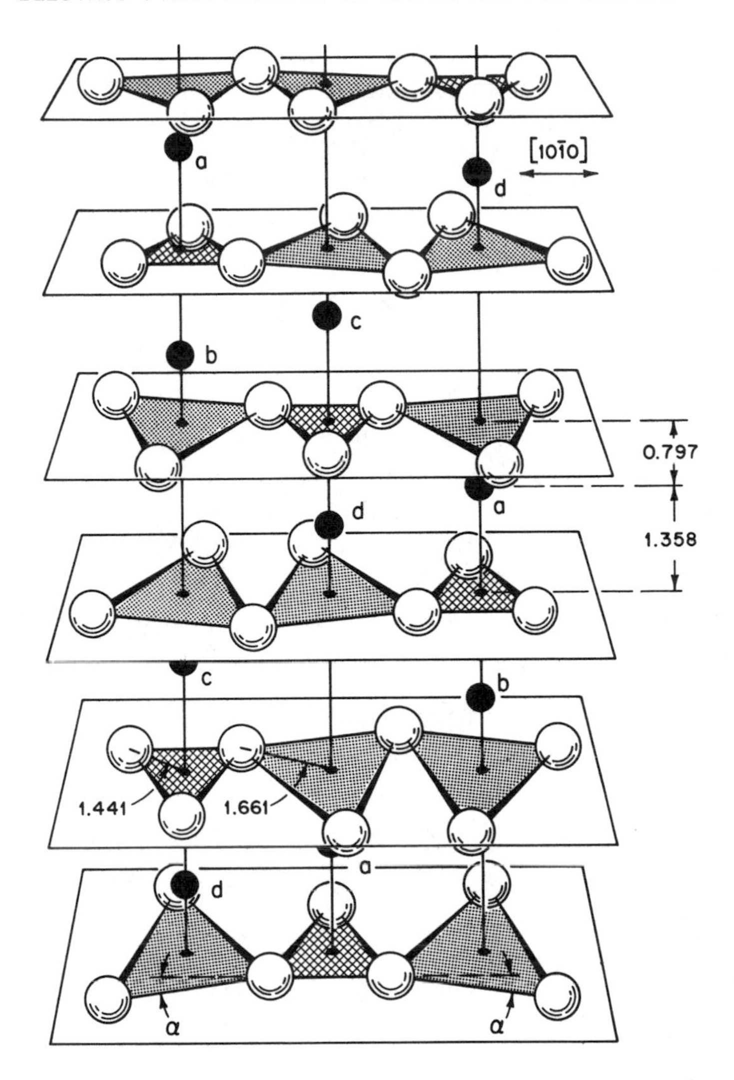

FIG. 8.4. Diagram of Al_2O_3 lattice showing the four Al^{3+} sites at which Cr^{3+} substitution occurs. Sites a,d are inversion images of one another as are also sites b and c. Sites a and b are related by a small rotation of the oxygen nearest neighbours about the crystal c-axis. (After Geschwind and Remeika, 1961).

sites a,b or between sites c,d, and the only shift parameter concerned here is R_{3D}.† Ions at sites a or b and in states $M_S = |\pm\frac{3}{2}\rangle$ undergo shifts $E_z R_{3D}$, those in states $M_S = |\pm\frac{1}{2}\rangle$ undergo shifts $-E_z R_{3D}$ according to the spin Hamiltonian eqn (3.10)(p.51). Ions at sites c,d undergo the same shifts with reversed sign.

If the exchange coupling is small (i.e. $J \ll D$), as it is for some more distant neighbours it will mix some states but not others. It will for example, mix the $M_S = |\pm\frac{1}{2}\rangle$ states of two Cr^{3+} ions, in sites a, b, yielding three symmetric states $|(a,\frac{1}{2}),(b,\frac{1}{2})\rangle$, $(\frac{1}{\sqrt{2}})\{|(a,\frac{1}{2}),(b,-\frac{1}{2})\rangle + |(a,-\frac{1}{2}),(b,\frac{1}{2})\rangle\}$, $|(a,-\frac{1}{2}),(b,-\frac{1}{2})\rangle$, and an antisymmetric state $(\frac{1}{\sqrt{2}})\{|(a,\frac{1}{2}),(b,-\frac{1}{2})\rangle - |(a,-\frac{1}{2}),(b,\frac{1}{2})\rangle\}$ separated from the symmetric states by J. Similar combinations will be formed between ions in $M_S = |\pm\frac{1}{2}\rangle$ states in sites a and c, a and d, etc. The shifts for these states can be derived from the shifts for isolated ions, as long as the electric field is not strong enough to alter the state mixture. (The criterion here is that $J \simeq |E_z R_{3D}|$ and is not likely to be met for any pair lines which are clearly resolved from the line due to isolated Cr^{3+} ions). Thus the states $|(a,\frac{1}{2}),(b,\frac{1}{2})\rangle$, $|(a,-\frac{1}{2}),(b,-\frac{1}{2})\rangle$, $(\frac{1}{\sqrt{2}})\{|(a,\frac{1}{2}),(b,-\frac{1}{2})\rangle + |(a,-\frac{1}{2}),(b,\frac{1}{2})\rangle\}$ have shifts $-2E_z R_{3D}$, whilst the states $|(a,\frac{1}{2}),(d,\frac{1}{2})\rangle$, $|(a,-\frac{1}{2}),(d,-\frac{1}{2})\rangle$, $(\frac{1}{\sqrt{2}})\{|(a,\frac{1}{2}),(d,-\frac{1}{2})\rangle \pm |(a,-\frac{1}{2}),(d,\frac{1}{2})\rangle$ $(\frac{1}{\sqrt{2}})\{|(a,\frac{1}{2}),(b,-\frac{1}{2})\rangle - |(a,-\frac{1}{2}),(b,\frac{1}{2})\rangle\}$ have zero linear shifts.

Provided that $J \ll D$ the pair states corresponding to one ion in a $|\pm\frac{1}{2}\rangle$ state and one in a $|\pm\frac{3}{2}\rangle$ state merely consist of

---

† The g-shifts are negligible since $g \simeq 2$ and is little affected by changes in the crystal field environment. For the D-shift parameters see Fig. 3.3 (p.42) (C_3 point symmetry) and Table 10.7 (p.253).

products of the isolated ion states, and the shifts can be obtained by summing the shifts for the isolated ions. Thus, for example, the shift for $|(a,\frac{3}{2}),(d,\frac{1}{2})\rangle$ will be $2E_zR_{3D}$ and the shift for $|(a,\frac{3}{2}),(b,\frac{1}{2})\rangle$ will be zero. The same holds true for pair states for which both ions are in $|\pm\frac{3}{2}\rangle$ states or in other pairs of states such as $|\pm\frac{3}{2}\rangle$, $|\mp\frac{1}{2}\rangle$ which are not coupled by the exchange operator. If however $J \gg D$ the eigenstates will consist of symmetric and antisymmetric combinations of the $|\pm\frac{1}{2}\rangle$ and $|\pm\frac{3}{2}\rangle$ substates.† The resultant spin $S = 3$, etc. is a good quantum number of the coupled system which is centrosymmetric about a point midway between the two Cr^{3+} ions if the ions are at inversion image sites such as a, d, etc. and is effectively centrosymmetric if the ions occupy sites such as a, c, which yield equal and opposite shifts under the conditions of the experiment. In this case there will be no linear electric field effect. There may be an effect if the coupled system is non-centrosymmetric as for example if the ions are at sites a and b. Full calculations have been made by Nikiforov (1965) in the $J \ll D$ and $J \gg D$ regimes and have been verified experimentally by Sherstkov et al. (1966) and by Parrot and Roger (1968). In both of these experimental studies the electric field effect was used to distinguish between different types of pair configuration. Parrot and Roger employed electric field modulation (§2.4) to detect non-centrosymmetric combinations of Cr^{3+} ions.

No mention has been made above of the possibility that the exchange coupling constant itself might undergo modification in the applied electric field. A shift in this parameter could also

---

† In the present discussion symmetric and antisymmetric refer to the form of the quantum-mechanical combination and not to the overall symmetry of the coupled pair which will be partly determined by whether the ions are in sites a, b, c, d.

contribute to the observed linear electric field effect for non-centrosymmetric coupled pairs. Other complications might also arise in the general situation when the magnetic field is not applied along a simple symmetry axis and when the exchange coupling contains anistropic terms. Some of these difficulties would perhaps have to be faced in any attempt to explain the bulk magneto-electric effect (see §7.3 for references) in terms of the shifts observed for isolated paramagnetic ions. Studies of polynuclear complexes of more than two coupled spins as suggested by Nikiforov, Mitrofanov, and Krotkii (1973), might also be useful for this purpose.

9. The application of linear electric field effect measurements

As understanding of the paramagnetic resonance phenomenon has progressed and as the body of detailed systematic knowledge has grown, so numerous ways have been found to apply resonance techniques in different areas of physics, chemistry, and biology. Most applications involve straightforward measurements of the resonance spectrum. These can now be performed in a routine manner with commercially available instruments. But an increasing number of problems call for more specialized resonance techniques such as ENDOR, studies of line-narrowing, and measurements of the spin lattice relaxation time T_1.

Linear electric field effect measurements may be considered as one such specialized resonance technique, although comparatively little use has been made of it up to the present. Given the difficulties of the measurements and the relatively recent introduction of these techniques this is hardly surprising. The situation may be expected to change, however, as the phenomena become better understood and as attention is directed towards possible applications. We shall therefore attempt to indicate briefly some of the ways in which linear electric field effect measurements might be used to complement other experimental techniques or to open up new areas of investigation.

9.1. INVESTIGATION OF LOCAL SYMMETRY AND OF THE LIGAND FIELD

Resonance experiments are often performed in order to find the local symmetry at a paramagnetic site. Standard measurements involving the determination of the g-tensor or the D-tensor do not, however, afford a very sensitive probe. It is impossible to distinguish between the non-centrosymmetric point groups and the equivalent centrosymmetric point groups (Table 5.1, p.141), and it is usually not possible to go beyond general classifications such as cubic, axial, or rhombic according to the number of principal values in the g- or D-tensor. These categories each include a number of point groups. The axial category, for instance, comprises the 15 non-centrosymmetric point groups D_2, C_{2v}, C_3, D_3, C_{3v}, C_4, D_4, C_{4v}, S_4, D_{2d}, C_6, C_{6v}, C_{3h}, D_{3h} and the 7 centrosymmetric point groups D_{2h}, S_6, D_{3d}, C_{4h}, D_{4h}, C_{6h}, D_{6h}. In contrast with this the information obtained from linear electric field effect measurements can be quite detailed. Not only does the observation of an effect serve at once to establish the point group as odd, but, in addition, it is often possible to identify the point group unambiguously by finding out which parameters are required in order to describe the effect. Perusal of Figs 3.1 and 3.3 (pp 46 and 52) will show that the only odd point groups having g-shift (or D-shift) tensors of the same form are the pairs (T,T_d), (D_6,D_4), (C_{4v},C_{6v}), (C_4,C_6).

Apart from helping to identify the site symmetry the EPR parameters can yield a great deal of valuable information regarding the immediate environment of the paramagnetic ion. Even a cursory survey is sometimes useful. For instance, if two out of three principal g-values lie close together (or if $E \ll D$) it can be tentatively inferred that the geometry of the ligands nearest to the paramagnetic ion is approximately axial. Linear electric field effect measurements can be even more informative than the normal EPR parameters in this respect since they generally give a more detailed characterisation of the centre. Thus it has been pointed out by Bichurin, Volkov, Zakharov, Kovalenko, Sen'kiv, Soldatov and Chunyaeva (1971) that for Mn^{2+} and Fe^{3+} ions in $CdWO_4$ the D-shift parameters suggest that the local symmetry does not deviate greatly from S_4, although the point symmetry is strictly C_2. This conclusion is based on the near equality of two pairs of coefficients R_{ij}. (In order to make the comparison, the coordinate systems must be chosen so that the twofold C_2 axis and the fourfold rotation inversion S_4 axis are the same.) In a similar manner, it has been argued by Royce and Bloembergen (1963) that, although the point symmetry for Cr^{3+} ions in Al_2O_3 is strictly C_3, the D-shift tensor is approximately that which one would expect for C_{3v} point symmetry. Two out of the five coefficients (i.e. R_{1E}, R_{14}) almost vanish when the axis system is rotated approximately 5° about the crystal c-axis. This latter result suggests that the ligand field is due primarily to the 6 nearest oxygen atoms in the Al_2O_3 lattice which are known from X-ray studies to subtend C_{3v} symmetry at the Al_2O_3 site with the C_{3v} mirror plane oriented at about 5° to the crystal b-axis. It will be apparent that some facility with the techniques of co-ordinate rotation (see §A.4) is useful when attempting to approximate low point symmetry site with a higher symmetry one in this way.

A more detailed analysis of the ligand field usually involves the construction of a model for the paramagnetic centre and the calculation of a set of theoretical parameters. It is, however, often difficult to obtain very conclusive evidence from EPR studies only, since the number of physical variables tends to exceed the number of experimental parameters. Linear electric field effect measurements can reduce the degree of arbitrariness here by providing a number of extra quantities to test against the theory. Such studies need not only concern the form of the crystal field, but can extend to an examination of the quantum mechanical model used to describe the centre. For example, several mechanisms have been suggested to account for the interaction of the Mn^{2+} ($S = \frac{5}{2}$) ion with crystal fields. (Since the ground state is an orbital S-state all these involve higher-order perturbations.) Comparisons between theoretical and experimental values of the D-parameter and of the R_{ij} parameters have been made for a number of centres, e.g. Mn^{2+} in $CaWO_4$ (Kiel and Mims 1967, Kovalenko 1971); Mn^{2+} in CdS (Kiel and Mims 1972a); Mn^{2+} Td sites in ZnS (Buch and Gelineau 1971); Mn^{2+} C_{4v} sites in NaCl (Dreybrodt and Silber 1969). In the last-mentioned reference a relativistic mechanism is invoked in order to explain the data.

9.2. THE MEASUREMENT OF INTERNAL ELECTRIC FIELDS

A paramagnetic centre whose behaviour in applied electric fields has been determined experimentally can be used to indicate the presence of electrostatic fields generated by lattice defects, crystal impurities, etc., in its immediate neighbourhood. Such fields are often quite large in comparison with the fields applied in a linear electric field effect experiment and they can give rise to distinct EPR spectal lines.[†] For instance, according to the Coulomb law $E = q/\varepsilon_r r^2$ a singly charged defect at a distance

---

[†] The discussion here concerns ions which, in the absence of any perturbation, would occupy non-centrosymmetric sites, and show a linear electric field effect. The introduction of a charged defect in the vicinity of an ion at a centrosymmetric site would presumably induce a quadratic shift, but shifts induced in this way will be proportional to $1/r^4$ and are likely to be smaller than shifts due to mechanical strains. Strains due to point defects are proportional to $1/r^3$.

$r = 5$ Å in a medium with relative permittivity $\varepsilon_r = 5$ generates a field of $1{\cdot}15 \times 10^7$ V cm^{-1}. This would be enough to produce g-shifts $\approx 0{\cdot}1$ for many of the centres listed in Chapter 10. Moreover, even when defects are more remotely situated and the resulting fields an order of magnitude smaller than the field estimated above, their effects may still be detected in the EPR spectrum as a broadening of the resonance lines (see Appendix B).

Although these properties have not yet been used to any significant degree for the purpose of investigating new types of centre, their existence has been demonstrated in a number of situations where the physical characteristics of the system were already reasonably well understood. Electrostatic broadening of the resonance lines has been observed for various ions in the scheelite lattice $CaWO_4$, and in the related monoclinic $ZnWO_4$ lattice (for references see Appendix B). It has also been proposed as a major determinant of the linewidth for Ti^{3+} in Al_2O_3 (Bates, Bentley, Jones, and Moore 1970). An attempt to use the line-broadening to measure the distribution of Li^+ defects in $ZnWO_4$ doped with Cr^{3+} has been made by Blazha, Bugai, Maksimenko, and Roitsin (1972). An estimate for the magnitude of the electrostatic dipoles generated by the substitution of Zn^{2+} in a CdS lattice has also been made by Deigen, Geifman, Maevskii, Kodzhespirov, Bulanyi, and Mozharovskii (1970) using Mn^{2+} as the paramagnetic ion to sense the resulting electrostatic fields.

The generation of satellite EPR spectra by lattice defect fields has been studied by Mims and Gillen (1967) in the $CaWO_4$: Ce^{3+} system. The EPR spectrum consists of one strong line associated with Ce^{3+} ions substituted at axial Ca^{2+} sites and a number of weaker lines which are produced when a vacancy or a charge compensating impurity ion such as Na^+ occurs at nearby points in the lattice. One of these centres consists of a Ce^{3+} ion and a vacancy located at adjacent Ca^{2+} sites. (The vacancy compensates for the excess positive charge at a remoter 'axial' Ce^{3+} site as well as for the excess charge of the nearby Ce^{3+}.) It is found that this centre has g-values close to those which one would estimate by considering the local electric field $E = -2e/\varepsilon_r r^2$ in conjunction with the measured shift parameter for the axial Ce^{3+} site. It is also found that in this case the compensation sites and the axial site respond to laboratory applied electric fields in ways which are recognizably similar. The study has been extended by Abdulsabirov, Antipin, Kurkin, Tsvetkov, Chirkin, and Shlenkin (1972) who explain the satellite spectra observed for Er^{3+} in $CaWO_4$ in the same way. They are able to interpret one set of lines as being due to vacancies at the adjacent Ca^{2+} site and another set as being due to Na^+ impurities. A third set of lines is attributed to O^{2-} interstitial ions.

Some caution is perhaps needed in applying the same arguments to other cases until more evidence for the generality of this mechanism accumulates, especially in cases where the lattice defect is situated as closely as in the above illustration. Defects also give rise to strain fields which, although they fall off more rapidly with distance than electrostatic fields, may not always turn out to be unimportant. It should also not be assumed without further demonstration that the correct results can be obtained by using the bulk relative permittivity to calculate the local electrostatic field when the charge is located only a few ångströms away. This assumption appears to be more or less satisfactory in the case of the centres in $CaWO_4$ which have been examined, but it might have to be revised in other cases.

9.3. ELECTRIC FIELD EFFECTS IN FERROELECTRIC MATERIALS

Linear electric field effect measurements have been used to study the internal field in ferroelectric materials. The nature of the information obtained from these studies can be appreciated by considering the results of Blinc and Sentjurc (1967) and Völkel and Windsch (1971) on Cu^{2+}-doped Rochelle salt ($KNaC_4H_4O_6.4H_2O$). The Cu^{2+} ion, which substitutes for Na^+ with the additional loss of H^+ to maintain charge balance, has C_{2v} point symmetry. Unlike most ferroelectrics Rochelle salt is ferroelectric only in a narrow temperature range (255-297K).

In this material g-shifts $\simeq 10^{-4}$ are obtained by applying fields $\simeq$ 7 kV cm^{-1}. The g-shifts are not proportional to the applied field, however. The reason for this behaviour is apparent when we consider the internal field E_{int} (eqns (4.5)-(4.7)) seen by Cu^{2+} ion. This field is determined largely by the relative permittivity of the bulk material which is a non-linear function of the applied field and which is strongly dependent on the temperature. A plot of the magnitude of the g-shifts against the bulk polarization shows that the two are proportional to one another as one would indeed expect in a case where the applied field (due to charges on the electrodes themselves) is small compared with the Lorentz field arising from the displacement of charges in the dielectric. A linear electric field effect spin Hamiltonian (eqn (3.2) p.39) can be set up for such a ferroelectric material by taking the E_i as the components of the internal field $\underline{E}_{int}$ (eqn (4.7), p.101) rather than of the applied field $\underline{E}_{app}$. Outside the ferroelectric range, where the relative permittivity falls off to values more typical of non-ferroelectric materials, the g-shifts become small and hard to detect.

Some similar experiments have been reported on Fe^{3+} and Gd^{3+} in $SrTiO_3$ (Sakudo, Unoki, and Fujii 1966 , Unoki and Sakudo 1970, 1973). This material is not ferroelectric but has an anomalously high polarizability associated with a structural phase transition at about 105 K. Below this temperature the Sr^{2+} sites have D_{2d} point symmetry, and the Gd^{3+} ion which substitutes at these sites can therefore undergo a linear electric field effect. As in the case of Cu^{2+}-doped Rochelle salt the effect is not proportional to the applied field, but to the internal field and therefore involves the non-linearity of the relative permittivity (Müller 1971).

The large electric field enhancement in $S_rT_iO_3$ makes it possible also to observe shifts for Fe^{3+} ions in this material, although these ions substitute at sites which remain centrosymmetric above and below the phase transition. (The point symmetry is O_h above and C_{4h} below the transition temperature). The effect is in this case quadratic and can be described by a spin Hamiltonian of the form

$$\mathcal{H}_{elec} = R_{ijkl}P_iP_jS_kS_l \quad ,$$

where P_i, P_j are the Cartesian components of bulk polarization. There are seven independent parameters R_{ijkl} below the transition temperature and three independent parameters above it.

The experiments described above differ somewhat from those discussed elsewhere in this monograph in that they are mainly concerned with a bulk property of matter rather than with a property of isolated centres. It should also be possible, however, to study internal electric fields on the microscopic scale by making linear electric field effect measurements. Experiments of this kind might, for instance, be made to discover the polarizability of various types of impurity ion or to investigate cooperative interactions between two or more impurity ions. Such experiments could be used to study mechanisms involved in ferroelectric behaviour just as paramagnetic resonance measurements have been used to elucidate problems in ferromagnetism and antiferromagnetism.

9.4. LINEAR ELECTRIC FIELD EFFECT STUDIES IN MOLECULAR BIOLOGY

EPR measurements are used extensively in biology both to

investigate radicals with g ≃ 2 and to study paramagnetic centres which involve ions such as Fe^{3+}, Cu^{2+}, Mn^{2+}.†‡ In the latter case the object is usually to identify the centre or examine its symmetry and probe the ligand field. Much of the discussion in §9.1 is applicable here. Linear electric field effect measurements provide a direct test for the non-centrosymmetric property and, where this is found, a means of studying the odd portion of the ligand field. A detailed ab initio calculation of the kind presented in Chapter 6 has not been attempted for any such complex centres and would probably be difficult to make in view of the large measure of covalent bonding which generally characterizes 3d ions in biological molecules. But a great deal of useful information can often be obtained by comparing the behaviour of a biological material with that of its chemical derivatives†† and with a range of related 'model compounds'. This approach

---

† For a recent text dealing with applications in biology see e.g. Swartz, Bolton, and Borg (1972). Signals due to radicals will show small or negligible linear electric field shifts for the reason given in §2.1.

‡ These ions occur naturally in many enzymes and cytochromes. In others the diamagnetic ion Zn^{2+} can be replaced by a paramagnetic ion with only partial loss of enzymatic activity. Ca^{2+} which plays an important part in many biological mechanisms can also be replaced by rare earth ions.

†† Derivatives may be obtained by changing the pH of the sample or by changing its oxidation state (e.g. $Fe^{2+} \rightarrow Fe^{3+}$). In other cases derivatives are formed by introducing new ligands such as CN^- or N_3^- which do not occur naturally.

has already been extensively used in conjunction with g-value measurements. Sets of comparative EPR measurements have been used as a means of identifying the ligands in a molecule whose structure is unknown.

Measurements of the linear electric field effect tend to be considerably more difficult to make for biological molecules than for paramagnetic centres in ionic crystals. Most samples are only available in amorphous form as frozen glasses and, even where single crystals have been grown, the resonance lines are usually wide.† No attempt has been made to perform measurements by the direct method (§2.3), and it would seem from the information at present available regarding the magnitude of the shifts that the method is unlikely to succeed here. The spin echo method (§2.5) has, however, been used to measure shift parameters $\delta g \leq 10^{-9}\ V^{-1}$ cm. (Peisach and Mims 1973; Mims and Peisach 1974). The width of an individual spin packet in biological materials is typically 100 mG as deduced from the electron spin echo phase memory time. This homogeneous width is probably associated with random flip-flop motions of neighbouring protons in the material.

A resonance experiment performed on a sample consisting of Kramers doublet centres randomly oriented in a powder or in an amorphous material yields at most the three principal g-values, the parameters which describe the orientation of the principal axis system being indeterminate. The principal values can be derived from an EPR spectrum of the form shown in Fig. 3.8 (p.74).

---

† It has been suggested that the line-broadening observed in metal protein systems may be due to internal electric fields (Appendix B) generated by ionic charges on the surface of the protein (Mims and Peisach 1974).

A linear electric field effect experiment for a sample of this kind is likewise limited in the information which it can provide by the lack of order in the material. Its properties can be specified by two measurements of the shift as a function of Zeeman field setting, one with $\underline{E}$ parallel to $\underline{H}_0$ and one with $\underline{E}$ perpendicular to $\underline{H}_0$ as shown in Fig. 3.10 (p.81). Some of the shift parameters in the linear electric field effect Hamiltonian can be derived from measurements made at either end of the spectrum as indicated in §3.7, but most of the parameters are involved in a complex fashion in the shifts observed between these two extremes. A detailed analysis of the situation would seem to require some form of numerical computation and fitting procedure, but nothing of this kind has yet been attempted.

Much remains to be done before it is possible to define the scope or assess the usefulness of linear electric field effect measurements in biology. Measurements have hitherto only been reported for Fe^{3+} $S = \frac{1}{2}$ centres. No measurements have been reported on ions with D-shifts or on ions where the EPR spectrum is complicated by large nuclear hyperfine splittings. From what little is known it seems unlikely that a full theoretical calculation of all third-rank tensor parameters B_{ij} or R_{ij} would, even if feasible, provide the best means of interpreting the data since most centres whose structure has been determined from X-ray measurements have a very low point symmetry (C_s or C_1). More might perhaps be accomplished by attempting to fit the data with some kind of simplified model.

10. Experimental data

Results are classified according to the point group of the site. This differs from the classification commonly used for paramagnetic resonance data but is more convenient here since the number of tensor coefficients to be tabulated varies considerably with the point symmetry. Many of the original papers cited contain some form of theoretical interpretation. In addition to this a number of papers have been published which deal exclusively with the calculation of the electric field effect for a particular paramagnetic centre. For example: Mn^{2+} in NaCl (Dreybrodt and Silber 1969); d^5 ions in ZnS (Buch and Gelineau 1971); Cu^{2+} in tetrahedral fields (Bates 1968); Cr^{3+} in Al_2O_3 (Artman and Murphy 1963a, 1963b, 1964); Ce^{3+} and Nd^{3+} in $CaWO_4$ (Kovalenko and Bichurin 1969, 1970).

The coefficients R_{ij} (which describe shifts in the 'D'- and 'E'-like terms) are given in units of Megahertz shift per 10^6 V cm^{-1} applied field (i.e. Hz cm V^{-1}). Published results have, where necessary, been multiplied by a factor of 2 to bring them into accord with the traceless practical notation as defined in eqn (3.10)-(3.12)(pp.51-53). The coefficient R_{123} ($=R_{132}$) is, for example, represented as R_{14} and not $\frac{1}{2}R_{14}$. The term $E_x(R_{123}S_yS_z+R_{132}S_zS_y)$ in the expansion of eqn (3.2) is thus condensed to $E_xR_{14}(S_yS_z+S_zS_y)$ and not to $\frac{1}{2}E_xR_{14}(S_yS_z+S_zS_y)$ as in some publications. The coefficients R_{iE} and R_{iD} describe shifts in the terms $E(S_x^2-S_y^2)$ and $D\{S_z^2-\frac{1}{3}S(S+1)\}$.

The coefficients T_{ij} are in units of g-shift per 10^9 V cm^{-1} and are also tabulated in Voigt notation with $T_{14} = T_{123} = T_{132}$, etc. As pointed out in §3.5 the Voigt notation is of questionable value here since it is not generally possible to define g_{jk} and T_{ijk} so that they are simultaneously symmetric in j,k. A set of equivalent symmetric T_{ij} parameters can, however, be derived from the g^2-shift parameters B_{ij} as in Table 3.2 (p.67) and have been used to describe data in many publications. These parameters lead to the correct frequency shifts, although they do not correctly describe the results of a paraelectric resonance experiment (§7.2). The g^2-shift parameters B_{ijk} are intrinsically symmetrical in j,k (eqn (3.32)) and can always be written in the contracted Voigt notation with $B_{14} = B_{123} = B_{132}$, etc. In cases where the data has been published in terms of the parameters B_{ij} no attempt has been made to convert them into an equivalent T_{ij} form.

We begin with the point symmetries which involve fewest coefficients.

10.1. T AND T_d POINT SYMMETRY

The term $R_{ijk}E_iS_jS_k$ in eqn (3.2) reduces to $R_{14}\{E_x(S_yS_z+S_zS_y) + E_y(S_zS_x+S_xS_z) + E_z(S_xS_y+S_yS_x)\}$. The x-,y-,z-axes are the C_2 axes of the tetrahedron and are all equivalent. The shifts in g are given by $\delta g_{yz}/E_x = \delta g_{zx}/E_y = \delta g_{xy}/E_z = T_{14}$. (The shift in g^2 can be written $\delta(g^2) = B_{14}(E_x\sin 2\theta \sin\phi + E_y\sin 2\theta\cos\phi + E_z\sin^2\theta \sin 2\phi)$, where $B_{14} = 2T_{14}g$ and g is isotropic.)

Experimental results are shown in Table 10.1. The effects for $3d^6$ and $3d^8$ ions are large since these ions have orbital degeneracy in the ground state in T_d symmetry. It is interesting to note that in spite of the relatively high sensitivity of these

TABLE 10.1

Linear electric effect coefficients for ions in Td sites

Ion	Configuration	S	Host lattice	R_{14}	T_{14}	Ref
Cr^{+}	$3d^5$	$\frac{5}{2}$	Si	59±9		1
Cr^{0}	$3d^6$	1	Si	$(16{\cdot}2\pm0{\cdot}9) \times 10^3$	500±70	1
Mn^{+}	$3d^6$	1	Si	$(75\pm12) \times 10^3$	850±20	1
Mn^{0}	$3d^7$	$\frac{1}{2}$	Si		120±30	1
Fe^{+}	$3d^7$	$\frac{1}{2}$	Si		730±50	1,2
Fe^{0}	$3d^8$	1	Si	$(1{\cdot}5\pm0{\cdot}12) \times 10^3$		1,2
Co^{2+}	$3d^7$	$\frac{3}{2}$	CdTe†	$\sim3 \times 10^3$		3
Mn^{2+}	$3d^5$	$\frac{5}{2}$	ZnS†	28		4
Fe^{3+}	$3d^5$	$\frac{5}{2}$	ZnS†	390		5

† Zincblende structure.

Refs 1. Ludwig and Ham (1962).
2. Ludwig and Woodbury (1961).
3. Christensen (1969).
4. Marti, Parrot, Roger and Herve (1968).
Marti, Parrot, and Roger (1970).
5. Parrot, Tronche, and Marti (1969).

ions to electric fields, the resonance lines are not always very broad. For example, the resonance line of Fe^0 in silicon has a halfwidth at half height of 3·5 G, which is equivalent to the shift produced by ∿7 kV cm^{-1}. The large, randomly oriented electric fields which characterize many ionic lattices are clearly absent here. Broader lines were found for Co^{2+} in CdTe.

Since ZnS is piezoelectric, there is a possibility of the shifts being partly due to bulk mechanical strains in the lattice. This effect has been calculated by Lambert, Marti, and Parrot (1970) and found to be ∿7 times smaller than the observed linear electric field effects for Mn^{2+}. Buch and Gelineau (1971) conclude as a result of a more detailed calculation that the indirect piezo-electric contribution is ∿20 times smaller than the primary effect in this material.

The magnitude of the linear electric shifts render some of the materials here suitable for the observation of paraelectric resonance (see Chapter 7). Ludwig and Ham (1962) and Christensen (1969) describe paraelectric resonance experiments for T_d centres. A linear electric field effect experiment performed in order to establish the tetrahedral symmetry of an Mn^{2+} centre in CaF_2 is reported by Reddy (1971).

10.2. C_{4v} POINT SYMMETRY

C_{4v} sites occur when a paramagnetic ion substituted in a cubic lattice is charge-compensated by a foreign ion or a vacancy lying along one of the 100 axes. Electric field effect experiments have been made for Mn^{2+} substituted for Na^+ in NaCl and compensated by an Na^+ vacancy, and also for a number of trivalent ions compensated by F^- interstitials in fluorite lattices.

The term $R_{ijk}E_iS_jS_k$ reduces to $R_{15}\{E_x(S_xS_z+S_zS_x) + E_y(S_yS_z+S_zS_y)\} + R_{3D}E_z\{S_z^2 - \frac{1}{3}S(S+1)\}$. The shift in g^2 is $\delta(g)^2 = B_{15}(E_x\sin 2\theta\cos\phi + E_y\sin 2\theta\sin\phi) + B_{31}E_z\sin^2\theta + B_{33}E_z\cos^2\theta$.

The equivalent symmetric g-shift parameters are given by $T_{15} = B_{15}/(g_{\|}+g_{\perp})$, $T_{31} = B_{31}/(2g_{\|})$, $T_{33} = B_{33}/(2g_{\|})$, where $g_{\|}$ and $g_{\perp}$ are the g-values along the C_{4v} axis and perpendicular to it. For an applied field along the z-axis the site remains axial, R_{3D} describing the shift in the D-parameter and T_{31}, T_{33} the shifts in $g_{\perp}$ and $g_{\|}$ which are induced in this way.

The experimental results are shown in Table 10.2. Due to experimental difficulties, only a limiting value of R_{3D} could be obtained for the Mn^{2+} C_{4v} sites in NaCl and no estimate was made for R_{15}. For the site geometry of the C_{4v} centres in the fluorite lattice see Fig. 6.2. (p.172). The table gives the g^2-shift parameters for the ground-state Kramers doublet of Ce^{3+}, Nd^{3+}, and U^{3+}. The absolute signs of the parameters B_{15}, B_{31}, B_{33} are not known, but it has been verified that B_{31}, B_{33} are opposite in sign. Parameters for Ce^{3+} in CaF_2 are calculated from first principles in Chapter 6.

10.3. C_{3v} POINT SYMMETRY

The term $R_{ijk}E_iS_jS_k$ reduces to $R_{15}\{E_x(S_xS_z+S_zS_x) + E_y(S_yS_z+S_zS_y)\} - R_{2E}\{E_x(S_xS_y+S_yS_x) + E_y(S_x^2 - S_y^2)\} + R_{3D}E_z\{S_z^2 - \frac{1}{3}S(S+1)\}$.

Experimental results are summarized in Table 10.3. Some of the determinations are incomplete, perhaps partly because of the difficulty of making measurements with the host lattices ZnS and CdS which tend to have poor insulating properties. The experimental problems arising from depolarization of the sample in the applied electric field are discussed by Marti, Parrot, Roger, and Herve (1968) and by Marti, Parrot, and Roger (1970). Experiments on Mn^{2+} in ZnS have also been made by Kozlov and Kovalenko (1969) who succeeded in applying a field of 300 kV cm^{-1}. The indirect piezoelectric contribution to the effect has not been calculated for the wurtzite form of ZnS but was calculated to be an order of magnitude smaller than the primary effect for Mn^{2+} in the zinc

TABLE 10.2

Linear electric effect coefficients for ions in C_{4v} sites. The g-values are given to two decimal places only.

Ion	Configuration	J	Host	R_{15}		R_{3D}			Ref.
Mn^{2+}	$3d^5$	$\frac{5}{2}$	NaCl			<5·5			1
		S'		B_{15}	B_{31}	B_{33}	$g_\perp$	$g_\parallel$	
Ce^{3+}	$4f^1$	$\frac{5}{2}$	CaF_2	5·5±1	-16±3	68±10	1·40	3·04	2
Ce^{3+}	$4f^1$	$\frac{5}{2}$	SrF_2	9±2	-25±4	120±18	1·47	2·92	2
Ce^{3+}	$4f^1$	$\frac{5}{2}$	BaF_2	31±6	-25±4	117±18	1·55	2·59	2
Nd^{3+}	$4f^3$	$\frac{9}{2}$	CaF_2	181±18	-17±2	133±13	1·30	4·41	3
Nd^{3+}	$4f^3$	$\frac{9}{2}$	SrF_2	230±23	-47±9	210±22	1·51	4·29	3
U^{3+}	$5f^3$	$\frac{9}{2}$	CaF_2	213±21	-28±3	48±5	1·87	3·50	3
U^{3+}	$5f^3$	$\frac{9}{2}$	SrF_2	275±27	-22±4	34±4	1·97	3·43	3
U^{3+}	$5f^3$	$\frac{9}{2}$	BaF_2	350±35	-35±6	78±8	2·11	3·23	3

Ref 1. Dreybrodt and Pfister (1969), 2. Kiel and Mims (1972a), 3. Kiel and Mims (1973).

TABLE 10.3

Linear electric effect coefficients for ions in C_{3v} sites

Ion	Configuration	J	Lattice	R_{2E}	R_{15}	R_{3D}	Ref.
Mn^{2+}	$3d^5$	$\frac{5}{2}$	ZnS†	-	2·8	39	1
Mn^{2+}	$3d^5$	$\frac{5}{2}$	CdS	40	1·2	23	2
Eu^{2+}	$4f^7$	$\frac{7}{2}$	CdS	-	-	90	3
Gd^{3+}	$4f^7$	$\frac{7}{2}$	CdS	-	-	14	3

† Wurtzite structure.

Refs 1. Marti, Parrot, Roger, and Herve (1968); Marti, Parrot, and Roger (1970).
2. Kiel and Mims (1972a).
3. Ludwig and Ham (1963).

blende form. Kiel and Mims (1972a) have also made some experimental observations which indicate that the piezoelectric contribution to the effect is small for Mn^{2+} in CdS.

10.4. C_{2v} POINT SYMMETRY

Measurements have been made on Mn^{2+} substituted in NaCl and charge compensated by a nearest-neighbour Na^+ vacancy in any one of 12 equivalent directions (110), (101), etc. (Dreybrodt and Pfister

1969). The term $R_{ijk}E_iS_jS_k$ here becomes $R_{15}E_x(S_xS_z+S_zS_x) + R_{24}E_y(S_yS_z+S_zS_y) + R_{3E}E_z(S_x^2 - S_y^2) + R_{3D}E_z\{S_z^2 - \frac{1}{3}S(S+1)\}$. The measured parameters were $R_{15} = -7{\cdot}7$, $R_{24} = -24{\cdot}4$, $R_{3E} = -16{\cdot}3$, $R_{3D} = 12{\cdot}2$. (These parameters have been obtained from those given in the reference by changing the axis system used so that the x-,y-,z-axes lie along the cubic (100), (01$\bar{1}$), (011) axes of NaCl, with the compensating vacancy along the z-axis.) An interesting feature of this experiment is the measurement of the absolute sign of the electric shift. It was possible to determine this by reorienting the Mn^{2+}-vacancy system in a strong electric field and thus increasing the number of centres corresponding to one of the inversion image sites. The signs are as given above when the electric field is taken as positive in the direction of the vacancy.

10.5. S_4 AND D_{2d} POINT SYMMETRY

In S_4 point symmetry the term $R_{ijk}E_iS_jS_k$ reduces to $R_{14}\{E_z(S_yS_z+S_zS_y) + E_y(S_xS_z+S_zS_x)\} + R_{15}\{E_x(S_xS_z+S_zS_x) - E_y(S_yS_z+S_zS_y)\} + R_{3E}E_z(S_x^2 - S_y^2) + R_{36}E_z(S_xS_y+S_yS_x)\}$. The g^2-shift is given by $\delta(g^2) = B_{14}\{E_x\sin 2\theta \sin\phi + E_y\sin 2\theta\cos\phi\} + B_{15}\{E_x\sin 2\theta\cos\phi - E_y\sin 2\theta\sin\phi\} + B_{31}E_z\sin^2\theta\cos 2\phi + B_{36}E_z\sin^2\theta\sin 2\phi$. The angular dependence of the g^2 shift for electric fields $E_a = E_x$, $E_b = E_y$, $E_c = E_z$ along the crystal a-, b-,c-axes can be shown better by rewriting this expression in the form $\delta g^2 = (B_{14}^2 + B_{15}^2)^{\frac{1}{2}}\{E_x\sin 2\theta\sin(\phi-\phi_1) + E_y\sin 2\theta\cos(\phi-\phi_1)\} + (B_{31}^2 + B_{36}^2)^{\frac{1}{2}}\{E_z\sin^2\theta\sin(2\phi-2\phi_3)\}$, where $\tan\phi_1 = -B_{15}/B_{14}$ and $\tan 2\phi_3 = -B_{31}/B_{36}$. The equivalent symmetric g-shift coefficients T_{ij} can be derived from the B_{ij} by means of the relations $T_{14} = B_{14}/(g_\parallel+g_\perp)$, $T_{15} = B_{15}/(g_\parallel+g_\perp)$, $T_{31} = B_{31}/2g_\perp$, $T_{36} = B_{36}/2g_\perp$.

TABLE 10.4

Linear electric effect coefficients for Kramers ions in S_4 sites. The amplitudes are accurate to ±10 per cent and the angles (see text) to ±2°. Equivalent symmetric g-shift parameters T_{ij} can be derived from the g-values and the B_{ij}.

Ion	Configuration	J	Host Lattice	$(B_{14}^2+B_{15}^2)^{\frac{1}{2}}$	$(B_{31}^2+B_{36}^2)^{\frac{1}{2}}$	ϕ_1	ϕ_3	$g_\perp$	$g_\parallel$	Ref.
Ce^{3+}	$4f^1$	$\frac{5}{2}$	$CaWO_4$	170	87	3°	8°	1·43	2·92	1
Ce^{3+}	$4f^1$	$\frac{5}{2}$	$SrWO_4$	160	95	4°	8°	1·45	2·87	2
Nd^{3+}	$4f^3$	$\frac{9}{2}$	$CaWO_4$	209	37	106°	72°	2·52	2·03	1
Nd^{3+}	$4f^3$	$\frac{9}{2}$	$SrWO_4$	310	43	98°	40°	2·56	1·53	2
Er^{3+}	$4f^{11}$	$\frac{15}{2}$	$CaWO_4$	1800	11 000	55°	31°	8·3	1·2	1
Er^{3+}	$4f^{11}$	$\frac{15}{2}$	$SrWO_4$	2020	16 700	71°	43°	8·47	0·83	2
Yb^{3+}	$4f^{13}$	$\frac{7}{2}$	$CaWO_4$	212	81	106°	47°	3·93	1·05	1
Yb^{3+}	$4f^{13}$	$\frac{7}{2}$	$SrWO_4$	340	500	97°	4°	3·88	0·58	3
Yb^{3+}	$4f^{13}$	$\frac{7}{2}$	$BaWO_4$	570	1180	97°	4°	3·82	0·3	3

Refs 1. Mims (1965), 2. Mims and Masuhr (1972), 3. Kiel and Mims (1970).

The B_{ij} parameters for a number of Kramers doublet rare-earth ions are shown in Table 10.4. The results are given in terms of the absolute magnitudes $(B_{14}^2 + B_{15}^2)^{\frac{1}{2}}$, $(B_{31}^2 + B_{36}^2)^{\frac{1}{2}}$ and the characteristic angles ϕ_1 and ϕ_3, since it is easier to specify the accuracy of the measurements when they are presented in this way.

The characteristic angles ϕ_1 and ϕ_3 for many of these ions do not appear to depend on the geometry of the nearest-neighbour oxygen atoms. This is in contrast to the results obtained for Mn^{2+} and Gd^{3+} in $CaWO_4$ in normal EPR where the symmetry of the fourth-degree term (i.e. the term in $S_4^{(4)}$; see §3.9) is clearly related to the geometry of the octahedron of nearest-neighbour oxygen atoms (Hempstead and Bowers 1960). The trend towards larger shifts in host lattices with a larger lattice constant (i.e. in $SrWO_4$ and $BaWO_4$) has been interpreted as being due to the enhanced ease with which the more loosely fitting paramagnetic ion can be displaced in an applied electric field (see §4.3).

Measurements have also been made on the hyperfine lines due to ^{143}Nd and ^{167}Er in $CaWO_4$ and $SrWO_4$ (Mims and Masuhr 1972). The results shown in Table 10.5 indicate that the ratios F_{ij}/T_{ij} are approximately the same as the ratios $A/g_{\parallel}$ and $B/g_{\perp}$ in the normal spin Hamiltonian. This is to be expected in the case of the rare earths for the same general reason that $A/g_{\parallel} \simeq B/g_{\perp}$ (see Elliott and Stevens 1953).

The D-shift parameters R_{ij} for some S-state ions in scheelite lattices are given in Table 10.6. In the first three cases these parameters have been combined to give two amplitudes $(R_{14}^2 + R_{15}^2)^{\frac{1}{2}}$, $(R_{3E}^2 + R_{36}^2)^{\frac{1}{2}}$ and two angles $\phi_1 = \text{arc tan}(-R_{15}/R_{14})$, $\phi_3 = \frac{1}{2}\,\text{arc tan}(-R_{3E}/R_{36})$ as was done in the case of the g^2-shift parameters B_{ij}. The increase in the Mn^{2+} shift in going from the $CaWO_4$ to the $SrWO_4$ host lattice has, like the corresponding changes for the Kramers ions in Table 10.4, been attributed to a reduction

TABLE 10.5

Parameters belonging to the shift term $E_i F_{ijk} S_j I_k$ associated with the electron nuclear coupling term $AS_z I_z + B(S_x I_x + S_y I_y)$ for ^{143}Nd and ^{167}Er in scheelite lattices. The F_{ijk} are given in Voigt notation ($F_{14} = F_{123} = F_{132}$, etc.) in units of Hz V^{-1} cm. It is found that $F_{ij}/T_{ij} \simeq A/g_{\parallel} \simeq B/g_{\perp}$. In order to facilitate this comparison the T_{ij} have here been taken in units of g-shift per 10^6 V cm^{-1}. A and B are in megahertz (Mims and Masuhr 1972.)

	^{143}Nd		^{167}Er
	$CaWO_4$	$SrWO_4$	$SrWO_4$
$\lvert F_{14}\rvert$	4·0	3·3	-
$\lvert F_{15}\rvert$	15	27	-
$\lvert F_{31}\rvert$	1·2	2·5	107
$\lvert F_{36}\rvert$	3·3	0·64	7
F_{14}/T_{14}	310	320	-
F_{15}/T_{15}	340	360	-
F_{31}/T_{31}	280	310	110
F_{36}/T_{36}	550	470	110
$B/g_{\perp}$	307	310	105
$A/g_{\parallel}$	315	287	103

TABLE 10.6

Linear electric effect coefficients for ions in S_4 sites. The spherical D-shift parameters $R^{(2)}_{i,j}$ in Refs. 5 and 6 may differ by a normalizing factor from those defined in §3.8 (see note in text).

Ion	Configuration	S	Host lattice	$(R^2_{14}+R^2_{15})^{\frac{1}{2}}$	$(R^2_{3E}+R^2_{36})^{\frac{1}{2}}$	ϕ_1	ϕ_3	Ref.
Mn^{2+}	$3d^5$	$\frac{5}{2}$	$CaWO_4$	58±5	126±10	40°	3°	1
Mn^{2+}	$3d^5$	$\frac{5}{2}$	$SrWO_4$	104±8	225±18	25°	8°	2
Mn^{2+}	$3d^5$	$\frac{5}{2}$	$PbMoO_4$	68±6	133±10	1°	44°	3
				R_{3E}	R_{36}	$R_{14}+R_{15}$		
Fe^{3+}	$3d^5$	$\frac{5}{2}$	YAG	80	200	-65		4
				$\lvert\text{Re } R^{(2)}_{0,2}\rvert$	$\lvert\text{Im } R^{(2)}_{0,2}\rvert$	$\lvert\text{Re } R^{(2)}_{1,1}\rvert$	$\{\lvert\text{Re } R^{(2)}_{1,1}-\text{Im } R^{(2)}_{1,1}\rvert\}$	
Gd^{3+}	$4f^7$	$\frac{7}{2}$	$CaWO_4$	4·4±0·3	-	-	-	5
Gd^{3+}	$4f^7$	$\frac{7}{2}$	$SrMoO_4$	5·7±0·3	7·6±0·7	22±2	30±4	5,6

Refs 1. Kiel and Mims (1967), 2. Kiel and Mims (1971), 3. Kiel, Mims, and Masuhr (1973), 4. Bichurin, Kozlov, Kovalenko, Tsinchik, and Shvartsman (1968), 5. Nepsha, Sherstkov, Legkikh and Meilman (1969), 6. Vazhenin, Sherstkov, Zolotareva, and Tryapitsyna (1973).

in lattice restoring forces and an enhanced ease of displacement of the Mn^{2+} ion in the applied electric field. It does not seem possible to fit the result for Mn^{2+} in $PbMoO_4$ into this simple picture, however.

The authors of Refs 5,6 (Table 10.6) define their measured coefficients as $|\mathrm{Re}\, R^{(2)}_{0,2}|$, etc. which, according to Table 3.3 (p.87) would be equivalent to $(2/\sqrt{6})|R_{3E}|$, etc. Other Soviet work using this notation suggests, however, that the coefficients refer to a set of spin operators normalized differently from those in eqn (3.58) and Table A.2.

10.6. C_3 POINT SYMMETRY

The term $R_{ijk}E_iS_jS_k$ reduces to $R_{1E}\{E_x(S_x^2 - S_y^2) -$
$- E_y(S_xS_y+S_yS_x\} - R_{2E}\{E_y(S_x^2 - S_y^2) + E_x(S_xS_y+S_yS_x)\} +$
$+ R_{14}\{E_x(S_yS_z+S_zS_y) - E_y(S_xS_z+S_zS_x)\} + R_{15}\{E_x(S_xS_z+S_zS_x) +$
$+ E_y(S_yS_z+S_zS_y)\} + R_{3D}E_z\{S_z^2 - \frac{1}{3}S(S+1)\}$.

The D-shift parameters for a number of ions substituted for Al^{3+} in Al_2O_3 are given in Table 10.7. Royce and Bloembergen (1963) have measured all five coefficients R_{ij}. (The published values of R_{14} and R_{15} have been halved to bring them into accord with the notation of eqn (3.10).) These parameters have been re-measured by Nepsha, Sherstkov, Gorlov and Shchetkov (1967), who obtain essentially the same values. Krebs (1964,1967) has measured the R_{3D}-parameter for a number of ions and attempted to correlate it with D (see Table 10.7), but the measurements on Fe^{3+} and the measurements of Adde and Pontnau (1970) on V^{3+} in Al_2O_3 seem to rule out the existence of any simple relationship between the two parameters. Royce and Bloembergen (1963) argue that large values of R_{3D}/D indicate the predominance of covalent bonding mechanisms.

Some additional measurements for Fe^{3+} in Al_2O_3, including

TABLE 10.7

Linear electric effect coefficients for ions in C_3 sites in Al_2O_3.

Ion	Configuration	J	R_{1E}	R_{2E}	R_{14}	R_{15}	R_{3D}	Ref
Cr^{3+}	$3d^3$	$\frac{3}{2}$	-20±3	73±3	20±10	45±10	269±5	1
			R_{3D}		D (GHz)	$\lvert R_{3D}/D \rvert$		
V^{3+}	$3d^2$	1	960		248·7	3·9		5
V^{2+}	$3d^3$	$\frac{3}{2}$	110·9±1·4		-4·806	23		2
Cr^{3+}	$3d^3$	$\frac{3}{2}$	269±5		-5·727	47		1
Mn^{2+}	$3d^5$	$\frac{5}{2}$	29·0		0·582	50		3
Fe^{3+}	$3d^5$	$\frac{5}{2}$	28·1		-5·03	5·6		3
Ni^{2+}	$3d^8$	1	1870		39·84	47		2
Cu^{3+}	$3d^8$	1	534		-5·652	95		2
			T_{111}	T_{113}	T_{131}	T_{311}	T_{333}	
Ti^{3+}	$3d^1$	$\frac{1}{2}$	125±40	195±40	0±10	0±20	0±20	4
					$g_{\parallel}$	$g_{\perp}$		
					1·07	0·14		

Refs 1. Royce and Bloembergen (1963), 2. Krebs (1967), 3. Krebs (1964), 4. Jones and Moore (1969), 5. Adde and Pontnau (1971).

some values for the linear shifts in the quartic spin operators are given by Sherstkov et al. (1968). The R_{11}, R_{12}, R_{14}, R_{15} are, however, given implicitly by 6 simultaneous equations which also contain 4 fourth-degree coefficients. The shift in the coefficient of the spin Hamiltonian operator $(S_+^4 + S_-^4)$ induced by fields E_x or E_y is given explicitly, and has the value 0·057 ± 0·006 MHz per 10^6 V cm^{-1}. (This paper employs a spherical tensor operator notation similar to that described in §§3.8-3.9, but it is not clear from the reference what normalizing factors have been used in defining the spin operators.)

Roitsin (1968) has made some observations on Cr^{3+} in Al_2O_3 in fields as high as $1{\cdot}5 \times 10^6$ V cm^{-1} and has been able to separate out shifts which are quadratic and cubic in the applied field. The quadratic shift is found by plotting the centre of gravity of the doublet corresponding to the two inversion image sites as a function of electric field (for a purely linear shift this centre of gravity would remain stationary). The cubic shift is derived by measuring the doublet splitting as a function of field and subtracting out the linear portion. Frequency shifts βE^2 and γE^3 were found with β = 60 MHz per $(10^6 \text{ V cm}^{-1})^2$ and γ = 19 MHz per $(10^6 \text{ V cm}^{-1})^3$. It is not clear whether these coefficients represent shifts in the coefficient D in $D\{S_z^2 - \frac{1}{3}S(S+1)\}$ or in some multiple of it, but they afford a useful indication of the magnitude of the higher-order electric effects. It is also pointed out by Roitsin that the randomly oriented electric fields or 'microfields' in the sample (see Appendix B) can combine with the applied field to produce a field-dependent line-broadening. This is observable in the range where quadratic electric effects become significant.

The measurements on the Ti^{3+} Kramers doublet in Al_2O_3 (Jones and Moore 1969) were made by comparing the signal due to paraelectric resonance for a sample placed in a microwave cavity at the point of maximum electric field with the signal due to magnetic resonance when the sample is placed in the conventional position (see Chapter 7). The experiment was made easier by smallness of $g_{\perp}$, which minimizes contributions due to residual components of the microwave magnetic field in the paraelectric resonance position. Only two out of the possible six T_{ij} coefficients could be measured in this way, lower limits being set for some of the other coefficients. A theoretical discussion of these results is given by Bates and Bentley (1969).

It may be noted that different values are given for g-shift parameters T_{113} and T_{131} and that they are not represented by a single Voigt parameter T_{15}. The parameters T_{ijk} and T_{ikj} can be measured separately in a paraelectric resonance experiment. Thus in the experiment described in the reference, the parameter T_{113} was obtained by orienting the Zeeman field $\underline{H}_0$ along the x-axis and the microwave electric field along the x-axis also. The transition inducing term in the Hamiltonian is then $T_{113}E_xH_xS_ze^{i\omega t}$. The parameter T_{131} was obtained by orienting $\underline{H}_0$ along the z-axis, the microwave electric field remaining along the x-axis. The transition-inducing term here is $T_{131}E_xH_zS_xe^{i\omega t}$. The composition of the eigenstates which are coupled by these transition operators is determined by the Zeeman term in the Hamiltonian. It is assumed that the state representation is chosen in such a way that the $\underline{g}$-matrix is symmetric (see §3.4).

10.7. C_2 POINT SYMMETRY

A number of measurements have been made in the $MgWO_4$, $ZnWO_4$, $CdWO_4$ series of host lattices where the point symmetry at the divalent anion site is C_2. For C_2 point symmetry it is customary to take the y axis as the C_2 rotation axis as indicated by the notation $C_2(y)$ in Figs 3.1 and 3.3 (p.46 and p.52). It is also a common practice in specifying the EPR parameters to define the x- and z-axes as the directions for which the spectrum passes through a maximum or minimum when the magnetic field is rotated in a plane perpendicular to the y-axis. In this coordinate system the D-term in the normal spin Hamiltonian can be written in the form $E(S_x^2 - S_z^2) + D\{S_z^2 - \frac{1}{3}S(S+1)\}$ and the Zeeman term has the form $g_xH_xS_x + g_yH_yS_y + g_zH_zS_z$. The x- and z-axes are assigned in such a way that $D > E$. This coordinate system is adopted purely as an experimental convenience and may be related to the crystal axes in a variety of ways for different paramagnetic centres. Thus, for example, the angle α between the x-axis and the crystal a-axis is given by $\alpha = 4{\cdot}2^\circ$ for Cr^{3+} in $CdWO_4$ (Kurtz and Nilsen 1962) and by $\alpha = 43{\cdot}6^\circ$ for Fe^{3+} in the same host lattice (Peter, Van Uitert, and Mock 1961). It should also be noted that the rotation of axes which eliminates the $S_xS_z + S_zS_x$ term from the normal spin Hamiltonian is not generally the same as the rotation which would eliminate the corresponding terms from $\mathcal{H}_{elec}$. The D-shift Hamiltonian can be written down from Fig. 3.3, giving the expression $R_{14}E_x(S_yS_z+S_zS_y) + R_{16}E_x(S_xS_y+S_yS_x) + R_{2E}E_y(S_x^2 - S_y^2) + R_{2D}E_y\{S_z^2 - \frac{1}{3}S(S+1)\} + R_{25}E_y(S_xS_z+S_zS_x) + R_{34}E_z(S_yS_z+S_zS_y) + R_{36}(S_xS_y+S_yS_x)$, where the crystal c-axis is the y-axis.

Some results for D-shift parameters are shown in Table 10.8. (The ion configurations and spin have been omitted to save space; they can be obtained from Table 10.7 if required.) The data is sometimes incomplete and it is difficult to draw any general conclusions from it. The increase in shift parameters with the increase in size of the ion which is replaced (the 'loose ion effect') occurs here for Cr^{3+} in $MgWO_4$, $ZnWO_4$, $CdWO_4$ as it did for a number of ions in the scheelite lattices $CaWO_4$, $SrWO_4$, $BaWO_4$ (§10.5) and also for certain ions in fluorite lattices (Table 10.2). The line-broadening appears to be due to randomly oriented internal electric fields ('microfields') in many cases. This may be partly due to the practice of adding Li^+ as a charge-compensating ion (substituting for Zn^{2+}, etc.) when growing crystals containing

TABLE 10.8

Linear electric effect coefficients for ions at C_2 sites.

Ion	Host lattice	R_{14}	R_{16}	R_{2E}	R_{2D}	R_{25}	R_{34}	R_{36}	Ref.
Cr^{3+}	$MgWO_4$	-	0	315 ±60	-	570 ±120	0	270 ±40	1
Cr^{3+}	$ZnWO_4$	380 ±40	-	165 ±15	10 ±15	600 ±30	0	410 ±40	2
Cr^{3+}	$ZnWO_4$	<300	88 ±10	135 ±5	0±5	500 ±25	-	335 ±35	3
Cr^{3+}	$CdWO_4$	350 ±60	<100	245 ±50	-	1450 ±100	540 ±60	410 ±60	4
Cr^{3+}	$CdWO_4$	-	-	300	-	-1230	-	-	5
Mn^{2+}	$ZnWO_4$	-	-	75	315	80	-	-	6
Mn^{2+}	$CdWO_4$	25	-60	120	45	-35	75	30	7
Fe^{3+}	$CdWO_4$	39	-60	120	45	-35	22	413	7

Refs 1. Bugai, Levkovskii, Maksimenko, Potkin, and Roitsin (1966) 2. Bugai, Levkovskii, Maksimenko, Pashkovskii, and Roitsin (1966), 3. Jones, Moore, and Neal (1968), 4. Levkovskii and Pashkovskii (1968), 5. Bichurin, Kovalenko, and Kozlov (1967), 6. Geifman, Glinchuk, Oganesyan, and Tsintsadze (1969), 7. Bichurin et al (1971).

trivalent paramagnetic ions. A detailed study for the case of Cr^{3+} in $ZnWO_4$ (Jones, Moore, and Neal 1968) indicates that the microfields $\simeq$ 100 kV cm^{-1}.

Some g-shift measurements have also been made for ions in the $CdWO_4$ lattice. Co^{2+} yields the g^2-shift parameters $B_{21} = 305$, $B_{22} = 230$, $B_{23} = 880$, $B_{25} = 210$, the g-values being $g_x = 3{\cdot}18$, $g_y = 3{\cdot}03$, $g_z = 6{\cdot}67$. (Galkin, Geifman, Deigen, Oganesyan, Prokhorov, Tsintsadze, and Shapovalov 1969). Measurements were made with the applied electric field along the y-axis only. Shifts in the hyperfine coupling parameters were also observed in these experiments. Cu^{2+} in $CdWO_4$ has been studied by Bugai et al. (1967). In this publication it is stated that the g-shifts are less than 10^{-10} V^{-1} cm. However, it seems possible that there may be a misprint since the graph accompanying the results indicates shifts which are considerably larger.

10.8. LOW POINT SYMMETRY SITES

Sites with C_1 point symmetry occur when trivalent rare-earth ions are substituted for Ca^{2+} in $CaWO_4$, and the additional positive charge is compensated by a vacancy or an Na^+ ion at a nearby Ca^{2+} site. (Vacancies or Na^+ ions at more remote Ca^{2+} sites are partially responsible for line-broadening (Appendix B) but do not give rise to discrete spectral lines.) Complete measurements of the eighteen g^2-shift parameters were made by Mims and Gillen (1967) for two such sites in Ce^{3+}-doped $CaWO_4$. It was shown that, for at least one of the two C_1 sites the g^2-shift behaviour is similar to that of the axial Ce^{3+} site which occurs when there are no nearby charge-compensating centres. An attempt was therefore made to treat the compensated sites as a modification of the axial site. A reasonably good estimate for the g values of the C_1 site was obtained by taking the local electrostatic field of the compensating centre as an applied field in conjunction with the g^2-shift parameters of the axial site (see §9.2). A similar attempt has been made to explain satellite EPR spectra for Er^{3+} in $CaWO_4$ by Abdulsabirov, Antipin, Kurkin, Tsvetkov, Chirkin, and Shlenkin, using linear electric field effect data measured for the axial site. No shift parameters for the C_1 sites were measured in the latter case.

The paramagnetic sites occurring in molecules of biological interest are also, in most cases, characterized by very low point symmetry. Although some measurements have been made on molecules of this type (Peisach and Mims 1973; Mims and Peisach 1974) no single-crystal studies have been attempted. Low spin ($S = \frac{1}{2}$) Fe^{3+}-centres in haeme give g-shifts $\delta g \simeq 10^{-9} V^{-1}$ cm. Measurements on amorphous samples yield relatively few of the g-shift parameters directly (§3.7), and a different approach may be required in such cases in order to interpret the data (see §9.4).

Appendix A: Mathematical

Material relating to spherical harmonics, 3j symbols, and coordinate rotations can be found in the following books:

'Theory of atomic spectra' by E. U. Condon and G. H. Shortley (Cambridge University Press, 1935).

'Elementary theory of angular momentum' by M. E. Rose (Wiley, New York, 1957).

'Angular momentum in quantum mechanics' by A. R. Edmonds (Princeton University Press 1960).

'Angular momentum' by D. M. Brink and G. R. Satchler (Clarendon Press, Oxford, 1968).

Short tables of 3j symbols are given in some of the above texts. For fuller tables see 'The 3j and 6j symbols' by M. Rotenberg, R. Bivins, N. Metropolis, and J. K. Wooton, (MIT, Cambridge, Massachusetts, 1959).

A.1. SPHERICAL HARMONICS[†]

The harmonics $C_k^q(\theta,\phi)$ can be defined in terms of the associated

---

† See e.g. Edmonds (1960), pp.22-25; Brink and Satchler (1968), pp.145-6.

Legendre polynomials $P_k^q(\theta)$ by the relation

$$C_k^q(\theta,\phi) = (-)^q \left\{\frac{(k-q)!}{(k+q)!}\right\}^{\frac{1}{2}} P_k^q(\cos\theta)e^{iq\phi}, \quad q \geq 0. \tag{A.1}$$

For negative q we have

$$C_k^{-q}(\theta,\phi) = (-)^q \left\{C_k^q(\theta,\phi)\right\}^* . \tag{A.2}$$

The associated Legendre polynomials $P_k^q(x)$ are solutions of the Legendre differential equation

$$(1-x^2)\frac{d^2y}{dx^2} - 2x\frac{dy}{dx} + \left\{k(k+1) - \frac{q^2}{1-x^2}\right\}y = 0, \tag{A.3}$$

and can be obtained from the relation

$$P_k^q(x) = \frac{(1-x^2)^{q/2}}{2^k k!} \frac{d^{k+q}}{dx^{k+q}}(x^2-1)^k . \tag{A.4}$$

Eqn (A.4) holds for positive k and for both positive and negative values of q in the range $|q| \leq k$. When $q = 0$, the polynomials $P_k^q(x)$ reduce to the Legendre polynomials $P_k(x)$. The $P_k^q(x)$ can be derived from the $P_k(x)$ by the relation

$$P_k^q(x) = (1-x^2)^{q/2} \frac{d^q P_k(x)}{dx^q}, \quad q \geq 0 . \tag{A.5}$$

The $P_k(x)$ can, in turn, be obtained from the generating function

$$(1-2xh+h^2)^{\frac{1}{2}} = P_0(x) + hP_1(x) + h^2P_2(x) + \ldots, \tag{A.6}$$

or by means of Rodrigues formula

$$P_k(x) = \frac{1}{2^k k!} \frac{d^k}{dx^k}(x^2-1)^k . \tag{A.7}$$

From eqns (A.1) and (A.5) we see that

$$C_k^0(\theta,\phi) = P_k(\cos\theta) \quad . \tag{A.8}$$

The harmonics $C_k^q(\theta,\phi)$ are related to the commonly used orthonormal spherical harmonics $Y_k^q(\theta,\phi)$ by†

$$C_k^q(\theta,\phi) = \left(\frac{4\pi}{2k+1}\right)^{\frac{1}{2}} Y_k^q(\theta,\phi). \tag{A.9}$$

This change in notation eliminates inconvenient normalizing factors in a number of calculations involving products of spherical harmonics. Thus, the spherical harmonic addition theorem becomes

$$\sum_q C_k^q(\theta,\phi)\, C_k^{-q}(\theta',\phi') = P_k(\cos\omega) \;, \tag{A.10}$$

where ω is the angle between the two directions defined by (θ,ϕ) and (θ',ϕ'). The factor $4\pi/2k+1$ appears however, in the orthonormality relation

$$\iint \{C_k^q(\theta,\phi)\}^* C_{k'}^{q'}(\theta,\phi)\sin\theta\, d\theta\, d\phi = \left(\frac{4\pi}{2k+1}\right)\delta(k-k')\delta(q-q'). \tag{A.11}$$

Harmonics up to $C_6^q(\theta,\phi)$ are shown in Table A.1. Further examples of the use of the harmonics C_k^q are given in the next section.

The spherical harmonics $C_1^q(\theta,\phi)$ transform under a rotation of the coordinate system in the same way as the spherical tensor components $E_q^{(1)}$ of the electric field (eqns (A.35),(A.38)). The spherical harmonics $C_2^q(\theta,\phi)$ transform in the same way as the spin operators

---

† The $Y_k^q(\theta,\phi)$ defined here are the same as those used by Condon and Shortley (1935). They differ by factors $(-1)^q$ from the harmonics used by some authors. See Edmonds (1960), p.21. The functions $Y_k^q(\theta,\phi) = (i)^k Y_k^q(\theta,\phi)$ are also sometimes used.

TABLE A.1

Spherical harmonics up to $C_6^q(\theta,\phi)$. The shorthand symbols C_θ, S_θ are used for cos θ and sin θ, respectively.

$$C_0^0 = 1;$$

$$C_1^0 = C_\theta;\; C_1^{\pm 1} = \mp\left(\frac{1}{2}\right)^{\frac{1}{2}} S_\theta e^{\pm i\phi};$$

$$C_2^0 = \frac{1}{2}\; 3\left(C_\theta^2 - 1\right);\; C_2^{\pm 1} = \mp\frac{1}{2}(6)^{\frac{1}{2}} C_\theta S_\theta e^{\pm i\phi};\; C_2^{\pm 2} = \frac{1}{4}(6)^{\frac{1}{2}} S_\theta^2\, e^{\pm 2i\phi};$$

$$C_3^0 = \frac{1}{2}\; 5\left(C_\theta^3 - 3\,C_\theta\right);\; C_3^{\pm 1} = \mp\frac{1}{4}(3)^{\frac{1}{2}}\left(5\,C_\theta^2 - 1\right) S_\theta e^{\pm i\phi};$$

$$C_3^{\pm 2} = \frac{1}{4}\,(30)^{\frac{1}{2}}\, S_\theta^2 C_\theta e^{\pm 2i\phi};\; C_3^{\pm 3} = \mp\frac{1}{4}(5)^{\frac{1}{2}}\, S_\theta^3 e^{\pm 3i\phi};$$

$$C_4^0 = \frac{1}{8}\left(35\,C_\theta^4 - 30\,C_\theta^2 + 3\right);\; C_4^{\pm 1} = \mp\frac{1}{4}(5)^{\frac{1}{2}}\left(7\,C_\theta^3 - 3\,C_\theta\right) S_\theta e^{\pm i\phi};$$

$$C_4^{\pm 2} = \frac{1}{8}\,(10)^{\frac{1}{2}}\left(7\,C_\theta^2 - 1\right) S_\theta^2 e^{\pm 2i\phi};\; C_4^{\pm 3} = \mp\frac{1}{4}\,(35)^{\frac{1}{2}} C_\theta S_\theta^3 e^{\pm 3i\phi};$$

$$C_4^{\pm 4} = \frac{1}{16}\,(70)^{\frac{1}{2}}\, S_\theta^4 e^{\pm 4i\phi};$$

$$C_5^0 = \frac{1}{8}\left(63\,C_\theta^5 - 70\,C_\theta^3 + 15\,C_\theta\right);$$

$$C_5^{\pm 1} = \mp\frac{1}{16}(30)^{\frac{1}{2}}\left(21\,C_\theta^4 - 14\,C_\theta^2 + 1\right) S_\theta e^{\pm i\phi};$$

$$C_5^{\pm 2} = \frac{1}{8}\,(210)^{\frac{1}{2}}\left(3\,C_\theta^3 - C_\theta\right) S_\theta^2 e^{\pm 2i\phi};$$

$$C_5^{\pm 3} = \mp\frac{1}{16}\,(35)^{\frac{1}{2}}\left(9\,C_\theta^2 - 1\right) S_\theta^3 e^{\pm 3i\phi};$$

$$C_5^{\pm 4} = \frac{3}{16}\,(70)^{\frac{1}{2}}\, C_\theta S_\theta^4 e^{\pm 4i\phi};\; C_5^{\pm 5} = \mp\frac{3}{16}\,(7)^{\frac{1}{2}}\, S_\theta^5 e^{\pm 5i\phi};$$

$$C_6^0 = \frac{1}{16}\left(231\,C_\theta^6 - 315\,C_\theta^4 + 105\,C_\theta^2 - 5\right);$$

$$C_6^{\pm 1} = \mp\left(\frac{1}{16}\right)(42)^{\frac{1}{2}}\left(33\,C_\theta^5 - 30\,C_\theta^3 + 5\,C_\theta\right) S_\theta e^{\pm i\phi};$$

$$C_6^{\pm 2} = \frac{1}{32}\,(105)^{\frac{1}{2}}\left(33\,C_\theta^4 - 18\,C_\theta^2 + 1\right) S_\theta^2 e^{\pm 2i\phi};$$

$$C_6^{\pm 3} = \mp\left(\frac{1}{16}\right)\,(105)^{\frac{1}{2}}\left(11\,C_\theta^3 - 3\,C_\theta\right) S_\theta^3 e^{\pm 3i\phi};$$

$$C_6^{\pm 4} = \frac{3}{32}(14)^{\frac{1}{2}}\left(11\,C_\theta^2 - 1\right) S_\theta^4\, e^{\pm 4i\phi};\; C_6^{\pm 5} = \mp\left(\frac{3}{16}\right)\,(77)^{\frac{1}{2}}\, C_\theta S_\theta^5 e^{\pm 5i\phi}\;;$$

$$C_6^{\pm 6} = \frac{1}{32}\,(231)^{\frac{1}{2}}\, S_\theta^6 e^{\pm 6i\phi}$$

$S_q^{(2)}$ (eqns (A.40)-(A.41). The general transforming equations for the harmonics $C_k^q(\theta,\phi)$ are

$$\underline{C}^{(k)\prime} = \underline{\tilde{\mathcal{D}}}^{(k)}\underline{C}^{(k)} ,$$

$$\underline{C}^{(k)} = \underline{\mathcal{D}}^{(k)*}\underline{C}^{(k)\prime} ,$$

where $\underline{C}^{(k)}$ is a column vector formed from the harmonics C_k^k, C_k^{k-1}, ...C_k^{-k}, and $\underline{\mathcal{D}}^{(k)}$ is a (2k+1) × (2k+1) rotation matrix whose elements are obtained as in eqn (A.37) using the substates m = k, k-1, ...-k, of a J = k manifold as a basis. The crystal field coefficients A_k^q, etc. (eqns (4.1),(4.2),(4.4)) transform contragrediently with respect to the $C_k^q(\theta,\phi)$, i.e. they transform according to the equations

$$\underline{A}^{(k)} = \underline{\mathcal{D}}^{(k)}\underline{A}^{(k)\prime} ,$$

$$A^{(k)\prime} = \underline{\mathcal{D}}^{(k)\dagger}\underline{A}^{(k)} ,$$

where $\underline{A}^{(k)}$ is a column vector formed from A_k^k, A_k^{k-1},....A_k^{-k}. The relationship between the transformation properties of the harmonics $C_k^q(\theta,\phi)$ and those of the coefficients A_k^q can be inferred in the same way as the relationship between the transformation properties of the spin operators $S_j^{(2)}$ and those of the coefficients $D_j^{(2)}$ (§A.4.4; see eqns (A.43)-(A.45).

A.2. HARMONIC POLYNOMIALS AND OPERATOR EQUIVALENTS

A set of harmonic polynomials $\mathcal{Y}_k^q(x,y,z)$ can be obtained from the spherical harmonics $Y_k^q(\theta,\phi)$ by substituting (x,y,z) for (r sin θ cos φ, r sin θ sin φ, r cos φ) in the products $r^k Y_k^q(\theta,\phi)$.

An alternative set of polynomials with different normalizing factors can be obtained by substituting in the products $r^k C_k^q(\theta,\phi)$. Polynomials of the latter type are closely related to the spherical tensor spin operators discussed in §§3.7-3.8 (see eqns 3.58) and Table 3.5). In simple cases they can be written down more or less directly by replacing (x,y,z) with spin operators (S_x,S_y,S_z) and by replacing non-commuting operators such as S_iS_j $(i \neq j)$ with commuting forms $\frac{1}{2}(S_iS_j+S_jS_i)$. The spin operator $S_1^{(2)}$ can, for example, be obtained from $C_2^1(\theta,\phi)$ as follows. Substitution of x,y,z, for (r sin θ cos φ, r sin θ sin φ, r cos θ) in $r^2C_2^1(\theta,\phi)$ yields the harmonic polynomial $-\frac{\sqrt{6}}{2}z(x+iy)$. Further substitution of (S_x,S_y,S_z) for (x,y,z) and the replacement of S_zS_x, S_zS_y by $\frac{1}{2}(S_zS_x+S_xS_z)$, $\frac{1}{2}(S_zS_y+S_yS_z)$ then yields the operator $S_1^{(2)} = -\frac{1}{2}\sqrt{\frac{3}{2}}\{S_z(S_x+iS_y)+(S_x+iS_y)S_z\}$. The operator $S_x^2+S_y^2+S_z^2 = S(S+1)$ is used to replace r^2. Thus from $r^2C_2^0(\theta,\phi) = \frac{1}{2}(3z^2-r^2)$ we obtain $S_0^{(2)} = \frac{1}{2}\{3S_z{}^2-S(S+1)\}$.

Angular-momentum operators corresponding to spin operators up to $S_q^{(6)}$ are shown in Table A.2. ($S_q^{(k)} \equiv \mathcal{O}_k^q$, $S \equiv J$). These operators are the same as those given by Smith and Thornley (1966). They can be derived† from the harmonics $C_k^q(\theta,\phi)$ and transform in the same way under coordinate rotations. Matrix elements are often given in terms of the Stevens operators O_k^q which have different normalizing factors and which are related to the $\mathcal{O}_k^q$ as shown in

---

†In the case of higher-order operators it is not always easy to introduce the commutation property (see e.g. Hutchings (1965), where the operator equivalent for $35z^4-30z^2r^2+3r^4$ is derived). The spherical harmonics cannot necessarily be recovered from the operators by substituting (x,y,z,r^2) for $(J_x,J_y,J_z,J(J+1))$.

TABLE A.2

Definition of operator equivalents $\tilde{O}_k^q$ and O_k^q. The $\tilde{O}_k^q$ are formed from the spherical harmonics $C_k^q(\theta,\phi)$ as indicated in A.2. The Stevens operators O_k^q differ by normalizing coefficients. The notation {...} indicates the continuation of the commuting expression. Matrix elements for O_2^0, O_2^2, O_4^0, O_4^2, O_4^3, O_4^4, O_6^0, O_6^2, O_6^3, O_6^4, O_6^6 are given by Abragam and Bleaney (1970), pp. 864-72. Matrix elements for $\tilde{O}_2^1$, $\tilde{O}_4^1$, $\tilde{O}_6^1$, $\tilde{O}_6^5$ are given by Buckmaster (1962).

$$\tilde{O}_2^0 = +\frac{1}{2}\, O_2^0 \equiv +\frac{1}{2}\,[3J_z^2 - J(J+1)]$$

$$\tilde{O}_2^{\pm 1} = \mp\frac{\sqrt{6}}{2}\, O_2^{\pm 1} \equiv \mp\frac{\sqrt{6}}{4}\,[J_zJ_\pm + J_\pm J_z]$$

$$\tilde{O}_2^{\pm 2} = +\frac{\sqrt{6}}{4}\, O_2^{\pm 2} \equiv +\frac{\sqrt{6}}{4}\, J_\pm^2$$

$$\tilde{O}_4^0 = +\frac{1}{8}\, O_4^0 \equiv +\frac{1}{8}\,[35J_z^4 - \{30J(J+1) - 25\}\, J_z^2 - 6J(J+1) + 3J^2(J+1)^2]$$

$$\tilde{O}_4^{\pm 1} = \mp\frac{\sqrt{5}}{4}\, O_4^{1} \equiv \mp\frac{\sqrt{5}}{8}\,[\{7J_z^3 - 3J(J+1)\, J_z - J_z\}\, J_\pm + J_\pm\, \{\ldots\}]$$

$$\tilde{O}_4^{\pm 2} = +\frac{\sqrt{10}}{8}\, O_4^{\pm 2} \equiv +\frac{\sqrt{10}}{16}\,[\{7J_z^2 - J(J+1) - 5\}\, J_\pm^2 + J_\pm^2\, \{\ldots\}]$$

$$\tilde{O}_4^{\pm 3} = \mp\frac{\sqrt{35}}{4}\, O_4^{\pm 3} \equiv \mp\frac{\sqrt{35}}{8}\,[J_zJ_\pm^3 + J_\pm^3J_z]$$

$$\tilde{O}_4^{\pm 4} = +\frac{\sqrt{70}}{16}\, O_4^{\pm 4} \equiv +\frac{\sqrt{70}}{16}\, J_\pm^4$$

$$\tilde{O}_6^0 = +\frac{1}{16}\, O_6^0 \equiv \frac{1}{16}[231J_z^6 - 105\{3J(J+1) - 7\}\, J_z^4 +$$

$$+ \{105J^2(J+1)^2 - 525J(J+1) + 294\}\, J_z^2 -$$

$$- 5J^3(J+1)^3 + 40J^2(J+1)^2 - 60J(J+1)]$$

TABLE A.2 (cont.)

$$\tilde{O}_6^{\pm 1} = \mp \frac{\sqrt{42}}{16} O_6^{\pm 1} \equiv \mp \frac{\sqrt{42}}{32} [\{33J_z^6 - 15(2J(J+1) - 1) J_z^3 + (5J^2(J+1)^2 - 10J(J+1) + 12) J_z\} J_\pm + J_\pm \{\ldots\}]$$

$$\tilde{O}_6^{\pm 2} = + \frac{\sqrt{105}}{32} O_6^{\pm 2} \equiv + \frac{\sqrt{105}}{64} [\{33J_z^4 - (18J(J+1) + 123) J_z^2 + J^2(J+1)^2 + 10J(J+1) + 102\} J_\pm^2 + J_\pm^2 \{\ldots\}]$$

$$\tilde{O}_6^{\pm 3} = \mp \frac{\sqrt{105}}{16} O_6^{\pm 3} \equiv \mp \frac{\sqrt{105}}{32} [\{11J_z^3 - 3J(J+1)J_z - 59J_z\} J_\pm^3 + J_\pm^3 \{\ldots\}]$$

$$\tilde{O}_6^{\pm 4} = + \frac{3\sqrt{14}}{32} O_6^{\pm 4} \equiv + \frac{3\sqrt{14}}{64} [\{11J_z^2 - J(J+1) - 38\} J_\pm^4 + J_\pm^4 \{\ldots\}]$$

$$\tilde{O}_6^{\pm 5} = \mp \frac{3\sqrt{77}}{16} O_6^{\pm 5} \equiv \mp \frac{3\sqrt{77}}{32} [J_z J_\pm^5 + J_\pm^5 J_z]$$

$$\tilde{O}_6^{\pm 6} = + \frac{\sqrt{231}}{32} O_6^{\pm 6} \equiv + \frac{\sqrt{231}}{32} J_\pm^6$$

---

the first two columns of Table A.2 (see e.g. Abragam and Bleaney (1970), pp. 864-72). The Stevens operators do not transform in the same way as the spherical harmonics $C_k^q(\theta,\phi)$ or $Y_k^q(\theta,\phi)$ under coordinate rotations.

A.3. VECTOR COUPLING COEFFICIENTS AND 3j SYMBOLS

The harmonic $C_k^q(\theta,\phi)$ can be expanded as a series of products $C_{k_1}^{q_1}(\theta,\phi)C_{k_2}^{q_2}(\theta,\phi)$ by means of the relation

$$C_k^q(\theta,\phi) = \sum_{q_1,q_2} (k_1 q_1 k_2 q_2 | k_1 k_2 k q) C_{k_1}^{q_1}(\theta,\phi) C_{k_2}^{q_2}(\theta,\phi). \qquad \text{(A.12)}$$

The summation is taken over all possible values of q_1, q_2 ($|q_1| \leqslant k_1$, $|q_2| \leqslant k_2$) such that $q_1 + q_2 = q$. The expansion can be made in a variety of ways by choosing different values of k_1, k_2 provided that k_1, k_2, and k obey the 'triangular rule' $k_1 + k_2 \geqslant k \geqslant |k_1 - k_2|$. The quantities $(k_1 q_1 k_2 q_2 \mid k_1 k_2 k q)$ are numerical coefficients, variously called the 'Wigner', 'Clebsch-Gordan', or 'vector-addition' coefficients. They can be derived from general formulae but are usually obtained from tables (see first paragraph of this Appendix). These coefficients automatically take on the value zero for arguments which violate the triangular rule or the rule $q_1 + q_2 = q$.

Eqn (A.12) is in essence merely a theorem in trigonometry. However, its chief applications are in quantum mechanics, where the harmonics $C_k^q(\theta,\phi)$ describe wavefunctions or are replaced by angular-momentum operators. In the former instance eqn (A.12) shows how a series of product wave-functions $\psi_{k_1}^{q_1}\,\psi_{k_2}^{q_2}$ belonging to two systems may be combined in such a way as to form a wave-function ψ_k^q having angular-momentum quantum numbers k,q. Conversely, eqn (A.12) can be used as a formula for resolving ψ_k^q into components. Combinations of this type are implied in the vector model of the atom where two angular momenta $\underline{k}_1$ and $\underline{k}_2$ add to form a resultant angular momentum $\underline{k}$.

Various notations have been used for the vector coupling coefficients.† Here we use the Wigner 3j symbols‡ which are

---

† The notation in (A.13) is that used by Edmonds (1960), (p.37). Brink and Satchler (1968) use $k_1 k_2 q_1 q_2 | k_q = (k_1 q_1 k_2 q_2 | k_1 k_2 k_q)$. Rose (1957) (p.85 et. seq.) uses $C(k_1 k_2 k | q_1 q_2 q) = C(k_1 k_2 k | q_1 q_2) = (k_1 q_1 k_2 q_2 | k_1 k_2 k q)$.

‡ Edmonds (1960), p.46. Brink and Satchler (1968), pp. 39-40, 136.

related to the Clebsch-Gordon coefficients by

$$\begin{pmatrix} k_1 & k_2 & k \\ q_1 & q_2 & q \end{pmatrix} = (-)^{k_1-k_2-q}(2k+1)^{-\frac{1}{2}}\,(k_1q_1k_2q_2|k_1k_2k{-q}). \tag{A.13}$$

It will be seen that the 3j symbols differ from the Clebsch-Gordan coefficients by a normalizing factor, a change in the sign of q and a possible change in the sign of the coefficient itself. The principal advantage of the 3j symbols is that they display the arguments clearly and make it easy to define the symmetry properties of the coefficients. In the 3j symbols, k_1, k_2, k, obey the triangular rule and $q_1 + q_2 + q = 0$. The 3j symbol is invariant under cyclic permutation of its columns and is multiplied by $(-)^{k_1+k_2+k}$ for non-cyclic ones, e.g.

$$\begin{pmatrix} k_1 & k_2 & k \\ q_1 & q_2 & q \end{pmatrix} = \begin{pmatrix} k_2 & k & k_1 \\ q_2 & q & q_1 \end{pmatrix} = (-)^{k_1+k_2+k}\begin{pmatrix} k_2 & k_1 & k \\ q_2 & q_1 & q \end{pmatrix}. \tag{A.14}$$

Also

$$\begin{pmatrix} k_1 & k_2 & k \\ -q_1 & -q_2 & -q \end{pmatrix} = (-)^{k_1+k_2+k}\begin{pmatrix} k_1 & k_2 & k \\ q_1 & q_2 & q \end{pmatrix}. \tag{A.15}$$

These relations reduce very considerably the space needed in order to tabulate the coefficients. General formulae are often too involved to be very useful, but the following special cases may be noted.

$$\begin{pmatrix} k_1 & k_2 & k \\ 0 & 0 & 0 \end{pmatrix} = 0 \text{ if } k_1 + k_2 + k \text{ is odd}, \tag{A.16}$$

$$\begin{pmatrix} k & k & 0 \\ q & -q & 0 \end{pmatrix} = (-)^{k-q}\,(2k+1)^{-\frac{1}{2}}\ , \tag{A.17}$$

$$\begin{pmatrix} k_1 & k_2 & (k_1+k_2) \\ q_1 & q_2 & (-q_1-q_2) \end{pmatrix} = \tag{A.18}$$

$$= (-1)^{k_1-k_2+q_1+q_2} \times \left\{ \frac{(2k_1)!(2k_2)!(k_1+k_2+q_1+q_2)!(k_1+k_2-q_1-q_2)!}{(2k_1+2k_2+1)!(k_1+q_1)!(k_1-q_1)!(k_2+q_2)!(k_2-q_2)!} \right\}^{\frac{1}{2}}.$$

The result (A.18) is used in §4.2. Recursion relations between the 3j symbols are discussed and some additional special cases are given in the texts cited earlier (see e.g. Edmonds (1960), pp. 48-50, Brink and Satchler (1968), pp. 136-140).

The 3j symbols obey the orthogonality relations

$$\sum_{k_1,k_2} (2k+1) \begin{pmatrix} k_1 & k_2 & k \\ q_1 & q_2 & q \end{pmatrix} \begin{pmatrix} k_1 & k_2 & k' \\ q_1 & q_2 & q' \end{pmatrix} = \delta(k-k')\delta(q-q'),$$

$$\sum_{k,q} (2k+1) \begin{pmatrix} k_1 & k_2 & k \\ q_1 & q_2 & q \end{pmatrix} \begin{pmatrix} k_1 & k_2 & k \\ q_1' & q_2' & q \end{pmatrix} = \delta(q_1-q_1')\delta(q_2-q_2') \tag{A.19}$$

Eqn (A.12) describing the decomposition of the spherical harmonic $C_k^q(\theta,\phi)$ becomes in 3j-symbol notation

$$C_k^q(\theta,\phi) =$$

$$= \sum_{q_1 q_2} (-)^{k_1-k_2+q}\,(2k+1)^{-\frac{1}{2}} \begin{pmatrix} k_1 & k_2 & k \\ q_1 & q_2 & -q \end{pmatrix} C_{k_1}^{q_1}(\theta,\phi) C_{k_2}^{q_2}(\theta,\phi). \tag{A.20}$$

$$C_{k_1}^{q_1}(\theta,\phi)C_{k_2}^{q_2}(\theta,\phi) =$$

$$= \sum_k (-)^q(2k+1)\begin{pmatrix} k_1 & k_2 & k \\ q_1 & q_2 & -q \end{pmatrix}\begin{pmatrix} k_1 & k_2 & k \\ 0 & 0 & 0 \end{pmatrix} C_k^q(\theta,\phi), \qquad \text{(A.21)}$$

where k takes on the values allowed by the triangle rule, and $q = q_1+q_2$ (note, however, that the second 3j symbol is zero if k_1+k_2+k is odd - eqn (A.16)). Some further addition theorems useful in manipulating spherical harmonics are given in Brink and Satchler (1968), p.146.

A.4. COORDINATE ROTATIONS

A.4.1. MATRICES. Let $\underline{M}$ be a matrix consisting of elements M_{ij} where i denotes the row and j the column. The symbol $\tilde{\underline{M}}$ denotes the 'transpose' of $\underline{M}$ obtained by interchanging rows and columns, i.e. $(\tilde{M})_{ij} = M_{ji}$. The transpose of a product is given by

$$\widetilde{(\underline{ABC})} = \underline{\tilde{C}}\,\underline{\tilde{B}}\,\underline{\tilde{A}} .$$

It is sometimes convenient to write a column vector (a matrix consisting of one column only) as the transpose $\tilde{\underline{v}}$ of a row vector (a matrix consisting of one row only).

If $\underline{M}$ is a square matrix and if the determinant $|M|$ is non-zero, an inverse matrix $\underline{M}^{-1}$ can be defined by

$$\underline{M}\,\underline{M}^{-1} = \underline{M}^{-1}\underline{M} = \underline{I} ,$$

where $\underline{I}$ is a unit matrix (i.e. a matrix consisting of diagonal elements only, each of them being unity). If $\underline{M}$ also has the property $\underline{M}^{-1} = \tilde{\underline{M}}$, i.e.

$$\underline{M}\tilde{\underline{M}} = \tilde{\underline{M}}\underline{M} = \underline{I} \ ;$$

it is called an 'orthogonal' matrix.

The symbol $\underline{M}^{\dagger}$ denotes the 'Hermitian conjugate' of $\underline{M}$ obtained by interchanging rows and columns and taking the complex conjugate of each element, i.e. $(M^{\dagger})_{ij} = (M_{ji})^*$. The Hermitian conjugate of a product is given by

$$(\underline{A}\underline{B}\underline{C})^{\dagger} = \underline{C}^{\dagger}\underline{B}^{\dagger}\underline{A}^{\dagger} \ .$$

If $\underline{M}$ has the property $\underline{M}^{-1} = \underline{M}^{\dagger}$, i.e.

$$\underline{M}\underline{M}^{\dagger} = \underline{M}^{\dagger}\underline{M} = \underline{I} \ ,$$

it is called a 'unitary' matrix. Unitary matrices represent a generalization of orthogonal matrices in the realm of complex numbers.

A.4.2. THE EULER ANGLES. Fig. A.1 indicates how the x,y,z Cartesian coordinate system may be rotated to give new Cartesian coordinates x''', y''', z''' by means of three steps performed in the following order:

(1) the x-,y-,z-axis system is rotated by α $(0 \le \alpha \le 2\pi)$ about the z-axis to give new axes x', y', z' ($z' \equiv z$ in this rotation);

(2) the x',y',z' system is rotated by β $(0 \le \beta \le \pi)$ about y' to give x'',y'',z'', ($y'' \equiv y'$ in this rotation);

(3) the x'',y'',z'' system is rotated by γ $(0 \le \gamma \le 2\pi)$ about z'' to give x''',y''',z''' ($z''' \equiv z''$ in this rotation).

The angles α,β,γ are known as the Euler angles. However, since conventions differ as to the sense of these angles, and the rotation axes chosen, it is essential before applying formulae

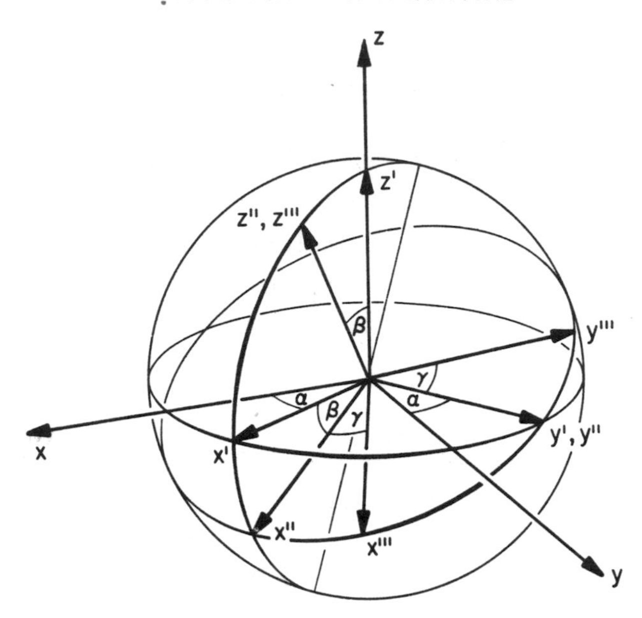

FIG. A.1. Rotation of a system of Cartesian axes x,y,z to new positions x''', y''',z''' is defined by the three Euler angles α,β,γ.

to verify the associated definitions.

The Euler angles enable us to specify the relationship between the coordinates (x,y,z), (x',y',z') of a point before and after an axis rotation. Let us suppose a point P is fixed in space and that its coordinates x,y,z in the original axis system form a column vector $\underline{r}$. Its new coordinates after the three rotations of axes will form a column vector $\underline{r}'$, where

$$\underline{r}' = \underline{\underline{M}}\underline{r} \tag{A.22}$$

and $\underline{\underline{M}}$ is the matrix

$$\begin{bmatrix} \cos\alpha\cos\beta\cos\gamma - \sin\alpha\sin\gamma & \sin\alpha\cos\beta\cos\gamma + \cos\alpha\sin\gamma & -\sin\beta\cos\gamma \\ -\cos\alpha\cos\beta\sin\gamma - \sin\alpha\cos\gamma & -\sin\alpha\cos\beta\sin\gamma + \cos\alpha\cos\gamma & \sin\beta\sin\gamma \\ \cos\alpha\sin\beta & \sin\alpha\sin\beta & \cos\beta \end{bmatrix} \tag{A.23}$$

$\underline{M}$ is an orthogonal matrix (§A.4.1). The elements of $\underline{M}$ consist of the cosines of the angles between the old and new coordinate axes. For instance, the element M_{13} is the cosine of the angle between the new x'''-axis and the old z-axis.

It is important to distinguish between the operation described above and the related operation of rotating a vector in space whilst the x,y,z coordinate system remains fixed. If we denote the vector before and after the rotation as $\underline{v}$ and $\underline{v}'$, then

$$\underline{v}' = \tilde{\underline{M}}\underline{v} \quad , \tag{A.24}$$

where $\tilde{\underline{M}}$ is the transpose (and also the reciprocal) of the matrix $\underline{M}$ in eqn (A.23). The rotations of the vector $\underline{v}$ (which can be visualized as an arrow embedded in a rigid body) are as follows:

(1) a rotation of $-\gamma$ about the z-axis;

(2) a rotation of $-\beta$ about the y-axis;

(3) a rotation of $-\alpha$ about the z-axis.

It will be noted that the angles are opposite in sign and the rotations are taken in the opposite order from those used to describe rotations of the coordinate system.

The rotation matrices as given in terms of Euler angles are somewhat cumbersome for the purpose of describing infinitesimal rotations. More convenient matrices can easily be derived, however. The matrix corresponding to a rotation of the coordinate axes by

$\Delta\phi_x$ about the x-axis is obtained by substituting $\alpha = -\pi/2$, $\beta = \Delta\phi_x$, $\gamma = \pi/2$ in (A.23). Matrices corresponding to coordinate axis rotations of $\Delta\phi_y$ about the y-axis or $\Delta\phi_z$ about the z-axis are obtained by substituting $\beta = \Delta\phi_y$ or $\alpha = \Delta\phi_z$ and setting the remaining Euler angles to zero. For a rotation of the coordinate axes by infinitesimal angles $\Delta\phi_x$, $\Delta\phi_y$, $\Delta\phi_z$ about the x-, y-, and z-axes, (the order of the operations is immaterial), the matrix $\underline{M}$ has the form

$$\underline{M}(\Delta\phi_x,\Delta\phi_y,\Delta\phi_z) = \begin{bmatrix} 1 & \Delta\phi_z & -\Delta\phi_y \\ -\Delta\phi_z & 1 & \Delta\phi_x \\ \Delta\phi_y & -\Delta\phi_x & 1 \end{bmatrix}$$

A.4.3. ORTHOGONAL TRANSFORMATIONS: principal axis transform. The term $\mathcal{H}_D = D_{jk}S_jS_k$ which enters into the spin Hamiltonian (3.1) can also be written in the form

$$\mathcal{H}_D = \underline{\tilde{S}}\underline{D}\underline{S} \; , \tag{A.25}$$

where $\underline{S}$ is a three-component column vector, made up of the operators S_x, S_y, S_z, and $\underline{D}$ is a 3 × 3 matrix. If we now rotate the coordinate system, the spin operators are transformed to $S_x', S_y'. S_z'$ as in eqn (A.22), i.e.

$$\underline{S}' = \underline{M}\underline{S} \; ,$$

where $\underline{M}$ is the matrix (A.23). The Hamiltonian $\mathcal{H}_D$ is a scalar operator, however, and will be unaffected by the change of coordinate system, so that

$$\mathcal{H}_D = \underline{\tilde{S}}\underline{D}\underline{S} \equiv \underline{\tilde{S}}'\underline{D}'\underline{S}' \; ,$$

where $\underline{D}'$ consists of a new set of coefficients belonging to the transformed spin operators $S'_jS'_k$.† From this identity we derive the relation

$$\underline{D} = \underline{\tilde{M}}\underline{D}'\underline{M} \;, \tag{A.26}$$

and the converse relation

$$\underline{D}' = \underline{M}\underline{D}\underline{\tilde{M}} \;, \tag{A.27}$$

which follows from the orthogonal property of the matrix $\underline{M}$. The transformations in eqns (A.26) and (A.27) are called orthogonal transforms, i.e. similarity transforms involving an orthogonal matrix. The same transformations

$$\underline{G} = \underline{\tilde{M}}\underline{G}'\underline{M} \;, \tag{A.28}$$

$$\underline{G}' = \underline{M}\underline{G}\underline{\tilde{M}} \;, \tag{A.29}$$

can be used to re-express the parameters of the g^2-matrix (eqns (3.25)) in a rotated coordinate system. They can also be used to transform the g-matrix provided that the Cartesian operators H_j, S_k in the spin Hamiltonian

$$\mathcal{H}_g = \beta \sum_{jk} g_{jk} H_j S_k = \beta \underline{\tilde{H}}\underline{g}\underline{S} \tag{A.30}$$

are transformed as in eqn (A.24). It is not essential here that the g-matrix should be symmetrical in j,k (see §3.4).

---

†This amounts to saying that the elements $(\mathcal{H}_D)_{pq}$ in the Hamiltonian matrix will remain unaltered provided that the basis wavefunctions are not changed when the coordinate system is rotated.

By means of a suitable orthogonal transformation, a real symmetric matrix can be transformed into a diagonal matrix. As an example we can take the g^2-matrix G_{jk}. The transforming equation giving a diagonal matrix $\underline{G}_D$ from G_{jk} is

$$\underline{G}_D = \underline{\tilde{N}}_D \underline{G} \underline{N}_D , \qquad (A.31)$$

where the matrix

$$\underline{N}_D = [\underline{v}_1, \underline{v}_2, \underline{v}_3] \qquad (A.32)$$

consists of three normalized column eigenvectors obtained by solving the matrix equation

$$\underline{G}\underline{v} = \lambda \underline{v} , \qquad (A.33)$$

and $\underline{G}_D$ consists of the three eigenvalues $\lambda_1, \lambda_2, \lambda_3$. Comparing eqns (A.29)-(A.31) we see that the transformation corresponds to a coordinate rotation by means of a matrix $\underline{M}_D = \underline{\tilde{N}}_D \equiv \underline{N}_D^{-1}$. The three new Cartesian axes are given in the old coordinate system by the vectors $\underline{v}_1, \underline{v}_2, \underline{v}_3$, these vectors being termed the 'principal axes' of $\underline{G}$. The transform is called a 'principal axis transform'.

The principal values g_1, g_2, g_3 of the g-tensor can be obtained by equating the eigenvalues of $\underline{G}$ to g_1^2, g_2^2, g_3^2 and taking square-roots.[†] g_1, g_2, g_3 are the values assumed by g in the equation $h = g\beta H_0$ when H_0 is oriented along each of the three principal axes $\underline{v}_1, \underline{v}_2, \underline{v}_3$. Experimental data on low-symmetry sites is usually expressed by giving the three principal g-values g_1, g_2, g_3, and the polar coordinates of the corresponding principal axes $\underline{v}_1, \underline{v}_2, \underline{v}_3$ with respect to some convenient set of crystallographic axes.

[†] It is not necessarily correct to take the positive roots (see Blume, Geschwind, and Yafet 1969).

By following a similar procedure with the matrix D_{ij}, we can obtain three principal values D_1, D_2, D_3 and thus re-express the D-term in the diagonal form

$$\mathcal{H}_D = D_1 S_x^2 + D_2 S_y^2 + D_3 S_z^2 \ .$$

A further simplification can then be made by requiring that $D_1 + D_2 + D_3 = 0$ (see §3.3), thus leaving $\mathcal{H}_D$ defined by two parameters D and E, as in

$$\mathcal{H}_D = D\left\{S_z^2 - \frac{1}{3}S(S+1)\right\} + E\left(S_x^2 - S_y^2\right) \ ,$$

and by three angles which give the orientation of the principal axis system. The principal axes obtained by solving the eigenvalue equation (A.33) for the matrix $\underline{D}$ can be assigned as x-, y-, z-axes in any arbitrary manner and three different sets of D- and E-parameters can therefore in principle be used to describe experimental data. The usual custom in order to avoid confusion is to choose the set which makes E positive and which makes D greater than E. (Conversion from one set of D,E-parameters to another can be made by changing to Cartesian coefficients D_1, D_2, D_3, permuting the subscripts, and then reverting to the D,E-form as in eqn (3.9).)

A.4.4. SPHERICAL TENSOR TRANSFORMATIONS OF THE ELECTRIC FIELD, OF THE D-TERM, AND OF THE QUARTIC TERM. Spherical tensor notation can be used as an alternative to Cartesian notation in formulating the spin Hamiltonian (see §§3.8–3.9). There is generally little to be gained by using this notation, however, unless it is necessary to specify higher-order terms in the spin Hamiltonian or to make coordinate transformations. For the transformation of second-rank tensors such as the D-tensor or the g-tensor the orthogonal transformations discussed in the previous section are usually convenient enough. But the spherical tensor notation possesses considerable advantages when it is required to change the coordinate system for the linear electric field effect terms. Since experimental data is customarily expressed in Cartesian notation, the transformation can be made in three steps: (1) conversion to spherical tensor form; (2) coordinate rotation; (3) reconversion to Cartesian form.

We begin with the transformation of the electric field operator (a first-rank Cartesian tensor) and of terms appearing as second- and fourth-rank Cartesian tensors in the standard form of spin Hamiltonian. As just pointed out, it may actually be easier in all cases save that of the fourth-rank term to use the methods of §A.4.3 and thus avoid the problem of converting to spherical tensor form, but it is necessary to understand these transformations in order to follow the argument in §§A.4.6-4.7.

Let us first consider the transformation of the electric field. The Cartesian components E_x, E_y, E_z can be converted to spherical tensor components $E^{(1)}_{\pm 1}$, $E^{(0)}$ as in eqn (3.56) and assembled to form a column vector

$$\underline{E}^{(1)} = \begin{bmatrix} E^{(1)}_{1} \\ \\ E^{(1)}_{0} \\ \\ E^{(1)}_{-1} \end{bmatrix} \tag{A.34}$$

If we now rotate the coordinate axes through Euler angles α, β, γ (Fig. A.1) leaving the electric field vector fixed in space we obtain new spherical tensor components $E^{(1)'}_{\pm 1}$, $E^{(1)'}_{0}$, forming a column vector $\underline{E}^{(1)'}$, where

$$\underline{E}^{(1)'} = \underline{\tilde{\mathscr{D}}}^{(1)} \underline{E}^{(1)} \quad . \tag{A.35}$$

The transforming matrix $\underline{\tilde{\mathscr{D}}}^{(1)}$ in (A.35) is the transpose of the matrix

$$\underline{\mathscr{D}}^{(1)} = \begin{bmatrix} e^{-i\alpha}\left(\frac{1+\cos\beta}{2}\right)e^{-i\gamma} & -e^{-i\alpha}\frac{\sin\beta}{\sqrt{2}} & e^{-i\alpha}\left(\frac{1-\cos\beta}{2}\right)e^{i\gamma} \\ \frac{\sin\beta}{\sqrt{2}}e^{-i\gamma} & \cos\beta & \frac{-\sin\beta}{\sqrt{2}}e^{i\gamma} \\ e^{i\alpha}\left(\frac{1-\cos\beta}{2}\right)e^{-i\gamma} & e^{i\alpha}\frac{\sin\beta}{\sqrt{2}} & e^{i\alpha}\left(\frac{1+\cos\beta}{2}\right)e^{i\gamma} \end{bmatrix} \tag{A.36}$$

The matrix $\underline{\mathscr{D}}^{(1)}$ can be obtained by calculating the elements

$$\mathscr{D}^{(1)}_{mm'} = \langle m \mid e^{-iJ_z\alpha}\, e^{-iJ_y\beta}\, e^{-iJ_z\gamma} \mid m' \rangle \tag{A.37}$$

in a J = 1 manifold of states.† (The 'substates' m = 1,0,-1 correspond to elements in the first, second, and third rows of $\underline{\mathscr{D}}^{(1)}$, and the 'substates' m' = 1,0,-1 to elements in the first, second, and third columns. The angular-momentum operators J_z, J_y are expressed in units of $\hbar$.) Since $\underline{\mathscr{D}}^{(1)}$ is a unitary matrix eqn (A.35) can be inverted to give $\underline{E}^{(1)}$ as a function of $\underline{E}^{(1)'}$ as in

$$\underline{E}^{(1)} = (\underline{\tilde{\mathscr{D}}}^{(1)})^{\dagger}\underline{E}^{(1)'} = (\underline{\mathscr{D}}^{(1)})^{*}\underline{E}^{(1)'} \quad . \tag{A.38}$$

---

†The definition given here is in accordance with the definition given by Rose (1957) and by Brink and Satchler (1968). The signs of α,β,γ are reversed in Edmonds (1960). Thus $D(\alpha,\beta,\gamma) = D_{\text{Edmonds}}(-\alpha,-\beta,-\gamma)$.

The spherical tensor components $E_{\pm1}^{(1)'}, E_0^{(1)'}$ in the new coordinate system can be converted to Cartesian components E_x', E_y', E_z' in the new system by means of eqn (3.57).

Next let us consider the spin operators appearing in the D-term of the spin Hamiltonian. The conversion to spherical tensor form is made by eqn (3.58), and the resulting spin operators $S_j^{(2)}$ are arranged to form a five-component column vector

$$\underline{S}^{(2)} = \begin{bmatrix} S_2^{(2)} \\ S_1^{(2)} \\ S_0^{(2)} \\ S_{-1}^{(2)} \\ S_{-2}^{(2)} \end{bmatrix} \qquad \text{(A.39)}$$

The transforming equations are

$$\underline{S}^{(2)'} = \underline{\mathscr{D}}^{(2)} \underline{S}^{(2)} , \qquad \text{(A.40)}$$

$$\underline{S}^{(2)} = \underline{\mathscr{D}}^{(2)*} \underline{S}^{(2)'} , \qquad \text{(A.41)}$$

where $\underline{\mathscr{D}}^{(2)}$ is the 5 × 5 unitary matrix obtained by evaluating the elements on the right-hand side of eqn (A.37) in a J = 2 manifold of states. (The 'substates' m = 2,1,0,-1,-2 correspond to elements in the first, second, third, fourth, fifth rows of $\underline{\mathscr{D}}^{(2)}$, etc.) The required matrix elements can be found by taking the parameters $d_{mm'}^{(2)}$ (i.e. the elements $\langle m \mid e^{-J_y\beta} \mid m' \rangle$) from Table A.3 and forming the product

$$\mathscr{D}_{mm'}^{(2)} = \exp\{-i(m\alpha + m'\gamma)\} d_{mm'}^{(2)} . \qquad \text{(A.42)}$$

TABLE A.3

The rotation matrix required to transform spherical tensors of the type $S_q^{(2)}$ consists of elements $\mathscr{D}_{mm'}^{(2)}(\alpha,\beta,\gamma) = \exp\{-i(m\alpha+m'\gamma)\}\, d_{mm'}^{(2)}$, where $d_{mm'}^{(2)}$ are the quantities given in the table below. The $d_{mm'}^{(2)}$ are interrelated by the equations $d_{mm'}^{(2)} = (-1)^{m-m'}\, d_{m'm}^{(2)} = d_{-m'-m}^{(2)}$.

$$d_{22}^{(2)} = d_{-2-2}^{(2)} = \cos^4(\beta/2)$$

$$d_{21}^{(2)} = -d_{12}^{(2)} = -d_{-2-1}^{(2)} = d_{-1-2}^{(2)} = -\frac{1}{2}\sin\beta(1+\cos\beta)$$

$$d_{20}^{(2)} = d_{02}^{(2)} = d_{-20}^{(2)} = d_{0-2}^{(2)} = \sqrt{\frac{3}{8}}\sin^2\beta$$

$$d_{2-1}^{(2)} = d_{1-2}^{(2)} = -d_{-21}^{(2)} = -d_{-12}^{(2)} = \frac{1}{2}\sin\beta(\cos\beta-1)$$

$$d_{2-2}^{(2)} = d_{-22}^{(2)} = \sin^4(\beta/2)$$

$$d_{11}^{(2)} = d_{-1-1}^{(2)} = \frac{1}{2}(2\cos\beta-1)(\cos\beta+1)$$

$$d_{1-1}^{(2)} = d_{-11}^{(2)} = \frac{1}{2}(2\cos\beta+1)(1-\cos\beta)$$

$$d_{10}^{(2)} = d_{0-1}^{(2)} = -d_{01}^{(2)} = -d_{-10}^{(2)} = -\sqrt{\frac{3}{2}}\sin\beta\cos\beta$$

$$d_{00}^{(2)} = \frac{1}{2}(3\cos^2\beta-1)\,.$$

Spin operators $S_j^{(2)'}$ in the new system can be converted to Cartesian spin operators in the old system by means of eqn (3.59).

In handling experimental data it is usually the coefficients of the operators that we wish to transform. The rules for transforming these coefficients can be derived from the rules for transforming the operators themselves as follows. In spherical tensor notation, the D-term becomes†

$$\mathcal{H}_D = \sum_j D_j^{(2)} S_j^{(2)} \quad (j = 0, \pm 1, \pm 2). \qquad \text{(A.43)}$$

If, as in the case of the spin operators $S_j^{(2)}$, we represent the coefficients $D_j^{(2)}$ by a column vector $\underline{D}^{(2)}$ the D-term can be then expressed in the form

$$\mathcal{H}_D = \underline{\tilde{D}}^{(2)} \underline{S}^{(2)} . \qquad \text{(A.44)}$$

Rotation of the coordinate system results in the transformation to new spin operators and coefficients $\underline{S}^{(2)'}$, $\underline{D}^{(2)'}$, but $\mathcal{H}_D$ remains unchanged since it is a scalar operator and we thus have

$$\mathcal{H}_D = \underline{\tilde{D}}^{(2)'} \underline{S}^{(2)'} = \underline{\tilde{D}}^{(2)} \underline{S}^{(2)} . \qquad \text{(A.45)}$$

Hence, substituting $\underline{S}^{(2)'} = \underline{\tilde{\mathcal{D}}}^{(2)} \underline{S}^{(2)}$ as in (A.40), we obtain the relation $\underline{\tilde{D}}^{(2)} = \underline{\tilde{D}}^{(2)'} \underline{\tilde{\mathcal{D}}}^{(2)}$. Transposing, we have

---

† The choice of the notation $D_j^{(2)}$ for the coefficients of the spherical spin operators leads to the inelegant apposition of the symbols $\underline{D}^{(2)}$ and $\underline{\mathcal{D}}^{(2)}$ in some of the succeeding equations. No real confusion is possible, however, and it seems preferable to retain a notation which indicates the relationship with the D-term in the spin Hamiltonian rather than adopt new symbols.

$$\underline{D}^{(2)} = \underline{\mathcal{D}}^{(2)}\underline{D}^{(2)'} \qquad (A.46)$$

and also the converse relation

$$\underline{D}^{(2)'} = \underline{\mathcal{D}}^{(2)\dagger}\,\underline{D}^{(2)} , \qquad (A.47)$$

which follows from the unitary property of $\underline{\mathcal{D}}^{(2)}$. It will be seen that conversion to spherical tensor form enables us to write Hamiltonian $\mathcal{H}_D$ as the product of the two vectors† instead of as the product of vectors and matrices as in eqn (A.25). This reduction in the algebraic order of the expression confers no especial benefits in the case of $\mathcal{H}_D$, but it can be very helpful when one has to transform the electric field shift terms.

The equations for transforming the fourth-degree spin operator term in the spin Hamiltonian are similar to those used to transform $\mathcal{H}_D$. Thus we have

$$\underline{S}^{(4)'} = \underline{\mathcal{D}}^{(4)}\underline{S}^{(4)} , \qquad (A.48)$$

where $\underline{S}^{(4)'}$, $\underline{S}^{(4)}$ are nine-component column vectors and $\underline{\mathcal{D}}^{(4)}$ is the 9 × 9 unitary matrix obtained by evaluating the matrix elements on the right-hand side of (A.36) in a J = 4 manifold of states. The elements of $\underline{\mathcal{D}}^{(4)}$ can be obtained from general formulae given in the textbooks listed at the beginning of the Appendix (see

---

† Not however the <u>scalar</u> product. The scalar product of two spherical tensor operators $\underline{U},\underline{V}$ has the form $\sum_j (-1)^j\, U_j V_{-j}$. This product has no relevance here since $D_j^{(2)}$ is not a tensor operator but is merely a vector made up of the coefficients of the tensor operators $S_j^{(2)}$.

e.g. Edmonds (1960), Chapter 4; Brink and Satchler (1968) §2.4). Conversion to or from Cartesian form is not usually needed here since it is the general practice to use spherical tensor operators for the fourth-degree term in the spin Hamiltonian. But the normalizing factors in the spin operators should be checked to see that they are the same as or in a constant proportion to those shown in Table A.2. The Stevens operators O_k^q cannot be transformed in this way.

Infinitesimal transformation matrices can be derived from the matrices expressed in terms of Euler angles by making the substitutions indicated at the end of §A.4.2. It is perhaps easier, however, to expand the exponential operators up to the first order and calculate the required matrix elements ab initio as in (A.37). The rotation matrix corresponding to infinitesimal rotations of the coordinate system by angles $\Delta\phi_x$, $\Delta\phi_y$, $\Delta\phi_z$ about the x-, y-, and z-axes consists of the elements

$$\mathscr{D}^{(k)}_{mm'} = \langle m|1-i(\Delta\phi_x J_x+\Delta\phi_y J_y+\Delta\phi_z J_z)|m'\rangle ,$$

where m, m' are magnetic substates in a J = k manifold and J_x, J_y, J_z are angular-momentum operators in units of $\hbar$ (see eqn 6.9).

A.4.5. SPHERICAL TENSOR TRANSFORMATION OF g. We can avoid the problems raised by possible lack of symmetry of the g matrix (§3.4) by framing the discussion in terms of the g^2-matrix G_{jk} (eqn (3.24)). The same arguments will apply to the g-matrix provided that it is made symmetric by a suitable choice of representation, and provided that the operators representing spin and the Zeeman field are both transformed when the coordinate system is rotated.

An additional problem arises here since the matrix G_{jk} is not traceless and contains an isotropic portion as well as a second-degree spherical tensor portion. Only the latter is changed by coordinate rotation. Thus, adopting the Voigt notation (§3.2), we can resolve G_{jk} into a trace

$$G^{(0)} = G_1 + G_2 + G_3 \tag{A.49}$$

and a traceless portion, in terms of which eqn (3.26) becomes

$$g^2 = G^{(0)} + \left(G_1 - \tfrac{1}{3}G^{(0)}\right)\ell^2 + \left(G_2 - \tfrac{1}{3}G^{(0)}\right)m^2 + \left(G_3 - \tfrac{1}{3}G^{(0)}\right)n^2 + 2G_4 mn + 2G_5 \ell n + 2G_6 \ell m. \tag{A.50}$$

In spherical tensor notation, (A.50) assumes the form

$$g^2 = G^{(0)} + \sum_j G_j^{(2)} C_2^j(\theta,\phi) \quad (j = 0, \pm 1, \pm 2)\ , \tag{A.51}$$

where the $C_2^j(\theta,\phi)$ are second-degree spherical harmonics, and the spherical tensor coefficients $G_j^{(2)}$ corresponding to the traceless portion of G_{jk} are related to the Voigt coefficients by

$$\begin{aligned} G_0^{(2)} &= G_3 - \tfrac{1}{3}G^{(0)}\ , \\ G_{\pm 1}^{(2)} &= \mp \sqrt{\tfrac{2}{3}}\,(G_5 \mp iG_4)\ , \\ G_{\pm 2}^{(2)} &= \tfrac{1}{2}\sqrt{\tfrac{2}{3}}\,\{(G_1 - G_2) \mp 2iG_6\} \end{aligned} \tag{A.52}$$

(cf. eqn (3.62)).

In matrix notation analogous to that used in (A.44), eqn (A.51) becomes

$$g^2 = G^{(0)} + \underset{\sim}{\underline{G}}^{(2)}\underline{C}^{(2)}\ , \tag{A.53}$$

where $\underset{\sim}{\underline{G}}^{(2)}$ is the row vector $\left[G_2^{(2)},\ G_1^{(2)},\ G_0^{(2)};\ G_{-1}^{(2)},\ G_{-2}^{(2)}\right]$,

$\underline{C}^{(2)}$ is the column vector

$$\begin{bmatrix} C_2^2 \\ C_2^1 \\ C_2^0 \\ C_2^{-1} \\ C_2^{-2} \end{bmatrix}$$

and $G^{(0)}$ is a scalar. When the coordinate system is rotated, $\underline{C}^{(2)}$ transforms in the same way as $S^{(2)}$, i.e.

$$\underline{C}^{(2)'} = \underline{\tilde{\mathscr{D}}}^{(2)}\underline{C}^{(2)} , \tag{A.54}$$

$$\underline{C}^{(2)} = \underline{\mathscr{D}}^{(2)*}\underline{C}^{(2)'} . \tag{A.55}$$

But $g^2 - G^{(0)}$ is a scalar and is independent of the coordinate system. Therefore by analogy with eqn (A.45) we have

$$g^2 - G^{(0)} = \underline{\tilde{G}}^{(2)'}\underline{C}^{(2)'} = \underline{\tilde{G}}^{(2)}\underline{C}^{(2)} , \tag{A.56}$$

where $\underline{C}^{(2)'}$ contains the transformed harmonics $C_2^j(\theta', \phi')$ and $\underline{G}^{(2)'}$ contains the transformed coefficients. Hence

$$\underline{G}^{(2)'} = (\underline{\mathscr{D}}^{(2)})^{\dagger}\underline{G}^{(2)} . \tag{A.57}$$

To complete the operation the new spherical tensor coefficients $G_j^{(2)'}$ can be reconverted into the Voigt form, and the trace $G^{(0)}$ added back into the result giving

$$G_1' = \frac{1}{3} G^{(0)} - \frac{1}{2} G_0^{(2)'} + \frac{1}{2} \sqrt{\frac{3}{2}} \left(G_2^{(2)'} + G_{-2}^{(2)'} \right) \quad ,$$

$$G_2' = \frac{1}{3} G^{(0)} - \frac{1}{2} G_0^{(2)'} - \frac{1}{2} \sqrt{\frac{3}{2}} \left(G_2^{(2)'} + G_{-2}^{(2)'} \right) \quad ,$$

$$G_3' = \frac{1}{3} G^{(0)} + G_0^{(2)'} \quad ,$$

$$\qquad\qquad\qquad\qquad\qquad\qquad\qquad\qquad\qquad\qquad \text{(A.58)}$$

$$G_4' = -\frac{i}{2}\sqrt{\frac{3}{2}} \left(G_1^{(2)'} - G_{-1}^{(2)'} \right) \quad ,$$

$$G_5' = -\frac{1}{2}\sqrt{\frac{3}{2}} \left(G_1^{(2)'} - G_{-1}^{(2)'} \right) \quad ,$$

$$G_6' = \frac{i}{2}\sqrt{\frac{3}{2}} \left(G_2^{(2)'} - G_2^{(2)'} \right) \quad .$$

(The essential steps in the transformation are embodied in eqns (A.49), (A.52), (A.57), (A.58).) It will be apparent that this procedure is quite cumbersome in comparison with the direct Cartesian transformation of $\underline{G}$ (eqn A.29)). The only reason for discussing it here is to prepare the way for the transformation of the g^2-shift parameters B_{ij} (§A.4.7).

A.4.6. SPHERICAL TENSOR TRANSFORMATION OF R_{ij} AND OF THE SHIFTS IN THE QUARTIC TERM. The third-rank Cartesian term $\mathcal{H}_{\text{D-shift}} = \sum_{i,j,k} R_{ijk} E_i S_j S_k$ can be rewritten in the spherical tensor form

$$\sum_{i,j} R_{i,j}^{(2)} E_i^{(1)} S_j^{(2)} \quad (i = 0, \pm 1;\ j = 0, \pm 1, \pm 2)$$

(see eqn (3.65)). Re-expressing this term as a product of matrices, we have

$$\mathcal{H}_{\text{D-shift}} = \underline{\tilde{E}}^{(1)}\underline{R}^{(2)}\underline{S}^{(2)} ,$$

where

$$\underline{R}^{(2)} = \begin{bmatrix} R^{(2)}_{1,2} & R^{(2)}_{1,1} & R^{(2)}_{1,0} & R^{(2)}_{1,-1} & R^{(2)}_{1,-2} \\ R^{(2)}_{0,2} & R^{(2)}_{0,1} & R^{(2)}_{0,0} & R^{(2)}_{0,-1} & R^{(2)}_{0,-2} \\ R^{(2)}_{-1,2} & R^{(2)}_{-1,1} & R^{(2)}_{-1,0} & R^{(2)}_{-1,-1} & R^{(2)}_{-1,-2} \end{bmatrix} \qquad \text{(A.59)}$$

and where $\underline{E}^{(1)}$, $\underline{S}^{(2)}$ are as in eqns (A.34), (A.39). Once again, since $\mathcal{H}_D$ is a scalar operator and independent of the coordinate system, we have an identity

$$\mathcal{H}_{\text{D-shift}} = \underline{\tilde{E}}^{(1)'}\underline{R}^{(2)'}\underline{S}^{(2)'} \equiv \underline{\tilde{E}}^{(1)}\underline{R}^{(2)}\underline{S}^{(2)} . \qquad \text{(A.60)}$$

Hence, from (A.35), (A.40),

$$\underline{R}^{(2)} = \underline{\mathcal{D}}^{(1)}\underline{R}^{(2)'}\underline{\tilde{\mathcal{D}}}^{(2)} \qquad \text{(A.61)}$$

and also

$$\underline{R}^{(2)'} = (\underline{\mathcal{D}}^{(1)})^{\dagger}\underline{R}^{(2)}\underline{\mathcal{D}}^{(2)*} . \qquad \text{(A.62)}$$

The transformation of Cartesian coefficients R_{ijk} to new coefficients R'_{ijk} is therefore made as follows. The Cartesian coefficients are (if need be) converted into traceless practical units by eqn (3.12). These are then converted into spherical tensor form by means of Table 3.3 (p.87). Rotation matrices $\underline{\mathcal{D}}^{(1)}$ and $\underline{\mathcal{D}}^{(2)}$ are constructed from eqn (A.36) and Table A.3 and the multiplication (A.62) is performed. Finally, the new spherical tensor coefficients are re-converted into Cartesian form by means of Table 3.4 (p.88).

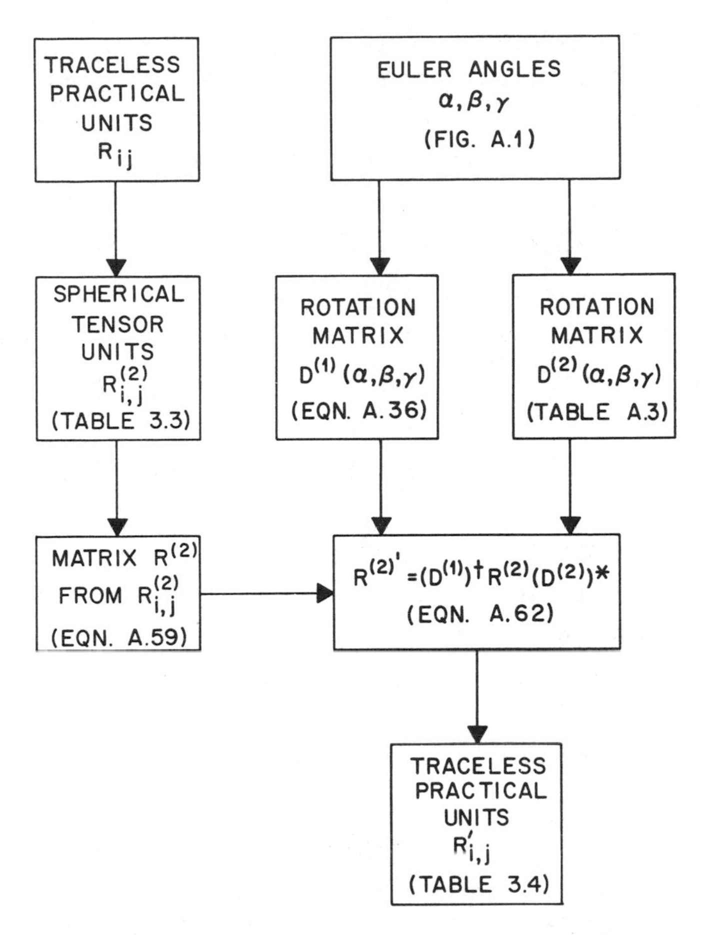

FIG. A.2. Flow chart showing the steps to be followed in order to transform the D-shift coefficients R_{ij} when the coordinate system is rotated. The coefficients are converted into spherical tensor form in order to make the transformation.

The steps in this calculation are shown schematically in Fig. A.2.

The advantage of using a spherical tensor transformation in place of a full Cartesian tensor transformation of the coefficients R_{ijk} (see e.g. Margenau and Murphy 1956, pp. 161-7) arises from the fact that the D-term can in this way be represented as a five-component vector rather than as a 3 × 3 matrix. There is, however, no particular advantage in specifying the electric field in spherical tensor components rather than in Cartesian components. In the one case the transformation is as in (A.35), in the other as in eqn (A.22), a 3 × 3 transforming matrix being required in both instances. Should it happen that the Cartesian transforming matrix $\underline{M}$ in Eqn (A.23) is appreciably easier to handle than the spherical tensor transforming matrix $\underline{\mathcal{D}}^{(1)}$ in eqn (A.36) the procedure indicated above can be modified as follows. The Cartesian coefficients (or traceless practical coefficients) are converted into the mixed form $R^{(C,2)}_{i,j}$ giving the D-shift Hamiltonian

$$\mathcal{H}_{\text{D-shift}} = R^{(C,2)}_{i,j} E_i S_j \qquad (i = x,y,z;\ j = 0,\pm 1,\pm 2)$$

(see eqn (3.66), (3.67)) in which the electric field remains in Cartesian components but spherical tensor operators are used for the spin. The new set of mixed coefficients in the rotated coordinate system can then be obtained from the matrix equation

$$\underline{R}^{(C,2)'} = \underline{M}\underline{R}^{(C,2)}\underline{\mathcal{D}}^{(2)*} , \tag{A.63}$$

where $\underline{R}^{(C,2)}$ is a 3 × 5 matrix analogous to $\underline{R}^{(2)}$ in eqn (A.59). Conversion to Cartesian form follows the same rule as conversion of the coefficients $D^{(2)}_q$ in Eqns (3.63), (3.64).

The transformation of the fourth-degree linear electric field shift term $R^{(4)}_{i,j} E_i S_j^{(4)}$ can be handled in the same way as the transformation of the D-shift term. In place of eqn (A.62) we have

$$\underline{R}^{(4)'} = (\underline{\mathcal{D}}^{(1)})^{\dagger}\underline{R}^{(4)}\underline{\mathcal{D}}^{(4)*} , \tag{A.64}$$

where $\underline{\mathcal{D}}^{(4)}$ is the 9 × 9 unitary matrix in eqn (A.48) and $\underline{R}^{(4)}$ is a matrix consisting of three rows and nine columns. (The first row of $\underline{R}^{(4)}$ will be $R^{(4)}_{1,4}$, $R^{(4)}_{1,3}$, $R^{(4)}_{1,2}$, $R^{(4)}_{1,1}$, $R^{(4)}_{1,0}$, $R^{(4)}_{1,-1}$, $R^{(4)}_{1,-2}$,

$R^{(4)}_{1,-3}, R^{(4)}_{1,-4}$.) The transformation will work equally well for mixed coefficients $R^{(C,4)}_{i,j}$, where the electric field is expressed in Cartesian components, provided that $\underline{\mathscr{D}}^{(1)}$ is replaced by the orthogonal matrix $\underline{M}$ (eqn (A.23)).

A.4.7. SPHERICAL TENSOR TRANSFORMATION OF B_{ij}. The coefficients B_{ij} can be transformed in the same manner as the coefficients R_{ij} provided that the quantities corresponding to the traces of the g^2-matrix are extracted and transformed separately (see §A.4.5). One possible procedure, shown diagrammatically in Fig. A.3, is as follows.

1. The coefficients B_{ij} are converted to a mixed set of coefficients $B^{(1,C)}_{i,j}$ for which the electric field is specified in spherical tensor form whilst the magnetic field remains specified by the Cartesian direction cosines. The conversion is made by means of the equations

$$B^{(1,C)}_{\pm 1,j} = \mp \frac{1}{\sqrt{2}} (B_{1j} \mp B_{2j}) ,$$

$$B^{(1,C)}_{0,j} = B_{3j} \qquad (j = 1,6). \tag{A.65}$$

2. The three traces

$$B^{(0)}_{i} = B^{(1,C)}_{i,1} + B^{(1,C)}_{i,2} + B^{(1,C)}_{i,3} \qquad (i = 0,\pm 1) \tag{A.66}$$

are extracted from the $B^{(1,C)}_{i,j}$ and the residual quantities are used to form spherical tensor coefficients $B^{(2)}_{i,j}$ ($i = 0,\pm 1;\ j = 0,\pm 1,\pm 2$). This step is analogous to the one taken in eqn (A.52) and is made by means of the relations

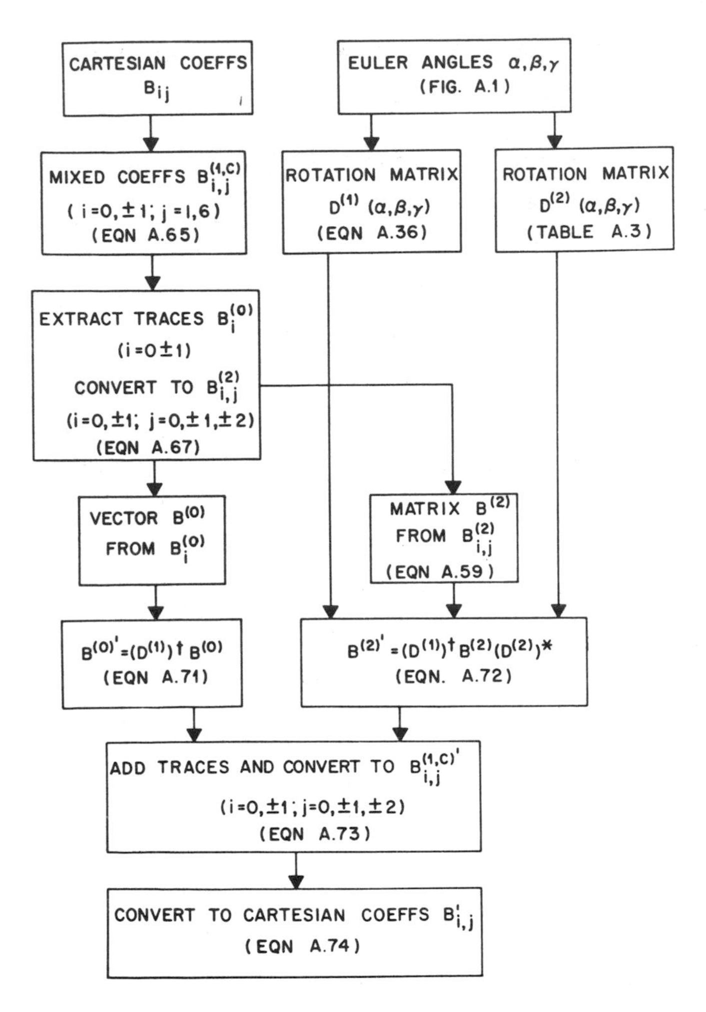

FIG. A.3. Flow chart illustrating one possible procedure for transforming the g^2-shift coefficients B_{ij} when the coordinate system is rotated. The coefficients are converted into spherical tensor form in order to make the transformation. Quantities which correspond to the trace of the g^2-matrix are extracted and transformed separately.

$$B^{(2)}_{i,0} = B^{(1,C)}_{i,3} - \frac{1}{3} B^{(0)}_{i} ,$$

$$B^{(2)}_{i,\pm 1} = \mp \sqrt{\frac{2}{3}} \left(B^{(1,C)}_{i,5} \mp iB^{(1,C)}_{i,4} \right) , \tag{A.67}$$

$$B^{(2)}_{i,\pm 2} = \frac{1}{2} \sqrt{\frac{2}{3}} \left\{ \left(B^{(1,C)}_{i,1} - B^{(1,C)}_{i,2} \right) \mp 2iB^{(1,C)}_{i,6} \right\} \; (i = 0,\pm 1) .$$

3. The three traces $B^{(0)}_{i}$ are assembled to give a column vector

$$\underline{B}^{(0)} = \begin{bmatrix} B^{(0)}_{1} \\ B^{(0)}_{0} \\ B^{(0)}_{-1} \end{bmatrix} \tag{A.68}$$

and the fifteen coefficients $B^{(2)}_{i,j}$ $(i = 0,\pm 1;\ j = 0,\pm 1,\pm 2)$ are assembled to give a matrix $\underline{B}^{(2)}$ having the same form as the matrix $\underline{R}^{(2)}$ in eqn (A.59). Eqn (3.28) can then be written in form

$$\delta(g^2) = \tilde{\underline{E}}^{(1)}\underline{B}^{(0)} + \tilde{\underline{E}}^{(1)}\underline{B}^{(2)}\underline{C}^{(2)} , \tag{A.69}$$

where $\underline{E}^{(1)}$ is as in eqn (A.34) and $\underline{C}^{(2)}$ is a five-component column vector made up of the spherical harmonics $C^{j}_{2}(\theta,\phi)$ as in eqn (A.53).

4. The coordinate system is rotated. Since $\delta(g^2)$ is a scalar quantity and cannot be affected by the rotation we have the identity

$$\tilde{\underline{E}}^{(1)'}\underline{B}^{(0)'} + E^{(1)'}\underline{B}^{(2)'}\underline{C}^{(2)'} \equiv \tilde{\underline{E}}^{(1)}\underline{B}^{(0)} + \tilde{\underline{E}}^{(1)}\underline{B}^{(2)}\underline{C}^{(2)} , \tag{A.70}$$

whence

$$\underline{B}^{(0)'} = (\underline{\mathscr{D}}^{(1)})^{\dagger}\underline{B}^{(0)} , \tag{A.71}$$

$$\underline{B}^{(2)'} = (\underline{\mathcal{D}}^{(1)})^{\dagger}\underline{B}^{(2)}\underline{\mathcal{D}}^{(2)*} , \tag{A.72}$$

5. The new coefficients in $B_q^{(2)'}$ are converted to a mixed form in which the electric field remains expressed in spherical tensor components and the three traces belonging to $\underline{B}^{(0)'}$ are added in. This is done by means of the relations.

$$B_{i,1}^{(1,C)} = \frac{1}{3} B_i^{(0)'} - \frac{1}{2} B_{i,0}^{(2)'} + \frac{1}{2}\sqrt{\frac{3}{2}} \left(B_{i,2}^{(2)'} + B_{i,-2}^{(2)'}\right) ,$$

$$B_{i,2}^{(1,C)} = \frac{1}{3} B_i^{(0)'} - \frac{1}{2} B_{i,0}^{(2)'} - \frac{1}{2}\sqrt{\frac{3}{2}} \left(B_{i,2}^{(2)'} + B_{i,-2}^{(2)'}\right) ,$$

$$B_{i,3}^{(1,C)} = \frac{1}{3} B_i^{(0)'} + B_{i,0}^{(2)} ,$$

$$B_{i,4}^{(1,C)} = -\frac{i}{2}\sqrt{\frac{3}{2}} \left(B_{i,1}^{(2)'} + B_{i,-1}^{(2)'}\right) ,$$

$$B_{i,5}^{(1,C)} = -\frac{1}{2}\sqrt{\frac{3}{2}} \left(B_{i,1}^{(2)'} - B_{i,2}^{(2)'}\right) ,$$

$$B_{i,6}^{(1,C)} = \frac{i}{2}\sqrt{\frac{3}{2}} \left(B_{i,2}^{(2)'} - B_{i,2}^{(2)'}\right) ,$$

$$(i = 0,\pm 1). \tag{A.73}$$

6. The mixed coefficients $B_{i,j}^{(1,C)'}$ are converted to the regular Cartesian coefficients B_{ij}' in the new coordinate system by means of the equations

$$B_{1j}' = -\frac{1}{\sqrt{2}} \left(B_{1,j}^{(1,C)} - B_{-1,j}^{(1,C)}\right) ,$$

$$B_{2j}' = -\frac{i}{\sqrt{2}} \left(B_{1,j}^{(1,C)} + B_{-1,j}^{(1,C)}\right) , \tag{A.74}$$

$$B_{3j}' = B_{0,j}^{(1,C)} \qquad (j = 1,6) .$$

(The essential steps in this transformation are embodied in eqns (A.65)-(A.67), (A.71)-(A.74).)

It will be apparent that there are several alternative procedures which are essentially equivalent to the above. For example, the traces can be extracted from the original Cartesian coefficients B_{ij} before any conversion is made to the spherical tensor form. Also, as pointed out earlier in connection with the problem of transforming the coefficients R_{ijk}, it is not essential to work with the electric field in spherical tensor form. Retaining the Cartesian form for the field we can at once extract the trace quantities

$$B_i^{(C,T)} = B_{i1} + B_{i2} + B_{i3} \quad (i = x,y,z) \tag{A.75}$$

and use the traceless residues to form a set of mixed coefficients $B_{i,j}^{(C,2)}$ (i = x,y,z' 0,±1,±2) analogous to mixed coefficients $R_{i,j}^{(C,2)}$ in eqns (3.66), (3.67). These coefficients yield a 3 × 5 matrix which is transformed as in (A.63) whilst the three traces $B_i^{(C,T)}$ yield a vector transforming as in (A.22). The choice of procedure will, of course, depend on the nature of the transformation to be made.

The g-shift tensor T_{ijk} can be transformed in the same manner of B_{ijk} provided that it is symmetric in j,k. However, as has been pointed out earlier (§3.4) it may not be possible to express it in a symmetric form, although an equivalent set of parameters symmetric in j,k and yielding the correct frequency shifts can be obtained from the B_{ij} by means of Table 3.2 (p.67). If it is necessary to handle an asymmetric tensor the methods described here are no longer applicable and more general forms of tensor transformation may have to be used.

Appendix B: Line-broadening due to internal electric fields

B.1. LINE-BROADENING DUE TO CHARGED POINT DEFECTS

Point defects in an ionic lattice can give rise to large internal electric fields and in this way lead to considerable broadening of the resonance line of paramagnetic centers which show a linear electric field effect. A very rough calculation will indicate the order of magnitude. If there are 10^{18} defects per square centimetre (a defect concentration ∿0.01 per cent) then on the average there will be one or more defects within a radius of 100 Å from any given lattice point. In a material such as $CaWO_4(\varepsilon_r \simeq 10)$ a single Ca^{2+} vacancy at this distance generates an electric field ≃ 30 kV cm^{-1}. This field leads to g-shifts ≃ 10^{-3} for some of the systems which have been studied experimentally (see Chapter 10) and is comparable with the applied fields often used in d.c. measurements of the linear electric field effect.

In some cases these internal randomly oriented fields (or microfields) may be the major factor responsible for line broadening. This is illustrated by the curve in Fig. B.1, which shows the electric field induced shifts and the linewidth plotted as a function of the angle of the Zeeman field H_0 in the ab-plane for a $CaWO_4$ sample doped with Er^{3+} (Mims and Gillen 1966). The line itself does not move in this experiment (the site is axial),

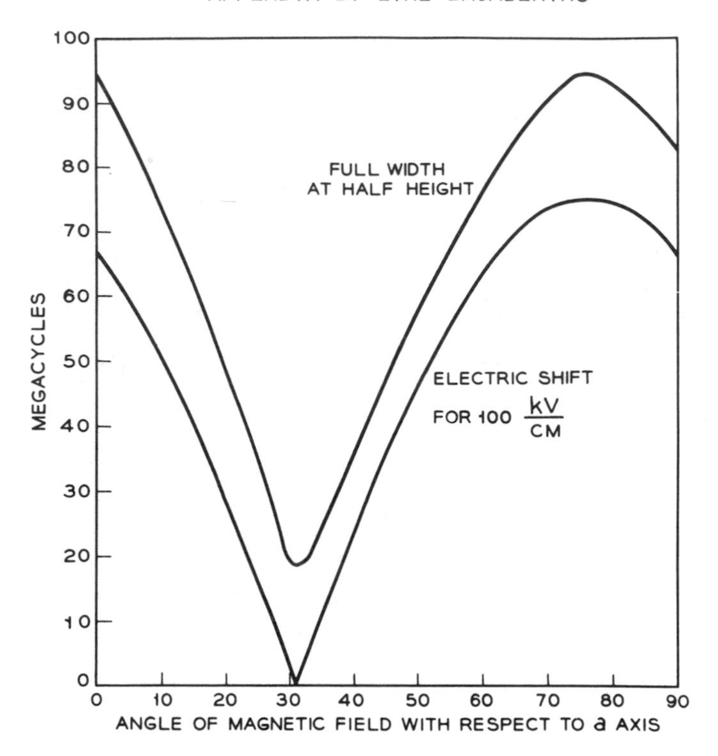

FIG. B.1. The upper curve shows the variation of linewidth with the azimuthal angle ϕ for a $CaWO_4$ sample doped with 4×10^{17} Er^{3+} ions per cubic centimetre. The Zeeman field $\underline{H}_0$ is in the ab-plane ($g = g_\perp$ = constant). The lower curve shows the shifts of resonance frequency which would correspond to a field of 100 kV cm^{-1} applied along the c-axis. (Electric fields along a- and b-axes produce no effect on the resonance frequency when $\underline{H}_0$ is in the ab-plane for this material.)

but the width of the line varies considerably, in a way which is directly correlated with the sensitivity of the Er^{3+} to an applied electric field. In this particular case (S_4 point symmetry, H_0 in the ab-plane) there is no shift for electric fields along the a- and b-axes, and the linewidth variation must therefore be due to components of the random internal electric fields parallel to the c-axis. The resonance lines for a number of ions in $CaWO_4$, and for Cr^{3+} in $ZnWO_4$ (Bugai et al. 1966). (Jones, Moore, and Neal 1968) have been shown to be broadened in a similar way. The list might indeed be a much longer one if it were as easy in other materials as it is in the tungstates to identify this source of line-broadening and to distinguish it from broadening due to mechanical strains.

A detailed calculation of the lineshape and the line-broadening due to a random distribution of point charges (or charge defects) can be made by means of the 'statistical theory of line-broadening'. Calculations of this type were first made by Holtzmark (1919) in order to explain the Stark broadening of optical lines in electrical discharges and the method has since been applied to a variety of problems including the broadening of paramagnetic resonance lines in dilute materials (see e.g. Stoneham 1969). The primary assumptions are as follows.

1. Each defect causes a shift $\varepsilon(\underline{z}_i)$ in the spectroscopic frequency, where $\underline{z}_i$ denotes the coordinates of the defect relative to the paramagnetic centre which is being observed. The contributions from a number of defects are additive, i.e.

$$\varepsilon(\underline{z}_1, \underline{z}_2, \ldots \underline{z}_N) = \sum_i \varepsilon(\underline{z}_i) \quad . \tag{B.1}$$

2. The positions at which the defects are found are not correlated with one another, and the probability $P(\underline{z}_1, z_2, \ldots . \underline{z}_N)$ of finding a given defect configuration can be expressed as the product of the individual probabilities $p(\underline{z}_i)$, i.e.

$$P(\underline{z}_1, \underline{z}_2, \ldots . \underline{z}_N) = \prod_i p(\underline{z}_i) \quad . \tag{B.2}$$

3. The lattice can be approximated by a continuous medium.

These assumptions tend to be well justified for low defect densities provided that the internal electric fields are not large enough to cause significant quadratic electric shifts.

If the probability of finding a defect over the range of positions $\underline{z}_i$ to $\underline{z}_i + d\underline{z}_i$ is $p(\underline{z}_i)d\underline{z}_i$, then by eqn (B.2) the probability of finding a configuration of N defects at coordinates $\underline{z}_i$ $(i=1,\ldots N)$ is given by

$$P(\text{config.}) = p(\underline{z}_1)p(\underline{z}_2)\ldots p(\underline{z}_N)\ d\underline{z}_1 d\underline{z}_2 \ldots d\underline{z}_N.$$

This configuration will result in a frequency shift of $\Delta\omega = \sum_{i=1}^{N} \varepsilon(\underline{z}_i)$. Our task is therefore to sum P(config.) over all possible configurations by integrating N times with respect to the variable $\underline{z}_i$, whilst selecting only those configurations which give shifts $\Delta\omega$ of a specified value. This will yield the intensity $I(\Delta\omega)$ of the resonance line at a frequency $\Delta\omega$ away from the unperturbed frequency. The required operation is performed by evaluating the multiple integral

$$I(\Delta\omega) = V^{-N} \int d\underline{z}_1\ p(\underline{z}_1) \int d\underline{z}_2\ p(\underline{z}_2)\ldots\int d\underline{z}_N p(\underline{z}_N)\ \delta\{\Delta\omega - \sum_i \varepsilon(\underline{z}_i)\}\ , \quad \text{(B.3.)}$$

where $\delta\{\ldots\}$ stands for the Dirac delta-function and the volume $V = \int^V dz\ p(\underline{z})$ normalizes $p(\underline{z})$. Writing the delta function in the integral form

$$\delta\{\Delta\omega - \sum_i \varepsilon(\underline{z}_i) = \frac{1}{2\pi} \int_{-\infty}^{+\infty} d\rho\ \exp[-i\rho\{\Delta\omega - \sum_i \varepsilon(\underline{z}_i)\}]\ , \quad \text{(B.4)}$$

substituting it in (B.3), dropping subscripts i, and rearranging, we have

$$I(\Delta\omega) = \frac{1}{2\pi} \int_{-\infty}^{+\infty} d\rho\{\exp(-i\rho\Delta\omega)\} \times [\frac{1}{V} \int^V p(\underline{z})\{\exp i\rho\varepsilon(\underline{z})\}d\underline{z}]^N\ . \quad \text{(B.5)}$$

We next take V and N to infinity, avoiding divergencies by rewriting $I(\Delta\omega)$ in the form

$$I(\Delta\omega) = \frac{1}{2\pi} \int_{-\infty}^{+\infty} d\rho\{\exp(-i\rho\Delta\omega)\}\{1-(J/V)\}^N\ , \quad \text{(B.6)}$$

where

$$J = \int^V \{1-\exp\ i\rho\varepsilon(\underline{z})\}\ p(\underline{z})d\underline{z}\ . \quad \text{(B.7)}$$

We thus obtain the lineshape function, as a Fourier transform

$$I(\Delta\omega) = \frac{1}{2\pi} \int_{-\infty}^{+\infty} d\rho \, \exp(-i\rho\Delta\omega)\exp(-nJ) \, , \tag{B.8}$$

where $n = N/V$ is the number of defects per unit volume.

Eqns (B.7)-(B.8) can be used to solve a number of line-broadening problems including the problem of line-broadening due to the magnetic dipolar interactions of electron spins in dilute materials. In the present instance we substitute the frequency shift function $\varepsilon(\underline{z})$ associated with a point electrostatic charge in the integral for J. If the lattice defects possess a charge Ze they will give rise to internal electric field components $E_i = Ze\,(x_i/r)/K_i r^2$, where the K_i are the principal relative permittivities and the x_i are the projections of the position vector $\underline{z}$ along the principal axes of the dielectric tensor. The frequency shift due to an individual defect is given by

$$\begin{aligned} \varepsilon(\underline{z}) &= \sum_i a_i E_i \\ &= Ze \sum_i a_i x_i / K_i r^3 \, , \end{aligned} \tag{B.9}$$

where the three parameters $a_i = \partial\omega/\partial E_i$ are the constants of proportionality which relate the frequency shift of the resonance line at a given magnetic field setting to the three components of the applied electric field resolved along the principal axes of the dielectric tensor.† Substituting

---

† When the dielectric is anisotropic it is usually easiest to solve the problem in the principal axis system of the dielectric tensor. For some paramagnetic centres this may not be the same as the axis system used in defining the linear electric effect spin Hamiltonian.

$$p(\underline{z})d\underline{z} = 2\pi r^2 dr\ d(\cos\theta) \tag{B.10}$$

in (B.7) and evaluating the integral in a coordinate system corresponding to these principal axes we obtain the result

$$J = \frac{4\pi}{15}\left[\ \left|\ \rho Ze\ \{\sum_i (a_i/K_i)^2\}^{\frac{1}{2}}\ \right|\ \right]^{\frac{3}{2}}\ . \tag{B.11}$$

Then, with some changes in the variables eqn (B.8) assumes the form

$$I(\Delta\omega) = \frac{1}{\pi\omega_0}\cdot\frac{1}{\pi}\int_0^\infty \cos\ (\rho\omega/\omega_0)\ \exp(-|\rho^{1\cdot 5}|)d\rho \tag{B.12a}$$

where

$$\omega_0 = (4/15)^{\frac{2}{3}}\ \pi n^{\frac{2}{3}}\ \ Ze\{\sum(a_i/K_i)^2\}^{\frac{1}{2}}\ . \tag{B.12b}$$

Eqn (B.12a) gives the lineshape.

Since J is real the line has no net shift, as indeed we might have anticipated from the fact that defects on opposite sites of the paramagnetic ion occur with equal probability and give rise to opposite frequency displacements. Numerical integration yields the form of the function in Fig. B.12. This function, sometimes described as a Holtzmark distribution†, is intermediate in form between a Lorentzian and a Gaussian. Its full width at half height is given by

†The distribution derived by Holtzmark (1919) is not in fact the one shown here, but is, instead, the distribution of the scalar magnitudes of the local electric field. The distribution function for each of the <u>components</u> E_i can easily be obtained from eqn (B.12) by substituting unity for the relevant shift parameter a_i and zero for the others.

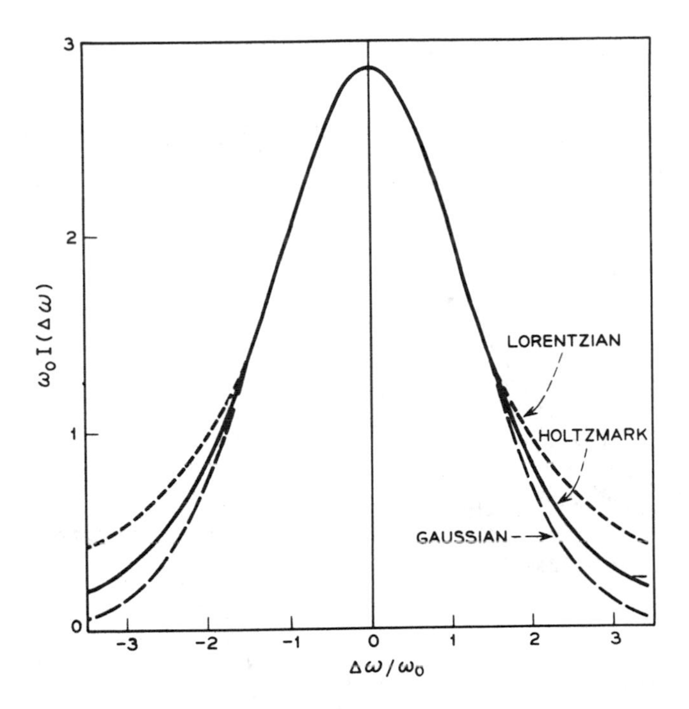

FIG. B.2. Theoretical lineshape function ('Holtzmark' function) for a paramagnetic resonance line broadened by internal electrostatic fields due to point charge defects. The linewidth is proportional to $n^{\frac{2}{3}}$, where n is the number of charge defects per cubic centimetre. Gaussian and Lorentzian curves are shown for comparison, these curves being scaled to give the same height and the same full width at the points of half height as the Holtzmark curve.

$$W = 2{\cdot}88\ \omega_0 = 3{\cdot}75\ n^{\frac{2}{3}}\ Ze\{\sum_i (a_i/K_i)^2\}^{\frac{1}{2}} \tag{B.13}$$

and depends on the $\frac{2}{3}$ power of the defect concentration. It may be noted that if the width W is required in radian frequency units the shift parameters a_i must be in units of rad $s^{-1}\ V^{-1}$. If the a_i are calculated in hertz the width W will also be in hertz.

Gaussian and Lorentzian lineshape functions, scaled so as

to have the same width W, are shown for comparison with the Holtzmark function in Fig. B.2. The Holtzmark lineshape function is also shown in differential form in Fig. B.3, the Gaussian and Lorentzian differential lineshapes being scaled in this case so as to have the same peak-to-peak distance.

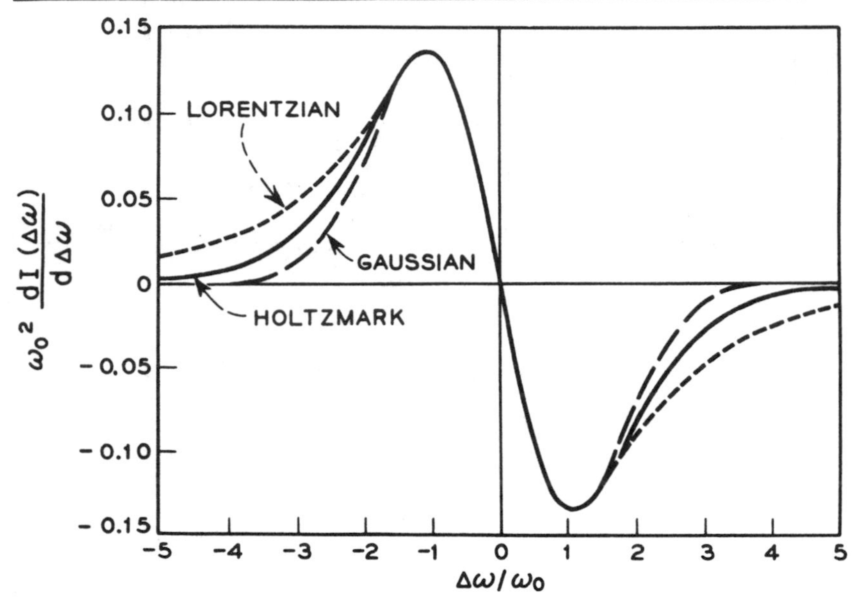

FIG. B.3. Differential lineshape functions for the three cases shown in Fig. B.2. The Gaussian and Lorentzian curves have been scaled to give the same height and the same peak-to-peak distance as the Holtzmark curve.

By an extension of the statistical theory Blazha et al (1972) have calculated lineshape functions corresponding to distributions of charged defects which are not uniformly random but which are weighted in a specified manner according to the distance from the paramagnetic centre. They have compared the resulting theoretical functions with experimental lineshapes for Cr^{3+} in $ZnWO_4$. The case of non-uniform defect distributions is also discussed briefly by Mims (see p.228 of Mims (1972)).

A procedure similar to the above can also be used to

calculate the broadening of paraelectric resonance lines, such as the lines associated with the tunnelling of Li^+ ions in KCl (Deigen, Glinchuk, and Vikhnin 1971), or the broadening of optical lines if this broadening is due to linear electric field induced shifts in the resonance frequencies.

B.2. LINE-BROADENING DUE TO ELECTRIC DIPOLES

A random array of electrostatic dipoles can also generate local electrostatic fields and lead to line-broadening. This mechanism may be of importance in organic systems where polar molecules are present, or in crystals where the substitution of an impurity causes a re-arrangement of local charges which is equivalent to the creation of new dipole moments in the lattice.[†] The latter case has been studied for the system $(Cd_{1-x}:Zn_x)S$ doped with Mn^{2+} by Deigen et al. (1971), who estimate the magnitude of the dipoles created by the substitution of Zn^{2+} in CdS from the known shift parameter for Mn^{2+} in CdS and from the observed broadening of the Mn^{2+} resonance lines.

The calculation can be made by means of the statistical theory outlined in the last section, but the problem is complicated by the fact that it contains two additional parameters, i.e. those needed to specify the orientations of the dipoles. Although a random distribution is assumed for the sites occupied by the dipoles in the statistical model the orientations of the dipoles need not themselves be random. Fortunately the lineshape is

---

[†] This situation may indeed be quite a common one. The lattice distortions caused by the substitution of a foreign atom or ion can always in principle result in the appearance of a local electrostatic moment if the substitution occurs at a non-centrosymmetric site.

independent of the dipolar orientations, and we can derive a general expression for it, leaving the orientational distribution to be substituted in the equation for the linewidth later on.

In place of the probability factor $p(\underline{z})d\underline{z}$ in eqn (B.10) we have

$$p(\underline{z}) = \frac{1}{3}\, d(r^3)\ d\Omega \times g_\mu(\Omega_\mu)d(\Omega_\mu) \quad , \tag{B.14}$$

where $\Omega \equiv (\theta,\phi)$ denotes the orientation of the line joining the dipole to the paramagnetic centre, $\Omega_\mu \equiv (\theta_\mu,\phi_\mu)$ denotes the orientation of the dipole, and $g_\mu(\Omega_\mu)$ is the probability of the dipolar orientation in question. $(\int g_\mu(\Omega_\mu)d\Omega_\mu = 1)$. As in §B.1 the perturbation $\varepsilon(\underline{z})$ represents the frequency shift induced by the electrostatic field of a single defect. Here this varies with distance as $1/r^3$ (see eqn (B.22)). We can therefore write

$$\varepsilon(\underline{z}) = (\mu/r^3)f(\Omega,\Omega_\mu,a_i,K_i) \quad , \tag{B.15}$$

where μ is the moment of the dipole and f a function depending on the two orientational parameters Ω,Ω_μ, on the frequency shift parameters $a_i = \partial\omega/\partial E_i$, and on the bulk relative permittivities K_i of the medium.

Since the basic statistical assumptions 1-3 (p.301) remain the same as in the last section, the lineshape function is still given by the same general eqn (B.8). The integral (B.7) must, however, be re-evaluated using the new expressions (B.14)-(B.15) for $p(\underline{z})d\underline{z}$ and $\varepsilon(\underline{z})$. Thus

$$J = \frac{1}{3}\iiint \{1-\exp(i\rho\mu f/r^3)\}g_\mu(\Omega_\mu)d(r^3)d\Omega d\Omega_\mu \quad . \tag{B.16}$$

In the general case J consists of a real and an imaginary part, the real part giving the lineshape function and the imaginary part representing a shift in the overall resonance frequency. Here we shall ignore the imaginary part, since it does not contribute to line broadening and retain only the real part

$$J_r = \frac{1}{3}\iiint (1-\cos\rho\mu f/r^3) g_\mu(\Omega_\mu) d(r^3) d\Omega d\Omega_\mu \quad . \qquad (B.17)$$

The integration with respect to r can be performed fairly straightforwardly, since r is not contained in the function f and is not correlated with the other variables. From (B.17) we have

$$J_r = (\pi/6)\mu|\rho|\iint |f| g_\mu(\Omega_\mu) d\Omega d\Omega_\mu \quad , \qquad (B.18)$$

which transforms analytically (eqn (B.8)), yielding the Lorentzian lineshape function

$$I(\Delta\omega) = \frac{(\Delta\omega_{dip}/\pi)}{(\Delta\omega)^2 + (\Delta\omega_{dip})^2} \quad , \qquad (B.19)$$

where

$$(\Delta\omega)_{dip} = \frac{\pi}{6} n\mu \int |f(\Omega,\Omega_\mu,a_i,K_i)| g_\mu(\Omega_\mu) d\Omega d\Omega_\mu \quad . \qquad (B.20)$$

It may be noted that for the dipolar case the linewidth is linear in the concentration n of the dipoles.

In order to calculate the function $f(\Omega,\Omega_\mu,a_i K_i)$ it is necessary to know the field components E_x, E_y, E_z at the paramagnetic site due to a dipole $\underline{\mu}$ in the environment. These fields can be derived from the formulae in Chapter 4 (e.g. eqns (4.19),(4.23)-(4.24), but are more readily obtained from the expression

$$U = (\mu\mu'/r^3)(\cos\psi - 3\cos\zeta\cos\zeta') \quad , \qquad (B.21)$$

in which U is the interaction energy of two dipoles $\underline{\mu},\underline{\mu}'$ making an angle ψ with each other and making angles ζ,ζ' with the vector

$\underline{r}$ joining their centres. Taking the Cartesian components μ_i, μ_j' as the dipoles in (B.21) we obtain a set of expressions for the interaction energies U_{ij} in terms of the direction cosines or $\underline{r}$. Rewriting these energies in the form $U_{ij} = -E_i\mu_j'$, where E_i is the field due to the dipole μ_i as seen by the dipole μ_j', and comparing the two expressions for U_{ij}, we thus obtain the results

$$E_x = (1/r^3)\Big\{\mu_x(3\sin^2\theta\cos^2\phi - 1) + \mu_y(\tfrac{3}{2}\sin^2\theta\sin 2\phi) + \mu_z(\tfrac{3}{2}\sin 2\theta\cos\phi)\Big\} ,$$

$$E_y = (1/r^3)\Big\{\mu_x(\tfrac{3}{2}\sin^2\theta\sin 2\phi) + \mu_y(3\sin^2\theta\sin^2\phi - 1) + \mu_z(\tfrac{3}{2}\sin 2\theta\sin\phi)\Big\} ,$$

$$E_z = (1/r^3)\Big\{\mu_x(\tfrac{3}{2}\sin 2\theta\cos\phi) + \mu_y(\tfrac{3}{2}\sin 2\theta\sin\phi) + \mu_z(3\cos^2\theta - 1)\Big\} , \tag{B.22}$$

where μ_x, μ_y, μ_z are the components of μ as given by

$$\mu_x = \mu\sin\theta_\mu\cos\phi_\mu, \quad \mu_y = \mu\sin\theta_\mu\sin\phi_\mu, \quad \mu_z = \mu\cos\theta_\mu . \tag{B.23}$$

The conversion from field components in vacuo as in eqn (B.22) to field components due to dipoles embedded in a dielectric medium is most easily made if the principal axis system of the dielectric tensor is chosen as the coordinate system. The frequency shift is then given by

$$\varepsilon = \sum_i a_i E_i / K_i . \tag{B.24}$$

The function $f(\Omega, \Omega_\mu, a_i, K_i)$ can be extracted by substituting

(B.22)-(B.23) in (B.24) and comparing the result with eqn (B.15). As in the previous analysis in §B.1 it should be noted that the shift parameters a_i must be expressed in radian frequency units to give the radian frequency linewidth. If the a_i are taken to be in hertz per unit field, $\Delta\omega_{dip}$ will be in hertz also.

Terminology and notation

A_{jk}	($j = 1,2,3$ or $j = x,y,z$, likewise k); coefficients of the electron-nuclear coupling operators $S_j I_k$ in the normal spin Hamiltonian.
A_K^Q, a_k^q, $a_k^q(E)$	Coefficients of the harmonics $C_K^Q(\theta,\phi)$, $C_k^q(\theta,\phi)$ in the crystal field potentials associated with the normal crystal field V, the induced crystal field δV (Chapter 4), and the equivalent even field δV_{EEF} (Chapter 5).
$A_K^Q(s)$, $a_k^q(s)$, $a_k^q(E,s)$	Spectroscopic crystal field parameters as defined in Chapter 4; usually expressed in cm^{-1} energy units ($1\ J = (5{\cdot}034020 \pm 0{\cdot}000036) \times 10^{22}\ cm^{-1}$).
B_{ijk}	($i = 1,2,3$ or $i = x,y,z$; likewise j,k); parameters describing the shift in g^2 induced by the applied field components E_i (§3.5); since $B_{ijk} = B_{ikj}$, the Voigt notation B_{ij} ($i = 1,2,3$ or x,y,z; $j = 1$ to 6), where $B_{i1} = B_{i11}$, $B_{i2} = B_{i22}$, $B_{i3} = B_{i33}$, $B_{i4} = B_{i23} = B_{i32}$, $B_{i5} = B_{i13} = B_{i31}$, $B_{i6} = B_{i12} = B_{i21}$, can also be used for these parameters.

$C_K^Q(\theta,\phi)$ — Spherical harmonics (§A.1).

c.c. — Complex conjugate.

centro-symmetric site — A site possessing inversion symmetry.

D — Coefficient of the operator $S_z^2 - \frac{1}{3}S(S+1)$ in the normal spin Hamiltonian.

D_{jk} — ($j = 1,2,3$ or $j = x,y,z$; likewise k); coefficients of the operator S_jS_k in the normal spin Hamiltonian; since $D_{jk} = D_{kj}$, the Voigt notation D_j ($j = 1$ to 6), where $D_1 = D_{11}$, $D_2 = D_{22}$, $D_3 = D_{33}$, $D_4 = D_{23} = D_{32}$, $D_5 = D_{13} = D_{31}$, $D_6 = D_{12} = D_{21}$, can also be used for these coefficients.

$D_q^{(2)}$ — ($q = 0,\pm1,\pm2$), coefficients of the spherical spin operators $S_q^{(2)}$ occurring in the term $D_q^{(2)}S_q^{(2)}$ in the normal spin Hamiltonian (eqn (3.60).)

$\mathcal{D}^{(k)}$ — Rotation operators (See §A.4.4)

debye — Unit of electrostatic dipole moment. 1 debye = 10^{-18} e.s.u. cm. = $3{\cdot}33 \times 10^{-30}$ C.m.

e — The electronic charge. $e = -(4{\cdot}803250\pm0{\cdot}000021) \times 10^{-10}$ e.s.u. $= -(1{\cdot}6021917\pm{\cdot}0000070)\times 10^{-19}$ C

E — Coefficient of the operator $S_x^2 - S_y^2$ in the normal spin Hamiltonian.

EEF — Abbreviation for 'equivalent even field' (§5.2).

EPR — Abbreviation for 'electron paramagnetic resonance'.

E_{ug}, E_{ij} — Energy denominators $E_u - E_g$, $E_i - E_j$, appearing in perturbation calculations (Chapters 5 and 7).

E_{app} — The applied electric field in parallel-plate geometry.

E_i — $(i = 1,2,3$ or $i = x,y,z)$; Cartesian components of E_{app}.

$E_i^{(1)}$ — $(i = 0,\pm1)$; spherical tensor components of E_{app} (eqns (3.56) and (3.57)).

F_{ijk} — $(i = 1,2,3$ or $i = x,y,z$; likewise $j,k)$; coefficients of the operators $E_iS_xI_k$ in $\mathcal{H}_{elec}$; if these operators are defined in such a way that $F_{ijk} = F_{ikj}$ (§3.4), the Voigt notation F_{ij} $(i = 1,2,3;\ j = 1$ to $6)$ can be used instead (see B_{ijk}).

g — The g-value; the constant of proportionality in the equation $\hbar\omega = g\beta H$.

g_{jk} — $(j = 1,2,3$ or $j = x,y,z$; likewise $k)$; the g-tensor; the coefficients of the operators βH_jS_k in the normal spin Hamiltonian; if these operators are defined in such a way that $g_{jk} = g_{kj}$ (§3.4), the Voigt notation g_j $(j = 1$ to $6)$ can be used instead (see D_{jk}).

G_{jk} — $(j = 1,2,3$ or $j = x,y,z$; likewise $k)$; parameters determining the quantity g^2 (eqn (3.23); since $G_{jk} = G_{kj}$, the Voigt notation G_j $(j = 1$ to $6)$ can also be used (see D_{jk}).

h — Planck's constant. $h = (6{\cdot}626196\pm0{\cdot}000050) \times 10^{-34}$ J s.

$\hbar$ — $h/2\pi = (1{\cdot}0545919\pm0{\cdot}000080) \times 10^{-34}$ J s.

h.c. — Hermitian conjugate.

H_0 — The Zeeman field.

H_1 — The amplitude of one circularly polarized component of the microwave resonance magnetic field.

H_j — (j = 1,2,3 or j = x,y,z); Cartesian components of H_0.

$\mathcal{H}_{elec}$ — The terms added to the normal spin Hamiltonian in order to provide a phenomenological description of the linear electric field effect (eqn (3.2)).

k — Restoring force constant for an atom or ion in a crystal lattice (§4.3).

K_i — Principal values of the dielectric tensor (Appendix B).

normal spin Hamiltonian — The spin Hamiltonian not including those terms associated with the electric field effect (eqn 3.1)).

normal crystal field — Crystal field not including perturbations due to applied electric fields.

M_k^q — Electrostatic multipole moments of degree k (eqn(4.13)).

P — Macroscopic polarization of a dielectric.

p_{ion} — Equivalent electrostatic dipole moment $p_{ion} = Zeu$ arising as a result of ionic displacements in an applied electric field (§4.3).

p_{el} — Electronic dipole moment induced in an ion or atom by the applied electric field (§4.3).

p_i — (i = x,y,z); Cartesian components of the electrostatic dipole moment.

p_μ — ($\mu = 0,\pm 1$); spherical tensor components of the electrostatic dipole moment (eqns (4.21) and (4.22)).

Q_{jk} — (j = 1,2,3 or j = x,y,z; likewise k); coefficients of the operators I_jI_k in the normal spin Hamiltonian. Since $Q_{jk} = Q_{kj}$ the Voigt notation Q_j(j = 1 to 6) may be used instead (see D_{jk}).

q_{ijk} — ($i = 1,2,3$ or $i = x,y,z$; likewise j,k); coefficients of the operators $E_i I_j I_k$ in $\mathcal{H}_{elec}$; since $q_{ijk} = q_{ikj}$, the Voigt notation q_{ij} ($i = 1,2,3$; $j = 1$ to 6) can be used instead (see B_{ijk}).

R, R_j — Radial distance from the centre of the paramagnetic ion to the centre of a neighbouring ion (§4.2).

$\langle r^K \rangle$ — Radial integrals occurring in the calculation of matrix elements (eqns (5.30) and (5.31)).

R_{ijk} — ($i = 1,2,3$ or $i = x,y,z$; likewise j,k); coefficients of the operators $E_i S_j S_k$ in $\mathcal{H}_{elec}$; since $R_{ijk} = R_{ikj}$, the Voigt notation R_{ij} ($i = 1,2,3$; $j = 1$ to 6) can be used instead.

R_{iD}, R_{iE} — Electric field induced shifts in D and E (eqns (3.11) and (3.12)).

$R^{(2)}_{i,j}$ — ($i = 0,\pm1$; $j = 0,\pm1,\pm2$); coefficients of the spherical tensor operators $E^{(1)}_i S^{(2)}_j$ (eqn (3.65); Tables 3.3 and 3.4).

$R^{(C,2)}_{i,j}$ — ($i = 1,2,3$ or $i = x,y,z$; $j = 0,\pm1,\pm2$); coefficients of the mixed Cartesian-spherical operators $E_i S^{(2)}_j$ (eqn (3.66)).

$R^{(4)}_{i,j}$ — ($i = 0, 1$; $j = 0,\pm1,\pm2,\pm3,\pm4$); coefficients of the spherical tensor operators $E^{(1)}_i S^{(4)}_j$ (eqn (3.71)).

$R^{(C,4)}_{i,j}$ — ($i = 1,2,3$ or $i = x,y,z$; $j = 0,\pm1,\pm2,\pm3,\pm4$); coefficients of the mixed Cartesian-spherical spin operators $E_i S^{(4)}_j$ (eqn (3.70)).

S_j — ($j = 1,2,3$); spin operators S_x, S_y, S_z.

$S^{(2)}_j$ — ($j = 0,\pm1,\pm2$); second-degree spin operators in spherical tensor notation (eqns (3.58)-(3.60)).

$S_j^{(4)}$ — ($j = 0,\pm1,\pm2,\pm3,\pm4$); fourth-degree spin operators in spherical tensor notation (Table 3.5).

T_{ijk} — ($i = 1,2,3$ or $i = x,y,z$; likewise j,k); coefficients of the operators $E_iH_jS_k$ in $\mathcal{H}_{elec}$. In general $T_{ijk} \neq T_{ikj}$ (§3.4). A set of equivalent symmetric coefficients can however be defined (§3.5). In this case the Voigt notation T_{ij}($i = 1,2,3$; $j = 1$ to 6) can be used instead (see B_{ijk}).

u — Displacement of a lattice ion due to the applied electric field (§4.3).

V — Crystal field potential in the absence of applied electric fields.

V_{odd}, V_{even} — Odd and even portions of V.

V_{app} — Voltage applied across a sample.

V_H — Perturbation operator associated with the Zeeman field.

$V_{k\ell}$ — Perturbation potentials used in the general formulae (5.1) to (5.7).

δV — Change in the crystal field potential caused by the applied electric field (Chapter 4).

$\delta V_{odd}, \delta V_{even}$ — Odd and even portions of δV.

δV_{EEF} — Equivalent even field derived from the odd harmonics in V and δV (§5.2).

Voigt notation — See D_{jk}, B_{ijk}, for an example.

Z — The number of electronic charges on an ion.

$\alpha_{e\ell}$ — Electronic polarizability of an atom or ion (§4.3).

α	Coefficient of the operator $I_{1z} + I_{2z}$ (eqn (8.8)). Euler rotation angle (§A.4.2).
β	The Bohr magneton $\beta = eh/2mc = -(0\cdot9274098\pm0\cdot0000065) \times 10^{-27}$ J G^{-1}. (β is also used as coefficient of $I_{1z}^2 + I_{2z}^2 - 5/2$ in §8.1.1 and as an Euler rotation angle in §A.4.2.)
γ	The gyromagnetic ratio $\gamma = -g(eh/2mc) = -g\beta/h$. If $g = 2$, $\gamma = (2\cdot79922\pm0\cdot00004)$ MHz G^{-1}. (γ is also used as the coefficient of $I_{1+}I_{2-} + I_{1-}I_{2+}$ in eqn (8.8) and as an Euler rotation angle in §A.4.2.)
Δ_x,Δ_y	Coefficients of the operators S_x, S_y, in the symmetry doublet Hamiltonian (3.74).
δ_{ij}	($i = x,y,z$; likewise j) coefficients of E_iS_j in the symmetry doublet doublet Hamiltonian (3.75).
ε	An energy perturbation function in §B.
ε_r	The relative permittivity.
η	Numerical factor entering into the point dipole calculation of δV (eqn (4.17)).
η_{EEF}	Numerical factor entering into the calculation of δV_{EEF} (eqn (5.26)-(5.27)).
ν	Frequency
$\Delta\nu$	Electric field induced shift in ν.
θ,ϕ	Polar and azimuthal angles (see Fig. 3.4).
σ	Shift parameter as defined in §3.7.
ψ_g	Ground-state wavefunction (Chapters 5-7).
ψ_u	Wavefunction belong to excited state of opposite parity to the ground state (Chapter 5-7).

τ Time between the two transmitter pulses in a two-pulse spin echo sequence (§§2.5;§3.7).

ω Radian frequency $\omega = 2\pi\nu$.

$\Delta\omega$ Electric field induced shift in ω.

$\overline{\Delta\omega}$ Shift in ω per unit applied field (§2.5).

Bibliography

ABDULSABIROV, R. YU, ANTIPIN, A. A., KURKIN, I. N., TSVETKOV, E. A., CHIRKIN, YU. K., and SHLENKIN (1972). FIZIKA tverd. Tela 14, 304 (transl. Soviet Phys. solid St. 14, 255).

ABRAGAM, A. and BLEANEY, B. (1970). Electron paramagnetic resonance of transition ions. Clarendon Press, Oxford.

ADDE, R. and PONTNAU, J. (1971). Magnetic Resonance (ed. I. Ursu), p. 762. Proceedings of XVI Congress Ampere.

ARMSTRONG J., BLOEMBERGEN, N., and GILL, D. (1961). Phys. Rev. Lett. 7, 11.

ARTMAN, J. O. and MURPHY, J. C. (1963a). J. chem. Phys. 38, 1544.

——— , ——— (1963b). In Paramagnetic resonance II (ed. W. Low), p. 634. Academic Press, New York.

——— , ——— (1964). Phys. Rev. 135, A1622.

ASTROV, D. N. (1959). J. exp. theor. Phys. 37, 881 (transl. Soviet Phys. JETP 10, 628).

BARAN, N. P., GRACHEV, V. G., ISHCHENKO, S. S., and CHERNENKO, L. I. (1973). FIZIKA tverd. Tela 15, 519 (transl. Soviet Phys. solid St. 15, 360).

BATES, C. A. (1968). J. Phys., C 1, 877.

BATES, C. A. and BENTLEY, J. P. (1969). J. Phys., C 2, 1947.

——— , ——— JONES, B. F., and MOORE, W. S. (1970). J. Phys., C 3, 570.

BENNETT, J. E. and INGRAM, D. J. E. (1956). Nature, Lond. 177, 276.

——— GIBSON, J. F., and INGRAM, D. J. E. (1957). Proc. R. Soc. A240, 67.

BICHURIN, M. I., KOVALENKO, E. S., and KOZLOV, V. G. (1967). Fizika tverd. Tela 9, 1518 (transl. Soviet Phys. solid St. 9, 1187).

——— KOZLOV, V. G., KOVALENKO, E. S., TSINCHIK, D. V., and SHVARTSMAN, G. I. (1968). Fizika tverd. Tela 10, 259 (transl. Soviet Phys. solid St. 10, 196).

——— VOLKOV, P. YA., ZAKHAROV, V. P., KOVALENKO, E. S., SEN'KIV, V. A., SOLDATOV, A. I., and CHUNYAEVA, S. I. (1971). Fizika tverd. Tela 13, 720 (transl. Soviet Phys. solid St. 13, 594).

BLAZHA, M. G., BUGAI, A. A., MAKSIMENKO, V. M., and ROITSIN, A. B. (1972). Fizika tverd. Tela 14, 2064 (transl. Soviet Phys. solid St. 14, 1779).

BLINC, R. and SENTJURC, M. (1967). Phys, Rev. Lett. 19, 1231.

BLOEMBERGEN, N. (1963). Magnetic and electric resonance and relaxation. Proceedings of XI Colloque Ampere (ed. J. Smidt), p. 39.

BLUME, M., GESCHWIND, S., and YAFET, Y. (1969). Phys. Rev. 181, 478.

BOTTCHER, C. J. F. (1952). Theory of electric polarisation. Elsevier, Amsterdam.

BRON, W. E. and DREYFUS, R. W. (1967). Phys. Rev. 163, 304.

BUCH, T. and GELINEAU, A. (1971). Phys. Rev. B 4, 1444.

BUCKMASTER, H. A. (1962). Can. J. Phys. 40, 1670.

BUEHLER, R. J. and HIRSCHFELDER, J. O. (1951). Phys. Rev. 83, 628

——— (1952). Phys. Rev. 85, 628.

BUGAI, A. A., DEIGEN, M. F., OGANESYAN, V. O., and PASHKOVSKII, M. V. (1967). Fizika tverd. Tela 9, 2450 (transl. Soviet Phys. solid St. 9, 1926).

——— DULIU, O. G., MAKSIMENKO, V. M., and SHEVCHENKO, YU. B. (1972). Fizika tverd. Tela 14, 572 (transl. Soviet Phys. solid St. 14, 475).

——— LEVKOVSKII, P. T., MAKSIMENKO, V. M., PASHKOVSKII, M. V., and ROITSIN, A. B. (1966). Zh. eksp. teor. Fiz. 50, 1510 (transl. Soviet Phys. JETP 23, 1007).

———, ———, ——— POTKIN, L. I., and ROITSIN, A. B. (1966). Fizika tverd. Tela 8, 3685 (transl. Soviet Phys. solid St. 8, 2954).

——— and ROITSIN, A. B. (1967). Zh. eksp. teor. Fiz. SSR, Pis'ma Redakt 5, 82 (transl. JETP Lett. 5, 67).

CARLSON, B. C. and RUSHBROOKE, G. S. (1950). Proc. Camb. Phil. Soc. 46, 626.

CHRISTENSEN, S. H. (1969). Phys. Rev. 180, 498.

COHEN, M. G. and BLOEMBERGEN, N. (1964). Phys. Rev. 135, A950.

CULVAHOUSE, J. W., SCHINKE, D. F., and FOSTER, D. L. (1967). Phys. Rev. Lett. 18, 117.

DATE, M., KANAMORI, J., and TACHIKI, M. (1961). J. phys. Soc. Japan 16, 2589.

DEIGEN, M. F. and ROITSIN, A. B. (1970). Zh. eksp. teor. Fiz. 59, 209 (transl. Soviet Phys. JETP 32, 115).

——— GLINCHUK, M. D., and VIKHNIN, V. S. (1971). Fizika tverd. Tela 13, 2714 (transl. Soviet Phys. Solid St. 13, 2270).

DEIGEN, M. F., GEIFMAN, I. N., MAEVSKII, V. M., KODZHESPIROV, F. F., BULANYI, M. F., and MOZHAROVSKII, L. A. (1970). Fizika tverd. Tela 12, 3336 (transl. Soviet Phys. solid St. 12, 2704).

DIEKE, G. H. (1968). Spectra and energy levels of rare earth ions in crystals (ed. H. M. Crosswhite and H. Crosswhite). Wiley Interscience, New York.

DREYBRODT, W. and PFISTER, G. (1969). Phys. Status Solidii 34, 69.

——— and SILBER, D. (1969). Phys. Status Solidii 34, 559.

ELLIOTT, R. J. and STEVENS, K. W. (1953). Proc. R. Soc. A218, 553.

FEDOTOV, YU. V., GRACHEV, V. G., and BAGMUT, N. N. (1973). Fizika tverd. Tela 15, 3128 (transl. Soviet Phys. solid St. 15, 2094).

FEHER, G., SHEPHERD, I. W., and SHORE, H. B. (1966). Phys. Rev. Lett. 16, 500.

FOLEN, V. J., RADO, G. T., and STALDER, E. W. (1961). Phys. Rev. Lett. 6, 607.

FREEMAN, A. J. and WATSON, R. E. (1965). Magnetism, Vol. IIA (ed. G. T. Rado and H. Suhl), p. 290-2. Academic Press, New York.

FROHLICH, H. (1958). Theory of Dielectrics. Clarendon Press, Oxford.

GALKIN, A. A., GEIFMAN, I. N., DEIGEN, M. F., OGANESYAN, V. O., PROKHOROV, A. D., TSINTSADZE, G. A., and SHAPOVALOV, V. A. (1969). Fizika tverd. Tela 11, 87 (transl. Soviet Phys. solid St. 11, 61).

GEIFMAN, I. N., GLINCHUK, M. D., OGANESYAN, V. O., and TSINTSADZE, G. A. (1969). Fizika tverd. Tela 11, 1702 (transl. Soviet Phys. solid St. 11, 1379).

GESCHWIND, S. G. and REMEIKA, J. P. (1961). Phys. Rev. 122, 757.

GOLDSCHVARTZ, J. M., OUWERKERK, A. C., and BLAISSE, B. S. (1970). Conference on dielectric materials, measurements and application. I.E.E. publications 67, p. 218.

GOLDSTEIN, H. (1950). Classical mechanics, p. 155. Addison Wesley, New York.

GOURARY, B. S. and ADRIAN, F. J. (1957). Phys. Rev. 105, 1180.

——— , ——— (1960). Solid St. Phys. 10 (ed. F. Seitz and D. Turnbull, 127.

GRAY, C. G. (1968). Can. J. Phys. 46, 135.

GRIFFITH, J. S. (1960). Molec. Phys. 3, 477.

——— (1971). The theory of transition metal ions. Cambridge University Press.

HAM, F. S. (1961). Phys. Rev. Lett. 7, 242.

——— (1963). Physics. Chem. Solids 24, 1165.

HEMPSTEAD, C. F. and BOWERS, K. D. (1960). Phys. Rev. 118, 131.

HOLTZMARK, J. (1919). Phys. Z. 20, 162.

HORNREICH, R. and SHTRIKMAN, S. (1967). Phys. Rev. 161, 506.

HOU, S. L. and BLOEMBERGEN, N. (1965). Phys. Rev. 138, A1218.

HUTCHINGS, M. T. and RAY, D. K. (1963). Proc. phys. Soc. 81, 663.

——— (1965). Solid St. Phys. 16 (ed. F. Seitz and D. Turnbull), 227.

JONES, B. F., MOORE, W. S., NEAL, J. (1968). J. Phys., D 1, 41.

——— , ——— (1969). J. Phys., C 2, 1964.

JUDD, B. R. (1962). Phys. Rev. 127, 750.

KAISER, W., SUGANO, S., and WOOD, D. L. (1961). Phys. Rev. Lett. 6, 605.

KAPLYANSKII, A. A. and MEDVEDEV, V. N. (1967). Fizika tverd. Tela 9, 2704 (transl. Soviet Phys. solid St. 9, 2121).

KIEL, A. (1966). Phys. Rev. 148, 247.

——— and MIMS, W. B. (1967). Phys. Rev. 153, 378.

KIEL, A. and MIMS, W. B. (1970). Phys. Rev. B1, 2935.

——, —— (1971). Phys. Rev. B3, 2878.

——, —— (1972a). Phys. Rev. B5, 803.

——, —— (1972b). Phys. Rev. B6, 34.

——, —— (1973). Phys. Rev. B7, 2917.

——, —— (1974). Phys. Rev. B10, 4795.

——, —— and MASUHR, G. J. (1973). Phys. Rev. B7, 1735.

KITTEL, C. H. (1956). Introduction to solid state physics (2nd edn). Wiley, New York.

—— (1971). Introduction to solid state physics (4th edn). Wiley, New York.

KOVALENKO, E. S. (1971). Fizika tverd. Tela 13, 2266 (transl. Soviet Phys. solid St. 13, 1901).

—— and BICHURIN, M. I. (1969). Fizika tverd. Tela 11, 1074 (transl. Soviet Phys. solid St. 11, 878).

——, —— (1970). Fizika tverd. Tela 12, 3383 (transl. Soviet Phys. solid St. 12, 2753).

KOZLOV, V. G. and KOVALENKO, E. S. (1969). Fizika tverd. Tela 11, 2651 (transl. Soviet Phys. solid St. 11, 2139).

KREBS, J. J. (1964). Phys. Rev. 135, A396.

—— (1967). Phys. Rev. 155, 246.

KUBLER, J. K. and FRIAUF, R. J. (1965). Phys. Rev. 140, A1742.

KURTZ, S. K. and NILSEN, W. G. (1962). Phys. Rev. 128, 1586.

KUSHIDA, T. and SAIKI, K. (1961). Phys. Rev. Lett. 7, 9.

LAMBERT, B., MARTI, C., and PARROT, R. (1970). J. Lumin. 3, 21.

LANDAU, L. D. and LIFSHITZ, E. M. (1958). Quantum mechanics, p. 133 et seq. Pergamon Press, London.

LEVKOVSKII, P. T. and PASHKOVSKII, M. V. (1968). Teor. eksp. Khim. 4, 135 (transl. Theor. exp. Chem. 4, 88).

LUCKEN, E. A. C. (1969). Nuclear Quadrupole Coupling Constants, Chapter 9. Academic Press, New York.

LUDWIG, G. W. and WOODBURY, H. H. (1961). Phys. Rev. Lett. 7, 240.

——— and HAM, F. S. (1962). Phys. Rev. Lett. 8, 210.

———, ——— (1963). Paramagnetic resonance II (ed. W. Low), p. 620 Academic Press, New York.

MANTHEY, W. J. (1973). Phys. Rev. B8, 4086.

MARGENAU, H. and MURPHY, G. M. (1956). Mathematics of physics and chemistry (2nd edn). van Nostrand, New York.

MARTI, C., PARROT, R., ROGER, G., and HERVE, J. (1968). C.r.hebd. Seanc. Acad. Sci., Paris 267B, 931.

———, ———, ——— (1970) Physics Chem. Solids 31, 275.

MIMS, W. B. (1964). Phys. Rev. 133, A835.

——— (1965). Phys. Rev. 140, A531.

——— (1972). Electron paramagnetic resonance (ed. S. Geschwind), Chapter 4, Plenum Press, New York.

——— (1974). Rev. scient. Instrum. 45, 1583.

——— and GILLEN, R. (1966). Phys. Rev. 148, 438.

———, ——— (1967). J. chem. Phys. 47, 3518.

——— and Masuhr, G. J. (1972). Phys. Rev. B5, 3605.

——— and Peisach, J. (1974). Biochemistry 13, 3346.

MOORE, C. E. (1949). Atomic energy levels, Vol. I. National Bureau of Standards.

——— (1952). Atomic energy levels, Vol II. National Bureau of Standards.

MOORE, W. S., BATES, C. A., and AL SHARBATI, T. M. (1973), J. Phys., C 6, L209.

MOTT, N. F. and GURNEY, R. W. (1940). Electronic processes in ionic crystals, p. 16. Oxford University Press (reprinted (1964) by Dover).

MUELLER, K. A. (1968). Phys. Rev. 171, 350.

MULLER, K. A. (1971). Solid State Commun. 9, 373.

NEPSHA, V. I., SHERSTKOV, YU. A., GORLOV, A. D., SHCHETKOV, A. A. (1967). Fizika tverd. Tela 9, 2433(transl. Soviet Phys. solid St. 9, 1907).

——— , ——— LEGKIKH, N. V., and MEILMAN, M. L. (1969). Phys. Status Solid 35, 627.

NIKIFOROV, A. E. (1965). Fizika tverd. Tela 7, 1248 (transl. Soviet Phys. solid St. 7, 1005).

——— MITROVANOV, V. YA., and KROTKII, A. I. (1973). Fizika tverd. Tela 15, 2852 (transl. Soviet Phys. solid St. 15, 1910).

NYE, J. F. (1957). Physical properties of crystals. Clarendon Press, Oxford.

OFELT, G. S. (1962). J. chem. Phys. 37, 511.

OWEN, J. and THORNLEY, J. H. M. (1966). Rep. Prog. Phys. 29, 675.

——— and HARRIS, E. A. (1972). Electron paramagnetic resonance (ed. S. Geschwind), Chapter 6. Plenum Press, New York.

PARROT, R. and ROGER, G. (1968). C.r.hebd. Seanc. Acad. Sci. 266B, 1628.

——— TRONCHE, G., and MARTI, C. (1969). C.r.hebd. Seanc. Acad. Sci. 269B, 321.

PARZEN, E. (1960). Modern probability theory and applications, p. 310. Wiley, New York.

PEISACH, J. and MIMS, W. B. (1973). Proc. natn. Acad. Sci. U.S.A. 70, 2979.

PETER, M., VAN UITERT, L. G., and MOCK, J. B. (1961). Advances in quantum electronics, p. 435. Columbia University Press.

PIRENNE, J. and KARTHEUSER, E. (1964). Physica 30, 2005.

POOLE, C. P. and FARACH, H. A. (1972). The theory of magnetic resonance. Wiley, New York.

RADO, G. T. (1961). Phys. Rev. Lett. 6, 609.

——— (1964). Phys. Rev. Lett. 13, 335.

REDDY, T. R. (1971). Phys. Lett. 36A, 11.

REICHERT, J. F. and PERSHAN, P. S. (1965). Phys. Rev. Lett. 15, 780.

ROITSIN, A. B. (1968). Fizika tverd. Tela 10, 948 (transl. Soviet Phys. Solid St. 10, 751).

——— (1971). Usp. fiz. Nauk 105, 677 (transl. Soviet Phys. Usp. 14, 766).

ROSE, M. E. (1958). J. Math. Phys. 37, 215.

ROYCE, E. B. and BLOEMBERGEN, N. (1963). Phys. Rev. 131, 1912.

SAKUDO, T., UNOKI, H., and FUJII, Y. (1966). J. phys. Soc. Japan 21, 2739.

SCHAFFER, C. E., (1973). Structure and Bonding 14, 69.

SHERSTKOV, YU. A., NEPSHA, V. I., NIKIFOROV, A. E., and CHEREPANOV, V. I. (1966). Zh. eksp. teor. Fiz. SSR, Pis'ma Redakt 3, 401 (transl. JETP Lett. 3, 262).

———, ——— VAGENIN, V. A., NIKIFOROV, A. E. and KROTKII, A. I (1968) Phys. Status Solidii 28, 269.

SIMANEK, E. and SROUBEK, Z. (1972). Electron paramagnetic resonance (ed. S. Geschwind), Chapter 8. Plenum Press, New York.

SMITH, C. S. (1958). Solid St. Phys. 6, (ed. F. Seitz and D. Turnbull), 175.

SMITH, D. and THORNLEY, J. H. M. (1966). Proc. phys. Soc. 89, 779.

SOCHAVA, L. S., TOLPAROV, YU. N., and KOVALEV, N. N. (1971). Fizika tverd. Tela 13, 1463 (transl. Soviet Phys. solid St. 13, 1219).

STONEHAM, A. M. (1969). Rev. mod. Phys. 41, 82.

STURGE, M. D. (1964). Phys. Rev. 133, A795.

SUGAR, J. and KAUFMAN, V. (1965). J. opt. Soc. Am. 55, 1283.

SWARTZ, H. M., BOLTON, J. R., BORG, D. C. (1972). Biological applications of electron spin resonance. Wiley, New York.

SZIGETI, B. (1949). Trans. Faraday Soc. 45, 155.

TESSMAN, J. R., KAHN, A. H., and SHOCKLEY, W. (1953) Phys. Rev. 92, 890.

UNOKI, H. and SAKUDO, T. (1970) J. phys. Soc. Japan 28, suppl., 125.

——, —— (1973). J. phys. Soc. Japan 35, 1128.

USMANI, Z. and REICHERT, J. F. (1969). Phys. Rev. 180, 482.

——, —— (1970). Phys. Rev. B1, 2078.

——, —— (1970). Phys. Rev. Lett. 24, 709.

VAZHENIN, V. A., SHERSTKOV, YU. A., ZOLOTAREVA, K. M., and TRYAPITSYNA, L. V. (1973). Fizika tverd. Tela 15, 951 (transl. Soviet Phys. solid St. 15, 663).

VOLKEL, G. and WINDSCH, W. (1971). Phys. Status Solidii 43, 263.

WEGER, M. and FEHER, E. (1963). Paramagnetic resonance II (ed. . W. Low), p. 628. Academic Press, New York.

WEIGHTMAN, P., DUGDALE, D. E., and HOLROYD, L. V. (1971). J. Phys., C 4, 3292.

WILLIAMS, F. I. B. (1967). Proc. phys. Soc. 91, 111.

ZAVOISKY, E. (1945). Fyzyol. Zh. 9, 211; 245.

Index